SOUTHWEST CONFERENCE on BOTANICAL MEDICINE

Lecture Notes

April 8 – 10, 2016

Southwest College of Naturopathic Medicine & Health Sciences

Tempe, Arizona

Produced by
Herbal Educational Services
555 Tyler Creek Rd
Ashland, OR 97520
Phone 541-482-3016
www.botanicalmedicine.org

© All rights reserved. Please email our website for permission to reproduce all or part of this book

Cover photo: *Larrea tridentata* (creosote) by Mimi Kamp

*Note: Power points in this book have been edited—the downloadable version offers full power point presentations. Order from: **www.botanicalmedicine.org***

Contents

Paul Bergner
    Common Lifestyle Patterns in Reproductive Disorders......................*1*
    Working with the Heavy Cannabis User....................................*6*
    Botanicals, Biofilms, and Chronic Infections............................*23*

Mary Bove, ND
    Herbal Galactagogues..*39*
    Luteal Phase Deficiency What is it all about?..........................*44*
    Exploring Botanicals Impacting Thyroid Function and Female
        Endocrine Health..*52*

Phyllis Hogan
    The Diamond of the Forest Chaga Mushroom Inonotus Obliquus.....*65*

Tori Hudson, ND
    Breast Cancer: Prevention, Breast Health Essentials Botanical &
        Nutritional Influences...*69*
    Abnormal Uterine Bleeding...*83*
    Endometriosis: A Comprehensive Approach............................*95*

Marianne Marchese, ND
    Infertility...*104*

Jason Miller, LAc, MAcOM
    Heart Arrhythmias, and Atrial Fibrillation: Balancing the
        Heart..*118*
    Chronic Prostate Conditions BPH, and Prostate Cancer................*134*

Rhonda PallasDowney
    The Doctrine of Signatures: Flower Essences to Support
        Reproductive Health..*152*

Kenneth Proefrock, ND
 Adolescent Angst: The Teenage Brain on Hormones......................171
 Modulating Neuroendocrine Responses to Stress with
  Botanical Agents...181
 The Troubled Trail of Testosterone: Social Expectation and the
  Search for Meaning along the Edge of Libido.......................191

JoAnn Sanchez & Sankar Jayavelu
 Three Ayurvedic Wonders — Ashwagandha, Brahmi and
  Holy Basil..201

Katie Stage, ND, RH (AHG)
 Multiphasic Dosing During a Woman's Cycle................................212

Jill Stansbury, ND
 Plant Intelligence a Garden Chat...220
 Androgenetic Alopecia..227
 The Lymphatic System and its Role in Fibrocystic Breast
  Disease..237

David Winston, RH (AHG)
 Autism Spectrum Disorders – The Search for Answers...................247
 Making Love – An Herbal/Nutritional Guide to Sexual Health........256
 Herbs and Nutrition for Cardiovascular Health and Disease..........269

Donald Yance, MH, CN, RH (AHG), SFO
 Reducing Estrogen Dominance in Men and Women for
 Optimizing Reproductive Health and Reducing Disease Risk..........279

SPEAKER CONTACT LIST

Paul Bergner
PO Box 13758
Portland, OR 97213
720-841-3626

Mary Bove, ND
515 Fish Pond Rd
Colebrook NH 03576
802-380-7355

Phyllis Hogan
107 N San Francisco St. #1
Flagstaff, AZ 86001
928-774-2884

Tori Hudson, ND
2067 NW Lovejoy
Portland, OR 97201
503-222-2322

Mimi Kamp
PO Box 447
Naco, AZ 85620
520-432-9094

Jeffrey Langland, PhD
SCNM- 2140 E Broadway Rd.
Tempe, AZ 85282
480-858-9100

Marianne Marchese, ND
13832 N. 32nd St. #126
Phoenix, AZ 85032
602-493-2273

Jason Miller, LAc, MAcOM
190 Oak St. Ste. #2
Ashland, OR 97520
541-482-2107

Rhonda PallasDowney
1131 S. 7th St.
Cottonwood, AZ 96326
928-639-3614

Kenneth Proefrock, NMD
14991 W. Bell Rd.
Surprise, AZ 85374
623-977-0077

JoAnn Castigliego Sanchez RH(AHG)
41921 North Central Ave.
New River, AZ 85086
623-465-7359

Katie Stage, ND, RH(AHG)
2164 E. Broadway Rd.
Tempe, AZ 85282
480-970-0000

Jill Stansbury, ND
408 E. Main St.
Battle Ground, WA 98604
360-687-2799

David Winston, RH(AHG)
PO Box 553
Broadway, NJ 08808
908-835-0822

Donald Yance, MH, CN
125 Clear Creek Drive
Ashland, OR 97520
541-488-0514

Common Lifestyle Patterns in Reproductive Disorders

Paul Bergner

Abstract: In reproductive therapeutics, broad patterns in the lifestyle, diet and constitution are often overlooked while focusing on interventions that may promote hormonal balance, either with hormone supplementation, or herbs or foods with actual or theoretical hormonal effects. We describe seven easy to identify patterns in the diet and lifestyle that lie at the root of many female or male reproductive complaints, and show interventions and herbal allies which may help correct those problems at their root.

Treatment vs. Cure

To treat a condition is to give some agent for it which is correct "by the book" and which modifies one or more of the symptoms of the condition. To cure a condition is to produce a state of health in which all of the symptoms are replaced by normal functioning. The skill set necessary to treat something, whether with drugs, supplements, or herbs involves memorizing patterns of symptoms, the names of these patterns, and the appropriate agent(s) to give for it. The skill set necessary for a cure involves being engaged with the patient to get their whole story, to explore with them the roots of their condition, and to invite them to a higher level of self mastery around the key discords in their lifestyle. It involves, education, knowledge of the psychology of behavioral change, inspiration, and communication, skills generally unnecessary for those who merely treat by the book. By extension, this implies that the healer will be one who is engaged in the mastery of the key determinants of health in their own lifestyle. The two skill-sets are radically different. A general rule of thumb is that a treatment which requires the patient to take a step into a high level of self mastery can lead to cure. A treatment which on the other hand makes them dependent, and requires no self mastery is unlikely to ever effect a cure.

Recognizing patterns

In **allopathic pattern recognition**, a particular set of symptoms leads to the diagnosis of a named disease. Then something which is correct "by the book" which modifies one or more of the symptoms in the pattern may be given. Examples in herbalism: Serenoa for prostate; Tanacetum parthenium for migraine; Lycopus for hyperthyroid, soy isoflavones for hyperestrogenic conditions.

In **physiological pattern recognition** a functional pattern is seen which may or may not correspond to an allopathic disease name. It may also be treated "by the book" and may or may not improve, but the root remains and continues to produce imbalance and drive pathology. Examples: Cinnamomum for insulin resistance; Curcuma for systemic inflammation; Agrimonia for leaky gut syndrome.

In **humoral or energetic pattern recognition**, a presentation of a set of combinations of hot/cold, most/dry, excess/deficient, hypertonic/hypotonic etc defines a humoral syndrome. The syndrome may be treated, again by the book. In some cases the condition may be cured, more often than not, it returns once the herbs are stopped, evidence that the root of the pattern remains.

In **Vitalist Pattern Recognition,** the full story reveals a pattern of living that promotes or facilitates the discordant condition. The normal functions of diet, activity, rest, etc are disrupted, causing a cascade of discordant humoral or physiological patterns, or diagnosable disease names. Identifying discords in the primary determinants of harmony in health, in the lifestyle, is the chief skill set.

The following are some of the key patterns in lifestyle and diet observed in approximately 3500 patient cases studied collaboratively in great detail at teaching clinics first at the Rocky Mountain Center for

Botanical Studies, continuing at the North American Institute of Medical Herbalism, and enduring at the Colorado School of Clinical Herbalism, between 1995 and the present. Identifying and recognizing these conditions is the core training of the pre-clinical advanced program at the school. The pattern names are used in case discussion and part of the culture of the school. Each pattern, understood at its root, suggests a rational cure in modification of the diet or lifestyle. Addressing these patterns often results in the improvement or cure a a wide variety of minor to major disorders of the female or male reproductive systems.

Dietary Patterns

The Standard American Diet (SAD Diet)

- Key Elements: low micro-nutrient density, bad oils, high glycemic index, chemical additives.
- Effects specific to reproductive system: Infertility due to malnutrition. Hormonal imbalances through poor functioning of higher regulatory center and poor liver clearance. Anything with an -itis. Insulin resistance diseases such as PCOS, precocious puberty, BPH.
- Interventions: Basic Paleo or Low Glycemic diet. Increase nutrient density, substitute protein snacks for carb snacks, replace sugary beverages with nutrient dense ones, "the oil change", prepare food from scratch a.m.a.p.

The Food Intolerance pattern

- A pattern of symptoms involving GI disturbance, Mood/Energy dysfunction, and musculoskeletal/skin complaints (the "food intolerance triangle")
- Effects specific to the reproductive systems: Anything with an -itis. Pelvic inflammation and prolapse. Possible blood deficiency/anemia. Hyperprolactinemia.
- Interventions: Basic Paleo diet without dairy or grains. Screen for offending foods with formal elimination and re-challenge. Treat malabsorption, GI inflammation, sluggish peristalsis, etc with herbal teas.

The Stress-Carbohydrate pattern

- A pattern of high stress throughout the day characterized by cravings for carbohydrates. Usually is indicative of insulin resistance.
- Effects specific to the reproductive systems: Insulin resistance diseases such as PCOS, precocious puberty, BPH.
- Interventions: High protein, low carb breakfast; supplementation with insulin sensitizing nutrients, low glycemic or ketogenic diet.

The Fast-Food vegetarian

- The diet is characterized by restriction of animal protein, but otherwise has the same problems, or worse, than the SAD diet. May include GI disturbance from soy protein, and often compensatory addictions to deal with the anguish of malnutrition.
- Effects specific to the reproductive systems: Blood deficiency/anemia; same as for sad diet but zinc deficiency aggravates estrogen-progesterone imbalances. Low EFA can affect fertility, anything with an -itis. May cause amenorrhea or oligomenorrhea through malnutrition or indirectly through subclinical or overt hyperprolactinemia.
- Intervention: Improve diet as with the above a.m.a.p. within the ethical framework of the patient. Supplement nutrients commonly deficient in vegetarians/vegans. EFA, iron, zinc, optimal rather than minimal protein.

Disordered Body Image pattern

- The diet is deficient, and the activity typically excessive. About 25% overlap with the fast-food vegetarian pattern. A most destructive pattern. Usually does not meet the criteria for diagnosis of an eating disorder, just a pattern to reduce calories and increase energy output, usually with the idea of losing or maintaining low weight.
- Specific effect to the reproductive systems: Everything in the SAD diet. The Female Athlete Triad. May cause amenorrhea or oligomenorrhea (common presenting symptoms in eating disorders) through malnutrition or indirectly through subclinical or overt hyperprolactinemia.
- Intervention: The most difficult patient for a nutritionist. Encourage nutrient density and moderation of exercise. Educate. Refer for therapy if appropriate to the case.

Sleep Debt

- Sleep studies over the last 100 years show a typical requirement for sleep for optimal health to be between 8-9 hours.
- Sleep less than 6 hours is definitely associated with a cascade of endocrine and immune disorders, including insulin resistance, cortisol disturbances, thyroid disruption.
- Effects specific to reproductive systems: Secondary through promotion of insulin resistance, as above.

Sedentary lifestyle

- More than 50% of the population does not meet the criteria for even light daily exercise.
- As little as 15 minutes of moderate walking exercise a day can reduce all-cause mortality by about 15%.
- 30 minutes a day of brisk moderate walking exercise five days a week can reduce all-cause mortality by 35%.
- Breaking daily exercise into 2-3 shorter periods provides more benefit than doing it all at once.
- Effects specific to reproductive system: pelvic stagnancy in females or males.
- Intervention: As above.

Drug Side Effects

- In one retrospective examination of my case files, 80% of patients had one or more presenting symptoms which was the side effect of a medication *which neither they nor their other providers recognized as such.*
- Side effects on reproductive function are common.
- Almost universal intestinal dysbiosis, impaired intestinal permeability or motility due in part to antibiotic history and NSAID.
- Intervention: must do at least do a rapid assessment of the possible presenting side effects of each medication taken. Include symptoms of withdrawal when relevant. Probiotic therapy and prebiotic-rich diet for most patients.

Pathophysiological patterns

Broad spectrum deficiencies of essential co-factors: protein, magnesium, zinc, iron, B-6, niacin, **vitamin C**, and **omega-3 fatty acids**. The bolded nutrients are commonly deficient in American women. The bolded nutrients are all necessary for normal dopamine function in the hypothalamus, at the top of the reproductive regulatory cascade. Magnesium, B6 and Zinc are necessary for liver processing of reproductive hormones. Zinc is essential for fertility in males or females.

Hyperestrogenism relative to progesterone

- Poor liver transformation
- Deficient fiber
- Deficient progesterone due to subclinical hyperprolactinemia and dopamine deficiency
- Effect of dietary estrogens (such as might occur in meat) is probably minor.
- Effect of xenoestrogens unknown. Usually responds quickly to simple natural medicine, arguing against major importance for xenoestrogens.
- Hyperestrogenism can induce subclinical hyperprolactinemia in a vicious cycle pattern.
- Endometrium is developed or overdeveloped, but vessels and secretory apparatus are
- underdeveloped or absent. Excessive menses, flooding. Lack of cramps in anovulatory
- cycle.
- Promotes breast growth and fibrocystic breast disease
- Promotes growth of uterine fibroids
- NOT known to be related to ovarian cysts.
- Promotes oxytocin, which may in turn worsen water retention and cramps

Hypo-estrogen relative to progesterone

- From deficient diet (micro-nutrients, fat) or malabsorption
- Depression as dominant PMS feature (PMS-D)

Decreased dopamine syndrome:

- Elevated prolactin and decreased GnRH
- Leads to hyperprolactinemia syndrome, see below.
- See nutritional co-factors and drug side effects above.
- **Dopamine** = neurotransmitter involved in production of norepinepherine in nerve synapses and adrenergic target organs, and also in adrenal epinepherine. Also produced in the hypothalamus.

    Phenylalanine Essential amino acid, protein in diet
    | phenylalanine hydroxylase
    Tyrosine cofactors: magensium, zinc, iron, B-6
    | tyrosine hydroxylase
    dopa
    | dopa decarboxylase
    dopamine
    = prolactin inhibiting hormone (PIH)
    Also inhibits GnRH

  - Many drugs inhibit dopamine production, block receptor sites, or cause depletion.
  - Excess stress and stress hormone production
  - **Vitex agnus castus is dopaminergic**, promoting dopamine inhibiting prolactin. It also promotes the production of progesterone from the corpus luteum, possibly through intermediary effects of prolactin, or possibly through GnRH and LH.

Hyperprolactinemia syndrome

Syndrome may be present with **normal levels of prolactin** if PGE 1 is deficient.
Symptoms (all may not be present)
- PMS that responds to evening primrose oil may indicate

- May or may not cause milk production
- Light or irregular periods
- Infertility
- Amenorrhea
- May cause low bone density with normal estrogen levels.
- -May- contribute to ovarian cysts

Causes
- Large tumors or small tumors (microadenoma) of the pituitary gland. Microadenoma
- may not be visible on scans.
- Hypothyroidism
- Also; excessive stress, including excessive exercise
- Prolonged breast stimulation (nursing, yoga techniques)
- *Many common drugs.*
- *Gluten sensitivity may cause*

Some humoral patterns

Stuck Liver Chi; Liver Fire Rising; False Cold

- Chief characteristic is tension with alterations of circulation; heat at the core as blood is congested there and cold at the periphery, hands and or feet as circulation is constricted there.
- A chief presentation of the Food Intolerance dietary pattern.
- May also be due to endogenous hormones
- May be due to alcohol abuse.
- May present as various kinds of heat in the pelvis.
- May present as on-again off-again menstrual flow as vascular system opens then shuts down.

Blood deficiency/Anemia

- A chief presentation of disordered body image pattern
- A chief presentation of the fast-food vegetarian pattern
- A chief presentation of malabsorption secondary to the Food Intolerance pattern, especially gluten.

Working with the Heavy Cannabis User
Side effects, withdrawal symptoms, and constitutional considerations

Paul Bergner
Southwest Conference on Botanical Medicine
April 2016
Tempe, AZ

"Give a man a fact which agrees with what he already believes, and he will accept it on the flimsiest of evidence. Give him a fact which goes against his current opinion and he will demand the most rigorous proof."

Bertrand Russell (paraphrased)

Science review

- Most of the science on adverse effects relies on epidemiology, which has its own inherent weakness.
- Better case-control and prospective trials have emerged more recently.
- Earlier literature seems divided into pro- and con- camps, each of which seems to spin the interpretation of science to their own bias.
- More recent literature (past 24-36 months), in the milieu of legalization of medical marijuana, seems more balanced, and aimed at improving the practice of medicine instead of arguing for or against legalization.

The package insert on a medical cannabis product needs to say more than
"But its safer than alcohol"

NAIMH Case series: Heavy Cannabis users
Colorado teaching clinics 2010 to 2015*

- 32 cases with 92 total visits
- Extensive history and intake (2-3 hours) and follow-ups (1+ hours)
- 9 Intake only; 23 others with average of 3 follow-up visits
- Follow-up range 2 weeks to 7 months.
- Self-reported Cannabis use
  - 25 >=4x/day
  - 2 = 1x per day
  - 5 >=4x/week and <1x/day

* 2010-2012 North American Institute of Medical Herbalism, Boulder
2012-2105 Colorado School of Clinical Herbalism, Boulder

General considerations

- Acute agonist effects on EC system cause altered function.
- Excessive acute agonist effects in EC system can produce acute crisis (overdose)
- Downregulation of EC in response to habitual stimulation resulting in deficient baseline function and *loss of initial benefits*.
- Withdrawal symptoms and consumption to avoid them in a vicious cycle pattern
- Possible permanent epigenetic effects during critical ages of development of the EC (adolescence, fetal?)

Acute effects

- Increased heart rate
- Increased appetite
- Dry mouth
- Decreased pupillary light reflex
- Impaired visual tracking
- Impaired concentration in irregular users.
- Normalizes deficient concentration in habitual users.
- Increased time to make decisions
- Impulsive behavior, impaired judgement
- Impaired working memory
- Impaired executive function

Subjective effects about 2-4 hours

May also produce, short term or chronically, depending on level of use:
- Anxiety
- Panic attacks (higher doses)
- Paranoia*
- Visual hallucinations*
- Auditory hallucinations*
- Difficulty thinking or concentrating*
- Difficulty speaking*

* Symptoms which overlap with those of psychosis

Intoxication as adverse effect

- Acute pleasurable intoxication may be harmless in some settings.
- In clinical trials intoxication is a frequent cause for discontinuing treatment. In trials with 2.5 mg THC, some participants typically drop out. In trials of 25mg THC, most participants drop out.
- In settings which may require attention and fast judgement in a rapidly changing situation, such as driving, child care, or some occupational pursuits, impairment could lead to injury of self or other.

Regular users, including medical patients, should be screened and educated about possible risks depending on the setting of use.

Driving impairment

Levels of evidence

- Epidemiology
- Evaluating measuring 11-nor-9-carboxy-THC (inactive long lasting metabolite) rather than THC in early epidemiology.
- Driving test in controlled area.
- Driving test on streets (equivalent to driver's license test)
- Blood levels taken after accident (under-report THC levels)
- Blood THC levels taken on autopsy after fatal accident.

- All levels of evidence point to some driver impairment.
- Measurable Impairment is present at all doses tested.
- Heavy users who have developed tolerance perform better than those who have not, but high level executive function and decision making remains impaired.

Odds ratio (adjusted) for driver culpability in fatal accidents at increasing concentrations of blood THC

Serum THC (ng/mL)	Odd Ratio
<1 ng/mL	1.57
1-2 ng/mL	1.54
3-4 ng/mL	2.13
>= 5 ng/mL	2.12

Hartman RL, Huestis MA. Cannabis effects on driving skills. *Clin Chem*. 2013 Mar;59(3):478-92

National and State Limits on blood THC

Colorado	5 ng/mL
Washington	5 ng/mL
Switzerland	2.2 ng/mL
Ohio	2.0 ng/mL
Nevada	2.0 ng/mL
Australia	0 ng/mL

THC is rapidly cleared from the bloodstream. Because no roadside THC blood test is available, the substantial delay between arrest and testing implies is the basis for those that argue for lower limits or zero tolerance. If someone has a level of 5 ng 2 hours after arrest, the implication is that the level was much higher while driving.

Side effects

THC dose range and effects

- 2.5 mg — Appetite stimulation, very low intoxication
- 2.5 to 5 — Appetite stimulation with very mild intoxication
- 5-10 — Intoxication in non-habituated users
- 5-25 — Nausea of chemotherapy (intoxicating)
- 10-25 — Typical intoxicating dose for habituated user
- 26-75 — Highly intoxicating dose or with Cannabis dependency and tolerance
- >75 mg — Extremely high dose suitable only for dependent users
- 800-1000 mg — Highest proposed doses for treating cancer.

Some THC doses for medical marijuana

Cancer pain	5 mg	TID or QID
Cancer: Nausea	5 mg-20mg	TID or QID
Cancer: cachexia	2.5 mg	BID or QID
Glaucoma	5 mg to 25 mg	5mg per 4-5 hours, 10 mg per 10 hours
Muscle spasm	20-25 mg	Divided doses

- A dose of 2.5 mg is typically not tolerated by some of the patients in a clinical trial.
- A dose of 25 mg is typically not tolerated by most patients in a clinical trial
- The exception is a patient who has developed tolerance from frequent high use.

"A Review of Medical Cannabis Studies relating to Chemical Compositions and Dosages for Qualifying Medical Conditions." Minnesota Department of Health, Office of Medical Cannabis. December 2014 http://www.health.state.mn.us/topics/cannabis/practitioners/dosage.pdf [Accessed 7/7/2015]

Dose range of Cannabis to obtain 2.5 to 90 mg of THC

THC strength of Cannabis (%)	Dosage of Cannabis
10%	.150 mg to 5.55 g
15%	120 mg to 3.69 g
20%	80 mg to 2.79 g
25%	40 mg to 2.25 g
30%	10 mg to 1.86 g

- Adverse effects increase with dose
- Inexperienced users may develop adverse effects at low doses
- Regular users develop tolerance of higher doses
- The presence and percentage of CBD in the strain moderates most side effects

Carter GT1, Weydt P, Kyashna-Tocha M, Abrams DI. Medicinal cannabis: rational guidelines for dosing. *IDrugs*. 2004 May;7(5):464-70.

Cannabis hyperemesis syndrome

- Among heavy chronic users, a syndrome of continuous nausea and uncontrollable vomiting may occur which does not respond to standard anti-nausea treatments in the emergency room.
- The full syndrome is characterized by relief from hot showers and baths, and sufferers who figure this out are found to seek relief as many as ten times a day.
- The onset can be insidious in long term heavy users.
- It may also appear intermittently during times of heavier use, such as increasing use for menstrual cramps.
- A lower grade and less severe nausea often cyclic and daily also may appear without the full syndrome.

NAIMH Case series
Nausea or emesis

- 25 heavy daily users (4x or more per day)
- 7 weekly (4 times or less) or light daily (1x only) users.
- 8/25 heavy daily users with nausea or vomiting most days, or a known history of Cannabis-related emesis.
- 4/8 from history, including 1 with 2 recent visits to ER
- 4/8 with resolution on lowering the dose (the others did not lower the dose).
- 0/8 recognized by patient or clinician as possible side effect of Cannabis.
- 0/7 of weekly or light daily users (=1x/day) reported nausea or vomiting as chief, secondary complaint, or in history.

Overdose

- Overdose may occur with any method of consumption.
- *More of a risk with edibles or concentrated forms*
- Dose of THC varies widely from plant to plant
- Dose amount may vary from lab to lab for the same product, and at the same lab with split samples.
- *Dose is much more unreliable on labels for edibles.*

Acute overdose

Presentation
- 8 (22.9%) Agitation/aggression
- 7 (20%) Psychosis
- 7 (20%) Anxiety
- 6 (17.1%) Vomiting

Outcome
- 71.4% received no treatment
- 85.7% were discharged/self-discharged
- 13.8% admitted
- 1 fatality

Fatality
18 year old male
- Collapsed with asystolic cardiac arrest while smoking
- Hypoxic brain injury due to extended cardiac arrest
- Blood tested positive for THC but not for any other drugs

See further discussion in Cardiovascular section

Dines AM, Wood DM, Galicia M, Yates CM, Heyerdahl F, et al. Presentations to the Emergency Department Following Cannabis use-a Multi-Centre Case Series from Ten European Countries. *J Med Toxicol.* 2015 Feb 5

Acute overdose continued

Case review
- Emergency room visits for drug overdose at 14 European medical centers
- 6 month period from October 2103 to March 2014 in Europe
- 2198 presentations
- 356 (16.2%) involved Cannabis
- 36 (1.6%) involved Cannabis alone.

Dose titration

- Advocate-researchers have promoted individual dose-titration as a method for individuals to determine the appropriate dose of the product they are using
- Users experienced in one form of Cannabis can usually do this without experiencing adverse effects.
- Inexperienced users, or those switching to high dose forms or edibles can experience overdose with this method.

Patients should be alerted to the fact that relying on dose titration when switching products or forms can produce significant adverse effects.

Dose inaccuracy in labeling

Lab variance in evaluating THC in Cannabis leaf

	THC (mg)	Variance from mean
Label (Lab 1)	16	-9.4
Lab 2	17.6	0.04
Lab 3	16.9	-4.4
Lab 4	13.9	-20.3
Lab 5	23.9	35.3

Mesh, A. "Testing Trainwreck" *Willamette Week*, Feb 25, 2015. Portland, OR

THC Lab variance in 15 edible products

THC (Label)	THC (Lab)	Variance
45.5	70	53.85%
75	97.8	30.40%
77	77.5	0.65%
79.3	75.6	-4.67%
12	8.7	-27.50%
100	57.8	-42.20%
105.6	58.6	-44.51%
10	5.2	-48.00%
32.1	16.2	-49.53%
75	32.6	-56.53%
150	61.5	-59.00%
197.3	50.1	-74.61%
25	5	-80.00%
17	3.28	-80.71%
350	52.5	-85.00%

Crombie, N. How potent are marijuana edibles? Lab tests yield surprising results. *Oregonian/Oregon-Live*. http://www.oregonlive.com/marijuana/index.ssf/2015/03/how_potent_are_marijuana_edibl.html

Reliability of CBD labels

- Cannabidiol content on label was 0.1%
- Values from the 4 Portland labs ranged from .003% to .66%.
- The extreme unreliability of CBD labeling may cause problems in individuals taking them to replace other drugs such as antispasmodic or anti-seizure medications

Patients seeking high-CBD strains for medical purposes cannot rely on values listed on the labels for either leaf/flower or edibles.

JAMA analysis of edibles

- ▶ Samples collected in Los Angeles, San Francisco, and Seattle in fall of 2014
- ▶ Large number of samples from each of baked goods, beverages, and candy.
- ▶ Whole product pulverized and divided for sampling

75 products THC	
Accurately labeled	17%
Under labeled	23%
Over labeled	60%

54 products CBD	
Labeled with CBD	13%
Under labeled	31%
Over labeled	69%

Vandrey R, Raber JC, Raber ME, Douglass B, Miller C, Bonn-Miller MO. Cannabinoid Dose and Label Accuracy in Edible Medical Cannabis Products. *JAMA*. 2015 Jun 23-30;313(24):2491-3.

THC:CBD ratio

- *High CBD products are less intoxicating and have fewer side effects than THC itself.*
- CBD has anti-anxiety, anti-psychotic, antispasmodic, and anti-seizure effects.
- Downregulation of system and tolerance effects has not been assessed for CBD
- CBD alone is available over the counter.
- THC:CBD products with ratio of 1:1 are also approved

Franjo Grotenhermen, Kirsten Müller-Vahl The Therapeutic Potential of Cannabis and Cannabinoids *Dtsch Arztebl Int.* 2012 July; 109(29-30): 495–501.

To minimize adverse effects Medical marijuana and to get appropriate effects, patients should select the most reliable product for accuracy of THC And CBD content.

FDA approved products with standard dosages:

    Marinol(dronabinol)   Pure THC analog
    Sativex (tincture)   Cannabis extract THC:CBD – 1:1

Pure CBD

Dependency

Addiction

- 4.3% of American estimated to have current or history of Cannabis Use Disorder.
- About 10% of Cannabis ever-users develop classical addiction.
- The figure is about the same as for alcohol addiction.
- It compares to 15% of people who ever try cocaine, and 25% of people who try heroin.
- Short and long term withdrawal symptoms lead to difficulty in quitting
- Inability to stop or cut down despite desire to do so.
- Second only to alcohol in number of admissions to drug treatment centers in the U.S.

SAMSHA. Results from the 2006 National Survey on Drug Use and Health: National Findings. Rockville, MD: Office of Applied studies, DHHS; 2007

Budney AJ, Roffman R, Stephens RS, Walker D. Marijuana dependence and its treatment. *Addict Sci Clin Pract.* 2007 Dec;4(1):4-16. Review

---

Treatments for Dependency(2013)

	Treatment	Inpatient	
Alcohol	2513*	1003	* thousands
Marijuana	845	485	
Cocaine	584	359	
Heroin	526	359	
Hallucinogens	303	206	
Inhalants	187	119	
Pain Relievers	746	421	
Tranquilizers	376	233	
Stimulants	461	247	
Sedatives	154	65	

Cannabis admission up 61% from 300,000 in 2007

SAMSHA. Results from the 2013 National Survey on Drug Use and Health: National Findings. Rockville, MD: Office of Applied studies, DHHS; 2014.

The patient seeking treatment

- 50% are over the age of 25.
- >10 years of near-daily use with > 6 serious attempts to quit.
- Recognize social, physical, and psychological consequences
  - Relationship and family problems
  - Guilt associated with use
  - Financial difficulties
  - Low energy, low self esteem,
  - Dissatisfaction with productivity levels, low life satisfaction
- Self-identify as unable to quit
- Memory problems
- Sleep disturbance and other physical withdrawal symptoms

Budney AJ, Roffman R, Stephens RS, Walker D. Marijuana dependence and its treatment. *Addict Sci Clin Pract.* 2007 Dec;4(1):4-16. Review

---

Mechanisms of dependency

- Downregulation of CB receptors and their sensitivity leads to relative cannabinoid deficiency when not using.
- Downregulation of dopamine system, via downregulated CB1 effects on dopamine, leads to craving and lack of motivation.
- Secondary effects on Mu-opioid receptors (similar to alcohol and nicotine)
- Epigenetic changes may cause permanent alterations in CB function (animal studies). The adolescent brain is especially susceptible (animal studies).

Fratta W, Fattore L. Molecular mechanisms of cannabinoid addiction. *Curr Opin Neurobiol.* 2013 Aug;23(4):487-92.

Withdrawal symptoms (DSM)

Psychological
- Irritability
- Anxiety
- Depressed mood
- Restlessness
- Insomnia, fatigue
- Reduced appetite/weight loss.

Physical
- Abdominal pain
- Sweating
- Shakiness
- Fever
- Chills
- Headache.

DSM5 (2013); Diagnostic code: 292.0

Withdrawal symptoms and duration*
(Marijuana Anonymous)

Psychological

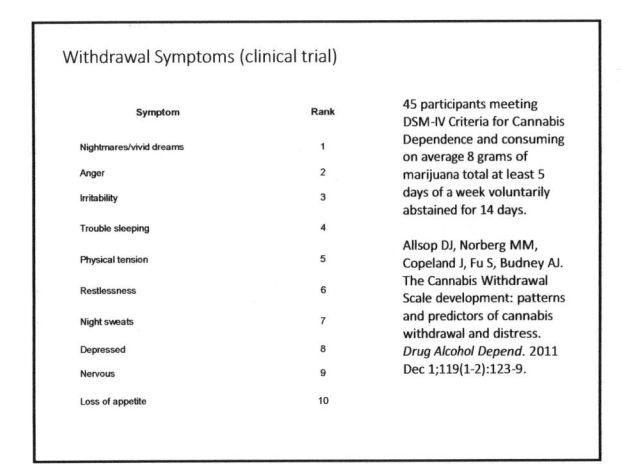

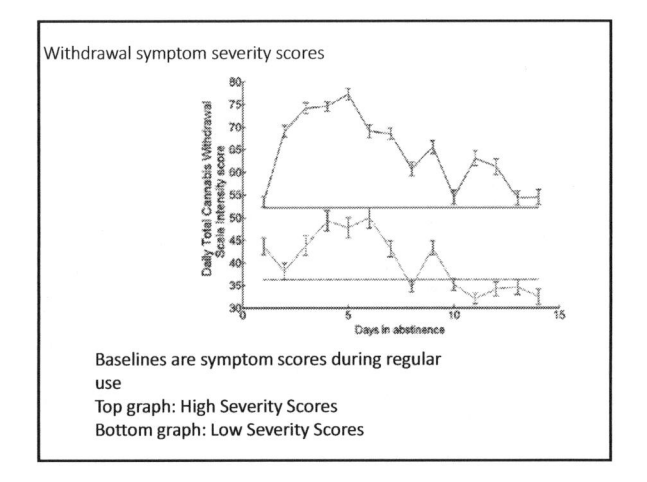

Insomnia	days (severe) to months
Depression	days (severe) to months
Nightmares/vivid dreams	Onset >1 week; last > 1 month
Anger	up to 3 months
Unstable mood	up to 3 months
Anxiety/Fear	up to 3 months
Loss of concentration	up to 1 month

Physical

Headaches	2 weeks to 2 months
Night sweats	2 nights to 1 month
Appetite loss	1-30 days
Vomiting	1-2 days
Tremors	Acute
Dizziness	Acute

* In order of frequency, from member questionnaire

Withdrawal Symptoms (clinical trial)

Symptom	Rank
Nightmares/vivid dreams	1
Anger	2
Irritability	3
Trouble sleeping	4
Physical tension	5
Restlessness	6
Night sweats	7
Depressed	8
Nervous	9
Loss of appetite	10

45 participants meeting DSM-IV Criteria for Cannabis Dependence and consuming on average 8 grams of marijuana total at least 5 days of a week voluntarily abstained for 14 days.

Allsop DJ, Norberg MM, Copeland J, Fu S, Budney AJ. The Cannabis Withdrawal Scale development: patterns and predictors of cannabis withdrawal and distress. *Drug Alcohol Depend.* 2011 Dec 1;119(1-2):123-9.

Withdrawal symptom severity scores

Baselines are symptom scores during regular use
Top graph: High Severity Scores
Bottom graph: Low Severity Scores

Cannabis Use Disorder (CUD)
Natural course in young individuals

- 816 individuals from Oregon Adolescent Depression Project
- 4 diagnostic assessments between ages 16 and 30
- 19.1% had CUD, average age of onset was 18.6 years.
- 81.8% achieved recovery by age 30
- Recidivism rate was 27.7% in first 36 months after stopping.
- Recidivism uncommon after 72 months of abstinence.

Interpretation: About 20% (3.7%) maintained dependence for about 11 years and did not quit.

Farmer RF, Kosty DB, Seeley JR, Duncan SC, Lynskey MT, et al Natural course of cannabis use disorders. *Psychol Med.* 2015 Jan;45(1):63-72.

NAIMH Case series
Signs of dependence

- 26 of 27 daily users with signs of dependence; insomnia, agitation, and/or anxiety on withdrawal

- 11 of 33 (9 daily, 2 weekly) seeking assistance to quit/cut down

- Significance for patients beginning to use medical Cannabis or beginning to experience tolerance

NAIMH Case series
Reasons for wanting to quit

- Anxiety
- *Sleep disturbance*
- Paranoia
- Isolation
- Respiratory
- Lack of motivation/inspiration
- *Aggravation of PTSD.*

NAIMH Case series
Outcomes at attempts to withdraw

- 3 of 11 successfully completely eliminated Cannabis, 1 with help of 12-step program.
- 8 of 11 did not reduce use below 1x/week after period of up to 7 months.
- Two successfully switched to conventional medications for PTSD and regained ability to sleep.

Patient education

- *Patients receiving a medical marijuana prescription for daily use should be informed of the likelihood of tolerance and withdrawal symptoms.*
- *Patients seeking assistance to withdraw should be informed of the likely symptoms and their duration*

Amotivational syndrome

- Recognized in scientific literature in chronic users in the 1970s.
- Subject of controversy because if difficult to evaluate motivation.
- Several decades of research link dopamine not only to reward but to motivation, and this coupled with identification of the dopamine deficiency in chronic Cannabis users, describes a mechanism.

Salamone JD, Correa M. The mysterious motivational functions of mesolimbic dopamine. Neuron. 2012 Nov 8;76(3):470-85.

NAIMH Case series
Some patient descriptions of amotivation

- Quitting pot due to "reduced motivation and inspiration." Wants to "stay in pjs all day"; "constant brain fog to tune out my meaningless life"
- "Feel like it's taking my vibrancy away, disconnecting me from my spirit. Like my potential is being stifled. It's keeping me from growing."
- She has not been employed since her now teenage daughter was born, this has led her to feel "lost" with an "overwhelming sense of apathy about life"; now "Feels no joy and has little focus or motivation to change her circumstances"
- In many of the patients, lack of motivation to make lifestyle changes is an obstacle to recovery typical in our clinic.

Long term cognitive effects

Effects on executive function

- Studies of various individual cognitive parameters in chronic Cannabis users are variable in their methodologies and outcomes.
- Negative effects on *executive function* are nearly universal in epidemiology (at least 9 studies) but suffer from the general weaknesses of epidemiology.
- See typical study, controlled for alcohol use and pre-morbid IQ by Thames et al. It shows a statistically significant lower executive function for current users (at least 1x in last month), former users (ever used but not in the past month), compared to non-users.
- Impairment among current users was dose dependent.

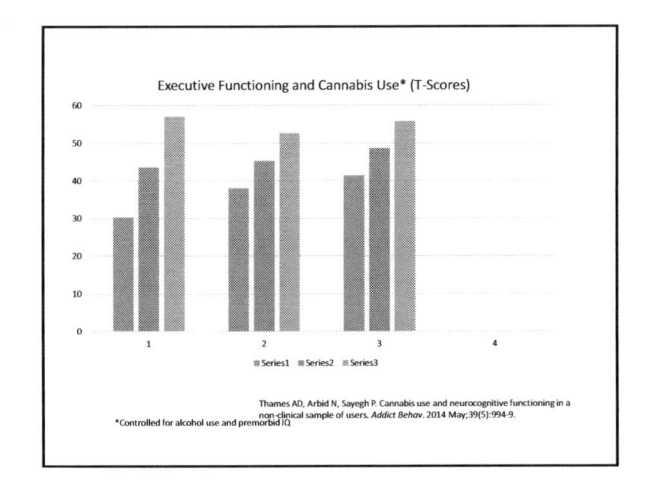

Executive Functioning and Cannabis Use* (T-Scores)

Thames AD, Arbid N, Sayegh P. Cannabis use and neurocognitive functioning in a non-clinical sample of users. *Addict Behav.* 2014 May;39(5):994-9.
*Controlled for alcohol use and premorbid IQ

Executive function

- Executive function = a synthesis of cognitive processes, including working memory, reasoning, task flexibility, and problem solving as well as planning and execution.
- Common test for evaluating is Trailmaking Part B.
- In most trials, chronic Cannabis users perform poorly on this test compared to matched controls.

Trailmaking Part B

The task is to draw a line from 1 to A, then to 2 to B, 3 to C, etc. Any errors are identified to patient, who continues until it is complete. Evaluation is measured by completion time.

Chronic cannabis users score lower than matched controls on the test even after 30 days of abstinence.

Dunedin cohort study

- The only prospective longitudinal study of cognitive function with pre-Cannabis cognitive scores.
- Birth cohort of 1037 individuals born in 1972-1973
- Assessed every 2 years until age 15, then at ages 18, 21, 26, 32, and 38
- Received psychological testing in 1985-6 (pre-Cannabis use) and again in 2010-2012.
- IQ scores were evaluated for age of onset of use (pre- and post- 18 y.o.) and for current use in 2010-2012.

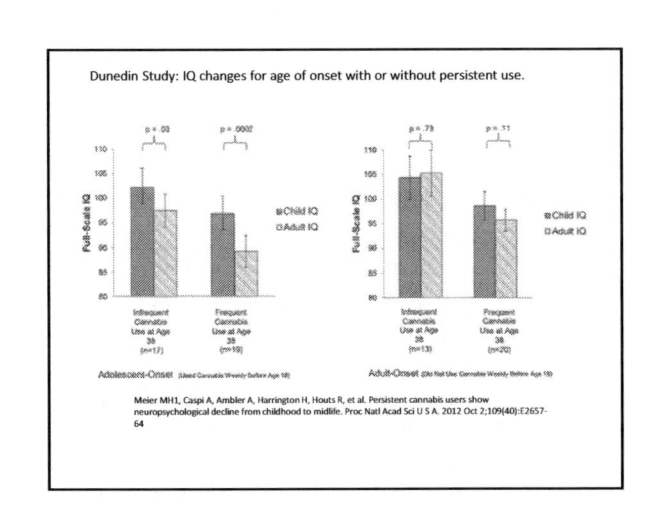

Dunedin Study: IQ changes for age of onset with or without persistent use.

Meier MH1, Caspi A, Ambler A, Harrington H, Houts R, et al. Persistent cannabis users show neuropsychological decline from childhood to midlife. Proc Natl Acad Sci U S A. 2012 Oct 2;109(40):E2657-64

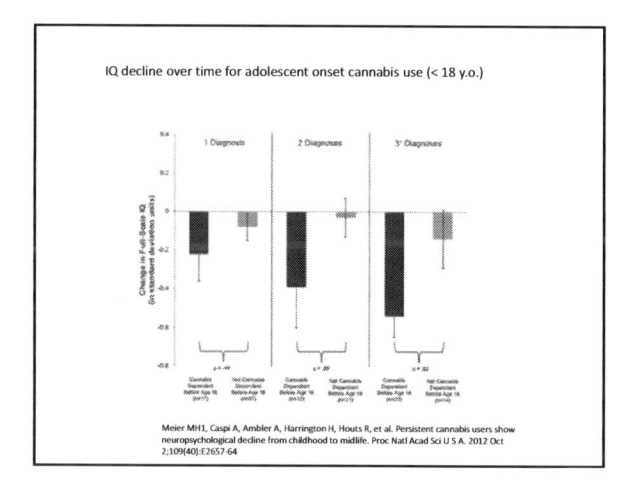

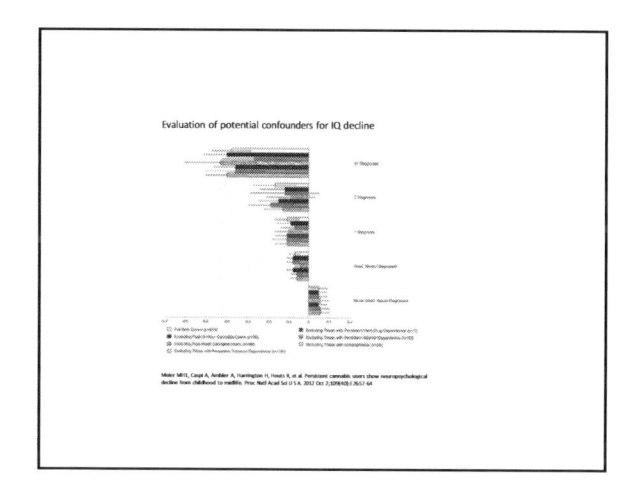

IQ decline over time for adolescent onset cannabis use (< 18 y.o.)

Meier MH1, Caspi A, Ambler A, Harrington H, Houts R, et al. Persistent cannabis users show neuropsychological decline from childhood to midlife. Proc Natl Acad Sci U S A. 2012 Oct 2;109(40):E2657-64

Evaluation of potential confounders for IQ decline

Meier MH1, Caspi A, Ambler A, Harrington H, Houts R, et al. Persistent cannabis users show neuropsychological decline from childhood to midlife. Proc Natl Acad Sci U S A. 2012 Oct 2;109(40):E2657-64

Adverse effects in adolescents

- Nearly half of 12th graders have tried marijuana, and 6% use daily (2009).
- Adolescents who use marijuana heavily tend to show disadvantaged attention, learning, and processing speed
- Abnormalities in brain structure
- Compromised objective indicators of sleep quality.
- Some abnormalities persist beyond a month of abstinence; may resolve within three months of cessation.
- Adolescent use also increases risk and earlier onset of psychosis and bipolar disorder

Jacobus J1, Bava S, Cohen-Zion M, Mahmood O, Tapert SF. Functional consequences of marijuana use in adolescents. Pharmacol Biochem Behav. 2009 Jun;92(4):559-65.

Effects on reproduction

Female
- Disrupted menstrual cycle
- Suppressed of oogenesis
- Impaired embryo implantation and development

Male
- Increased ejaculation problems
- Reducing sperm count and motility
- Loss of libido
- Impotence.

Bari M, Battista N, Pirazzi V, Maccarrone M. The manifold actions of endocannabinoids on female and male reproductive events. Front Biosci (Landmark Ed). 2011 Jan 1;16:498-516.

Patients being evaluated for infertility or other reproductive issues, whether male or female, should be investigated for the possible contribution that Cannabis might be making to the condition.

Psychosis symptoms and illness

- *Psychotic symptoms* are not the same as persistent *psychotic disorder*.
- 5-8% Prevalence in the general population. 75-90% are transitory.
- 9-14% in interview based studies of teenagers.
- 10-25% (.9% to 3.5%) of these develop persistent disorders.
- In Dunedin Study, 14% of 11 year-olds showed symptoms.
- In Dunedin study, symptoms in 11 years olds showed a 5-16x risk of persistent psychotic illness in adulthood related to severity.

van Os J, Linscott RJ, Myin-Germeys I, Delespaul P, Krabbendam L. A systematic review and meta-analysis of the psychosis continuum: evidence for a psychosis proneness-persistence-impairment model of psychotic disorder. Psychol Med. 2009 Feb;39(2):179-95.

Ian K, Jenner JA, Cannon M. Psychotic symptoms in the general population - an evolutionary perspective. Br J Psychiatry. 2010 Sep;197(3):167-9.

Psychosis symptoms

Symptoms of distorted function
- Delusions
- Hallucinations
- Feelings of paranoia and suspiciousness
- Disorganized thinking
- Disorganized speaking

Symptoms of Loss of normal function
- Loss of or decreased motivation
- Loss of or decreased in ability to take initiate or come up with new ideas
- Loss of or decreased talking
- Difficulties expressing emotion
- Difficulties thinking and/or concentrating

Cannabis and psychosis symptoms

- Higher doses of marijuana and overdoses produce symptoms that meet the criteria for a diagnosis of psychosis.
- Of Cannabis overdoses admitted for emergency care, 20% displayed psychotic symptoms.
- Possible confounder: a large percentage of patients with mental illness, especially schizophrenia and bipolar, abuse Cannabis.
- For most, Cannabis psychotic effects are very temporary.
- A more persistent Cannabis psychosis is described as a common cause for admission to mental hospitals in Africa and India, most patients being chronic abusers of hashish. The duration of the episode is typically > 30 days, but is shorter than other admissions for psychotic disorders.

Scientific studies

- Early prospective studies show early-onset Cannabis use to be associated with an increased risk of persistent psychosis-related outcomes.
- A recent meta-analysis of these studies adjusted for various methodological issues, and found the risk to be present, but greatly reduced.
- A sibling pair analysis found correlations closer to the early prospective studies.

Risk at six years since first use

Symptom	Odds ratio
Non-affective psychosis	2.2
Delusions	4.2
Hallucinations	2.8

Moore TH, Zammit S, Lingford-Hughes A, Barnes TR, Jones PB, Burke M, Lewis G Cannabis use and risk of psychotic or affective mental health outcomes: a systematic review. *Lancet* 2007;370 (9584) 319- 328.

McGrath J, Welham J, Scott J, Varghese D, Degenhardt L, et al. Association between cannabis use and psychosis related outcomes using sibling pair analysis in a cohort of young adults. *Arch Gen Psychiatry*. 2010 May;67(5):4407.

NAIMH Case series

- All patients heavy users, > 4x/day for >1.5 years
- One 50 y.o male patient with diagnosis of schizophrenia and multiple other diagnoses reported "continuous" use of Cannabis since teenage years (self medication).
- 21 year old female, daily heavy use for six years. Worsening symptoms of detachment from reality (her description). Similar symptoms in parent and sibling. (aggravation of familial risk)
- 21 year old female, severe PTSD. Cannabis dependence with hyperemesis, very heavy user for 2 years. Appearance of psychotic symptoms at same time as hyperemesis and menstrual disruption.

- *Cannabis patients should be screened for personal history or family history of psychosis, schizophrenia, or bipolar disorder.*
- *Adolescents should be systematically informed of long term risks*
- *Heavy users should be screened for appearance and aggravation of persistent symptoms.*

Post-traumatic stress disorder

- PTSD is a qualifying medical condition for medical Cannabis in AZ, CA, CT, ME, and NM.
- Cannabis Use Disorder is very high among patients with PTSD.
- Patients use it for hyper-arousal, negative affect, and sleep disturbances.
- Level of evidence to date is empirical, many patients self medicate, and report relief.
- No RCT on use of Cannabis for PTSD or long term assessment
- Review article concludes that use for PTSD is not yet based on evidence, especially for long term use, and *may worsen PTSD*.

Belendiuk KA, Baldini LL, Bonn-Miller MO. Narrative review of the safety and efficacy of marijuana for the treatment of commonly state-approved medical and psychiatric disorders. *Addict Sci Clin Pract*. 2015 Apr 21;10:10.

Cannabis, PTSD, and sleep

- Improving sleep and suppressing nightmares is most common reason for combat veterans use of Cannabis.
- After dependence and downregulation of CB system, symptoms may return, including an aggravation of both detachment/numbness and hyperarousal.
- Poor sleep and the reappearance of nightmares is biggest obstacle to withdrawal (additive effects of Cannabis sleep disturbance and PTSD symptom)
- **Cannabis use disorder predicts a poor outcome for recovery from PTSD.**

Bonn-Miller, Marcel O.; Boden, Matthew Tyler; Vujanovic, Anka A.; Drescher, Kent D. Prospective investigation of the impact of cannabis use disorders on posttraumatic stress disorder symptoms among veterans in residential treatment. *Psychological Trauma: Theory, Research, Practice, and Policy*, Vol 5(2), Mar 2013, 193-200.

NAIMH Case series

8 of 25 very heavy users had PTSD
3 of 8 quit Cannabis or wanted to quit due to aggravation of PTSD.

- Case 1: 29 y.o. Male. Medical cannabis for pain for 2+ years aggravated depression. Quit with help of conventional psych and sleep meds.
- Case 2 ; 28 y.o. Male. Cannabis eventually created sleep dependency and aggravated triggering/activation. Quit with conventional meds and 12 Step program.
- Case 3: 25 y.o. Female. Wants to quit due to sleep dependency and poor sleep.

4/8 exhibited signs of aggravation but did not relate it to Cannabis

- Case 4: 21 y.o. Female. Aggravation of withdrawal/numbness
- Case 5: 21 y.o. Female. Extreme aggravation of withdrawal/numbness for 2+ years. Nocturnal emesis. Menstrual disruption. Emerging psychotic symptoms.
- Case 6: 26 y.o. Female. Sleep dependence. Daily AM emesis.
- Case 7: 23 y.o. Trans. Sleep dependence/disturbance. Regular emesis.

Case 8: 2 years since last use, began using high THC Cannabis for insomnia and hyperarousal during case and reported good relief at 4-6 weeks.

- *PTSD patients using or wishing to use Cannabis for their symptoms should be informed of the possible loss of benefit after dependence and downregulation of the EC, and the possible adverse outcome of dependence on the course of PTSD.*

Respiratory effects

Lung cancer

- Epidemiological evidence is lacking that smoking Cannabis is associated with lung cancer.
- Smoking Cannabis initiates many of the same processes that are considered causative of lung cancer in tobacco smokers
  - Squamous metaplasia
  - Cellular disorganization
  - Nuclear variation
  - Mitotic features
  - Increased nuclear-to-cytoplasmic ratio

Auerbach O, Stout AP, Hammond EC, Garfinkel L. Changes in bronchial epithelium in relation to sex, age, residence, smoking, and pneumonia. *N Engl J Med* 1962; 267:111-119

Respiratory symptoms in Dunedin Study

- 1037 young adults had medical evaluation and were assessed for regular (>1x week for one year) Cannabis smoking at ages 18, 21, 26, 32, and 38.
- After quitting, odds ratios returned to normal.

Symptom	Odds ratio
Morning cough	1.97
Sputum production	2.31
Wheeze	1.55

Hancox RJ, Shin HH, Gray AR, Poulton R, Sears MR. Effects of quitting cannabis on respiratory symptoms. Eur Respir J. 2015 Apr 2. pii: ERJ-02289-2014.

Respiratory immunity

Cannabis smoke depresses the activity of alveolar macrophages in a dose-dependent manner (animal trial). The cytotoxic constituent was in the gaseous portion of smoke, and was water soluble.

Huber GL, Simmons GA, McCarthy CR, Cutting MB, Laguarda R, Pereira W. Depressant effect of marihuana smoke on antibactericidal activity of pulmonary alveolar macrophages. *Chest*. 1975 Dec;68(6):76973.

- Alveolar macrophages from Cannabis-only smokers (but not tobacco smokers) were found to be deficient in their ability to kill *Staphylococcus aureus*.
- In AIDS, marijuana smoking was associated (OR 2.24) with the first appearance of pneumonia.
- In AIDS patients (pre-1994), marijuana smoking was associated with a higher risk (OR 3.7) for progression to Kaposi's sarcoma.

Taskin, DP. Effects of Smoked Marijuana on the lung and its immune defenses: Implications for Medicinal use in HIV infected patients. In: Russo, E. *Cannabis Therapeutics in HIV and AIDS*. Haworth Press, New York: 2001

Medical Cannabis patients should be screened for lung health and risk factors for pneumonia or HIV related lung diseases, and advised if appropriate to use non-smoking forms of Cannabis.

Allergy
Patients may become sensitized to inhaled Cannabis

- 340 asthmatic patients who used drugs
- 61% sensitized to Cannabis
- 61-72% of patients previously sensitized to tobacco or tomato were sensitive to Cannabis.
- Prick tests and IgE for cannabis had a good sensitivity (92 and 88.1%, respectively) and specificity (87.1 and 96%) for cannabis sensitisation.

Armentia A, Castrodeza J, Ruiz-Muñoz P, Martinez-Quesada J, Postigo I, et al. Allergic hypersensitivity to cannabis in patients with allergy and illicit drug users. *Allergol Immunopathol (Madr)*. 2011 Sep-Oct;39(5):271-9

NAIMH case series

1 patient, a former smoker, was so sensitive to Cannabis that his lungs would be inflamed for up to seven days after taking a single hit.

Pesticide contamination

- A large number and variety of pesticides are typically used in commercial Cannabis production
- Pesticides in smoked Cannabis are rapidly absorbed without a first pass through the liver.
- The amounts of some pesticides found in testing labs is "astronomically high" in several cases 300x to 800x the amount allowed by the FDA in food.
- An analytical lab in Oregon has found the roach-killing pesticide in the product Raid in Cannabis samples.

Lab testing

- States with legalization have requirements for lab testing for pesticides. Best-defined today in Colorado and Washington.
- In Oregon some specific pesticides must be tested including *bifenthrin*.
- Lab owners report losing customers permanently if they report the presence of bifenthrin. Many labs have stopped testing for bifenthrin because they do not want to lose customers
- One lab found 40% of submitted concentrate samples were positive for the pesticide, and about 20% of flower.
- One lab reports that nearly all customers opt for a cheaper test for 15 pesticides than a comprehensive one for 44. Some only test for 8.

Crombie, N "It Doesn't pay to be honest: Labs test for pesticides but without oversight" Oregonian, June 11, 2015. http://www.oregonlive.com/marijuana-legalization/pesticides/chemhistory.html [Accessed 7-9-2015]

Glaucoma

- THC lowers intraocular pressure
- Effective in about 60-65% of individuals.
- 5 mg may lower pressure for about 4 hours. Requires 8x/day dosing to maintain lower pressure.
- 25 mg may lower pressure for about 10 hours; requires 3 doses per day to maintain pressure. The majority of patients at the 25 mg dose drop out of glaucoma trials due to intoxication.
- Tolerance develops at this level of dose and frequency
- A rebound increase in intraocular pressure beyond baseline can occur if doses are missed, or on withdrawal of the drug.

Belendiuk KA, Baldini LL, Bonn-Miller MO. Narrative review of the safety and efficacy of marijuana for the treatment of commonly state-approved medical and psychiatric disorders. *Addict Sci Clin Pract*. 2015 Apr 21;10:10.

Adverse cardiovascular effects

- Acute tachycardia
- Chronic reduced blood pressure and heart rate
- Rebound tachycardia (not clinically significant)
- Rebound hypertension clinically significant in subset of patients. About 1/3 of group had mean rebound of 23 mm systolic/12mm diastolic
- Could be significant in individuals with hypertension.

- Multiple case reports of myocardial infarction and atrial fibrillation in young heavy Cannabis users without recognized risk factors.
- 1 fatality out of 36 Cannabis-only emergency admissions in a series in Europe, acute MI in young otherwise healthy male.
- 8 case reports of atrial fibrillation in young otherwise healthy heavy Cannabis users.
- In a series of 88 AF patients in a British emergency center, in 3/88 Cannabis was the precipitating factor. 1 recurred on rechallenge.
- 1 fatality in young healthy male long term heavy user engaging in strenuous exercise.

Korantzopoulos P, Liu T, Papaioannides D, Li G, Goudevenos JA. Atrial fibrillation and marijuana smoking. Int J Clin Pract 2008;62:308e313.

Thomas G, Kloner RA, Rezkalla S. Adverse cardiovascular, cerebrovascular, and peripheral vascular effects of marijuana inhalation: what cardiologists need to know. Am J Cardiol 2014;113:187e190.

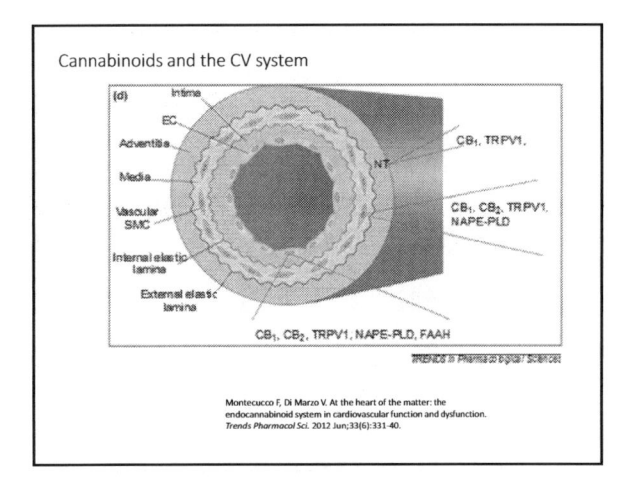

Cannabinoids and the CV system

Montecucco F, Di Marzo V. At the heart of the matter: the endocannabinoid system in cardiovascular function and dysfunction. Trends Pharmacol Sci. 2012 Jun;33(6):331-40.

Possible mechanisms

- High dose?
- Tolerance with rebound effects?
- Simultaneous use with tobacco?
- High demand on system when exercising with sedated CV system?

Acute coronary syndromes in heavy users who are young without other risk factors or precipitated by Cannabis use should be taken seriously, recognized as possibly related to Cannabis, and patients should be informed. Regular heavy users should be monitored for possible aggravation of hypertension.

Pregnancy and lactation

Pregnancy

- Studies of effects on standard measures of birth outcome, such as infant mortality and birth weight, are mixed.
- Some studies show no effect and others showing a small effect.
- Associations may be present for:
  - Infertility
  - Placental complications
  - Fetal growth restriction
  - Stillbirth.
- Difficult to separate Cannabis effect from confounders

Metz TD, Stickrath EH. Marijuana use in pregnancy and lactation: a review of the evidence. Am J Obstet Gynecol. 2015 May 15. pii: S0002-9378(15)00501-3.

- Other measures of more subtle effects show that fetal exposure can adversely effect neurodevelopment.
- This may occur not only in utero during critical periods of brain growth, but also later during critical phases in adolescent maturation.
- Discovery of permanent epigenetic effects with adolescents use (animal studies) raises alarm about exposure during fetal development

---

Associations with fetal exposure in later life

- Permanent changes in dopaminergic receptors
- Executive functioning skills
- Inattention
- Impulsivity
- Conduct and behavior problems
- Poorer school achievement

Pregnant women should be educated about possible adverse effects and counseled to avoid Cannabis use during pregnancy

---

Lactation

- Few studies: One case series of two women volunteers
- THC metabolites concentrate in human milk at a higher concentration than in the mother's serum.
- THC metabolites can be obtained from the feces of the nursing infant.

Lactating women should be informed of possible adverse effects, and counseled to avoid Cannabis use, or switch to another method of feeding.

Perez-Reyes M, Wall ME. Presence of delta9-tetrahydrocannabinol in human milk. *N Engl J Med*. 1982 Sep 23;307(13):819-20.

Constitutional effects

- Cannabis classified in Chinese medicine as hot and dry.
- Avicenna described it as hot and dry and "dessicant" and states that overuse "damages the semen."
- Contemporary Unani medicine describes it as cold and dry, (in that system cold means that it can reduce the consciousness or produce stupor) It is in the 3rd degree, meaning strong but non-lethal.
- In the Chinese system, prolonged use "injures the Yin"
- Disturbance of reproductive function in both females and males is considered very serious in Chinese medicine: prolonged high use "injures the Jing" or life essence.

NAIMH Case series
 Consitutional effects

- 27 of 28 users evaluated with dry constitution
- 18 had cold-dry constitution
- 9 had hot-dry constitution

Consider Western demulcents or Chinese Yin Tonics to counter effects.

All-cause mortality

- 2010 Systematic review of studies between 1990 and 2008
- Insufficient study to determine whether ACM is elevated among Cannabis users in the general population.
- Possible causes of elevated mortality are motor vehicle accidents, brain and lung cancers
- No evidence of risk of suicide.

Calabria B, Degenhardt L, Hall W, Lynskey M. Does cannabis use increase the risk of death? Systematic review of epidemiological evidence on adverse effects of cannabis use. *Drug Alcohol Rev.* 2010 May;29(3):318-30.

Wild from card safety issues from NAIMH case series

- A young woman and her husband, both dependent on Cannabis, moved to Colorado in order to obtain medical cards.
- She brought old medical records indicating a 2 year-old history of a dermoid Ovarian cyst.
- Without obtaining a new medical visit, she presented the records to an MD to obtain a card, complaining of chronic pelvic pain. She received the card and was medicating the pain with Cannabis.
- A few days later she came to the NAIMH clinic for an intake, was found to have high Cannabis daily intake (4x/day) which was not helping her pain, and also daily nausea.
- Several days later she was admitted to the ER with an Ectopic pregnancy.

Considerations for natural therapeutics to support withdrawal

- Dopaminergic nutrients: Mg, B6, Zn, C, EFA, protein, Fe (if deficient)
- NAC. Dopaminergic effects. Used successfully in multiple clinical trials for various addictions including Cannabis. Reduces cravings. 1.2 to 3.6 g/day.
- Consider nutritional and botanical formulas to support sleep.
- Consider nutritional and botanical formulas to moderate anxiety.
- For the future: What is the pathway and cofactors for production of endocannabinoids? Do these deficiencies produce endocannabinoid deficiency and predisposition to addiction?

Asevedo E, Mendes AC, Berk M, Brietzke E. Systematic review of N-acetylcysteine in the treatment of addictions. *Rev Bras Psiquiatr.* 2014 Apr-Jun;36(2):168-75.

All materials copyright Paul Bergner 2015. All rights reserved

Paul Bergner
Director
North American Institute of Medical Herbalism
Editor: Medical Herbalism journal
http://naimh.com

See files and supplemental readings at http://naimh.com/scbm

Botanicals, Biofilms, and Chronic Infections

Paul Bergner

Southwest Conference on Botanical Medicine

Tempe, AZ

April 2016

New Concepts in Microbiology

- Old Model. Freely mobile microbial invaders infect a sterile body. They can be cultured on lab plates. Antibiotics can kill and remove them.
- New methods of detection have increased not only the number of microorganisms we can recognize but have completely overthrown the previous model of infection.

The Great Plate Count Anomaly: Staley and Konopka

- Typically of bacteria observed in lake water in a microscope, only 0.1 to 1% can be cultured in media.
- The great majority of microbes in the human gut cannot be cultured, including some of the dominant species.
- We know a lot about *Escherichia coli* because it is easy to culture but It is a very minor part of the gut population, less than 0.1%.

DNA sequencing to identify bacteria

- DNA Extraction
- Polymerase Chain Reaction
- Sequencing

Phylogenetic tree

- Archaea distinguished from Bacteria on phylogenetic tree
- From 1980 to 2012, the number of known Bacterial families has grown from 12 to more than 100. Two-thirds have never been cultured or identified in a microscope, and their existence could not be detected through traditional methods.

- About ten times as many Viruses as Bacteria exist in an on the human body and its biome. A Fungome also exists in normal health.
- Most viruses are bacteriophages
- The community of bacteria, virus, and fungi has been called the "Third Arm of the Immune System" due to its barrier function, resistance to invasion, and secretion of antimicrobial compounds.

Some surprising results

- An estimated 40,000 different microbial species inhabit the human gut. No more than a few hundred of these have been seen on a microscope or been cultured. Collectively these comprise an essential metabolic and immune organ.
- More than 30 bacteria species have been found in the normal flora of the bladder which had never been detected on urine culture or microscopy.
- A microbiome has been discovered in the normal placenta. It is composed of bacteria similar to the oral microbiome with no similarity to the vaginal microbiome.

Respiratory Microbiome - Nose

Naris (R)

Despite the prescence of *Staphylococcus aureus*, infections don't occur

Staphylococcus

Naris (L)

Innocuous bacteria keep infectious bacteria at bay

In many conditions, establishment of colonies of pathogenic bacteria more likely to be due to disruption of the biofilms of the normal microbiome than to simple invasion and infection.

Biofilms

Bacteria live in a biofilm state

Planktonic form.
Free moving

Biofilm form.
Non-mobile, linked in a matrix

The biofilm for of bacteria is resistant to both antibiotic therapy and the immune system

Most bacteria in an on the human body exist in biofilm form. Most are beneficial commensal bacteria and provide barrier, immune, and metabolic functions

MRSA   Pseudomonas

Biofilms are part of normal microbiome defense of the body but pathological biofilms are nearly universally present in:

- Oral plaque, periodontal disease, abscess
- MRSA infections on skin
- Other skin infections
- Chronic wounds and ulcers
- Chronic sinus infection
- Upper GI disturbances
- Vaginal infection
- Bladder infection

- Biofilms are the normal life state for bacteria and some fungi
- Biofilms can be viewed as semi-independent multicellular organisms with specialized metabolism and immune defenses.
- They are interlinked by filaments of polysaccharide, protein, or strands of genetic material
- A gradient of metabolism from aerobic at the surface to anaerobic at the core develops, allowing resistance to substances which might attack the metabolism.
- In some species, an attached biofilm layer provides nutrients to a superficial layer, which may the secrete antibiotics, reproduce, etc.
- Once aggregated, bacteria in biofilms can dramatically change their functions and secretions.

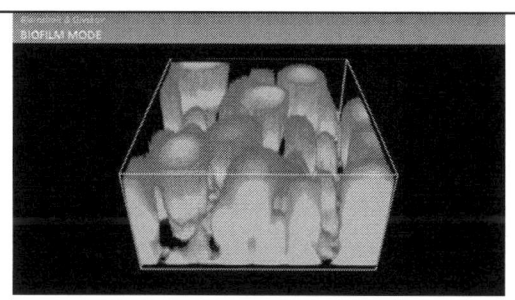

The biofilm "mushrooms" in the picture are about actual size, this only occurs in lab conditions

Biofilms have not been studied in the living organism.

Biofilms in infected wounds are typically in the range of 5 to 10 micrometers, or 1/100 of a millimeter. Requires about 100x magnification to be visible.

One sample of *Borrelia* biofilm in tissue samples required 400X magnification.

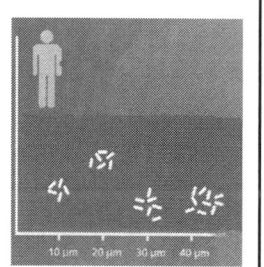

Biofilms Have Been Found

Vascular grafts and stents
Heart Valves
Pacemakers
Chronic osteomyelitis
Chronic otitis media
Foreign body associate infections
Chronic sinusitis
Chronic lung infection (cystic fibrosis
Artificial joints and pins
Implants
Endocarditis
Chronic wounds
Infectious kidney stone

Killed cells in the biofilm are red. Colistin* kills the anaerobes at the center of the biofilm, but leaves the metabolically active aerobes at the surface intact, and the biofilm is completely restored. Tobramycin kills the aerobes, but leaves the anaerobes intake. The combination can kill the biofilm.

Multispecies biofilms

Microorganisms frequently form which may also include fungi.

Below: Oral plaque is a multispecies biofilm with constantly changing and evolving components

Tolerance genes are most easily spread in multi-species biofilms. Multispecies biofilms evolve in their composition and their resistance with each dose of antibiotics

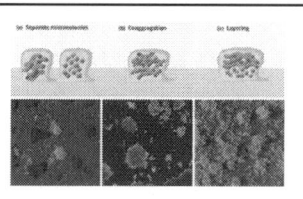

Burmølle M, Webb JS, Rao D, Hansen LH, Sørensen SJ, Kjelleberg S. Enhanced biofilm formation and increased resistance to antimicrobial agents and bacterial invasion are caused by synergistic interactions in multispecies biofilms. Appl Environ Microbiol. 2006 Jun;72(6):3916-23

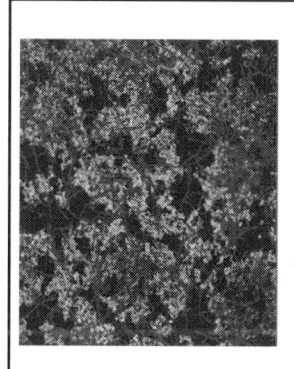

Right: A 3 species biofilm grown in saliva

Below: a "corncob" biofilm with cocci attached to bacilli

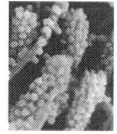

Bacterial vaginosis multispecies biofilm

"Currently, it is consensus that BV involves the presence of a dense, structured and polymicrobial biofilm, primarily constituted by *G. vaginalis* clusters, strongly adhered to the vaginal epithelium"

Machado D, Castro J, Palmeira-de-Oliveira A, Martinez-de-Oliveira J, Cerca N. Bacterial Vaginosis Biofilms: Challenges to Current Therapies and Emerging Solutions. Front Microbiol. 2016 Jan 20;6:1528.

Berberine and companion alkaloids

May act against biofilms by attacking both Aerobes and anaerobes

---

In this *ex vivo* trial both *Coptis* root and it constituent *berberine* significantly inhibit the growth of gut bacteria under both aerobic and anaerobic conditions. In *in vitro* trials, both RC and berberine significantly inhibit the growth of *Firmicutes* under anaerobic conditions.

Xie W, Gu D, Li J, Cui K, Zhang Y. Effects and action mechanisms of berberine and Rhizoma coptidis on gut microbes and obesity in high-fat diet-fed C57BL/6J mice. PLoS One. 2011;6(9):e24520

The Odwalla Juice E-coli epidemic

- Odwalla juice marketing unpasteurized juices during the 1990s.
- In 1996, a batch of their apple juice became infected with pathogenic E-coli bacteria. The apple juice is a component in most of their juices.
- An epidemic followed across the American West, with cases reported in Washington State, Colorado, and California. One child died in Colorado, and 13 more were hospitalized with kidney damage.
- A number of individuals in Boulder, CO became sick. None were ever recorded in the official statistics of the epidemic.
- A tincture formula of equal parts of *Hydrastis, Mahonia, Berberis v.*, and *Coptis chinensis* proved rapidly effective against a case with fever and bloody diarrhea (blood resolved after two moderate doses)

Alkaloids in some berberine-containing plants.

Most of these alkaloids have anti-microbial or other pharmacological effects in scientific trials

Alkaloid	Hydrastis	Mahonia	Berberis	Coptis
Berberine	x	x	x	x
Berbamine		x	x	
Berberastine	x			x
Berberubine			x	x
Canadine	x			
Chondocurine			x	
Columbamine			x	x
Coptisine			x	x
Epiberberine				x
Hydrastine	x			
Hydrastinine	x			
Jatrorrhizine		x	x	x
Oxicanthine			x	
Oxyacanthine		x	x	
Palmatine		x	x	x
Tetrahydroberberastine	x			

Hydrastis	H + M	H + M + B	H + M + B + C
Berberine	Berberine	Berberine	Berberine
Berberastine	*Berbamine*	Berbamine	Berbamine
Canadine	*Berberastine*	Berberastine	Berberastine
Hydrastine	Canadine	*Berberubine*	Berberubine
Hydrastinine	Hydrastine	Canadine	Canadine
OH-4-berberastine	Hydrastinine	*Chondocurine*	Chondocurine
	Jatrorrhizine	Columbamine	Columbamine
	Oxyacanthine	Hydrastine	*Coptisine*
	Palmatine	Hydrastinine	*Epiberberine*
	OH-4-berberastine	Jatrorrhizine	Hydrastine
		Oxicanthine	Hydrastinine
		Oxyacanthine	Jatrorrhizine
		Palmatine	Oxicanthine
		OH-4-berberastine	Oxyacanthine
			Palmatine
			OH-4-berberastine

Berberine compound formula
Potential synergistic alkaloids from *Hydrastis, Mahonia, Berberis,* and *Coptis* combination
New alkaloids with each addition are marked **bold italic**.
The possible synergistic auxiliary compounds in each plant may also be present.

FIGURE 3: Inhibiting ratios of different concentrations of cefoxitin and five berberine alkaloids on MRSA.

Luo J, Yan D, Yang M, Dong X, Xiao X. Multicomponent therapeutics of berberine alkaloids. *Evid Based Complement Alternat Med*. 2013;2013:545898. doi: 10.1155/2013/545898. Epub 2013 Mar 24.

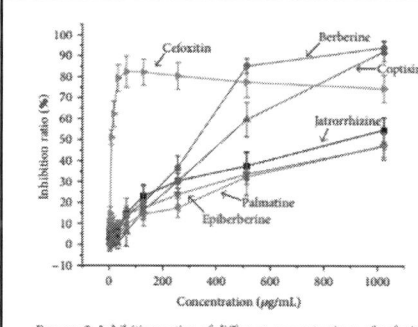

Berberine and its related alkaloids common in berberine-containing plants each inhibit bacteria individually

Pairs of alkaloids usually show synergistic effects against bacteria.

Microbial defenses

This Biofilm will now come to order
"Quorum sensing" by bacteria

- Planktonic bacteria secrete signaling molecules.
- As the population grows, the concentration of signaling molecules rises, and bind to surface receptors on the bacteria.
- This triggers bacterial DNA activation
- Increased production of the triggering molecule
- Expression of matrix materials to form a biofilm
- Production of antibiotics to protect the colony from other bacteria, fungi, etc.
- Production of adhesion molecules
- Production of proteases and other substances enabling invasion of tissues.

PUBMED search: (biofilm* OR quorum)

Some plants with anti-biofilm/quorum properties

- The discovery of the quorum-sensing property essential to formation and functioning of a biofilm has led to a research quest for plant constituents with anti-quorum or anti-biofilm properties.

Science + tradition
- *Allium*
- *Hydrastis* (leaf)
- *Commiphora myrrha*
- *Boswellia*
- *Achillea*
- *Aloe*
- *Hypericum*
- *Althaea*
- *Arctostaphylos*
- *Acalypha*
- *Quercus* and **tannins**

Traditional use
- *Anemopsis*
- *Larrea*
- *Baptisia*
- *Thuja*
- *Bursera*

Multiple Drug Resistant Efflux Pumps (MDR)

- Bacteria contain transporters in their membranes which actively pump harmful substances back out of the cell.
- The process is non-specific, evicting a wide variety of substances. It can result in complete inactivation of antibiotic substances.
- MDR activity is responsible for bacterial resistance to both plant and pharmaceutical antibiotics.
- A bacterial population will evolve to contain robust MDR pump activity in response to plant or pharmaceutical antibiotics.
- Bacteria of unrelated species can acquire the MDR pump resistance genes from each other.
- The pharmaceutical quest for effects MDR pump inhibitors (MDRi) has led to a flurry of research into plant compounds in the last few years.

Efflux pumps

- Efflux pumps allow microorganisms to expel many kinds of substances harmful to them.
- Genes coding for more efficient efflux pumps are part of bacterial resistance.
- Efflux pump inhibition is a potential target for antimicrobial therapy with plants or drugs.

MDR pump inhibitors in plants

- Most *isolated* plant antimicrobial substances are not effective against gram negative bacteria, due to membrane functions and MDR pumps, but the plants themselves may be very effective due to synergistic constituents, include MDR inhibitors.
- Addition of MDR constituents can multiply effectiveness dramatically 100-1000x.
- Many whole plants contain MDR pump inhibitors.
- Likewise, plant materia rich in MDR pump inhibitors may be added in formula to topical preparations or other herbs.

Some widely dispersed MDRi constituents

Luteolin	Apigenin	Kaempferol	Myricetin
Artemisia	Artemisia	Allium	Arctostaphylos spp.
Echinacea	Echinacea	Echinacea	Arbutus spp.
Plantago	Plantago	Althaea	Other Ericacaea
Baptisia		Berberis v	
		Calendula	

Some plants containing MDRi

- *Hydrastis* (leaf)
- Some *Berberis* species (leaf)
- *Allium sativum*
- *Allium spp.*
- *Calendula*
- *Plantago*
- *Echinacea*
- *Artemisia spp.*
- *Hypericum*
- *Althaea*
- *Achillea*
- *Commiphora*
- *Boswellia*
- *Baptisia*
- *Arctostaphylos*
- *Arbutus*

Plants and biofilms
Plants can do through multiple mechanisms what no drug can do

Many plants have developed mechanisms to kill bacteria, prevent or disrupt quorum-sensing in bacteria, or suppress efflux pumps. This is essential to their survival. Synergistic constituents may:

- Attack microbial cell wall
- Attack microbial metabolism
- Disrupt bacterial resistance functions (MDR pumps for instance)
- Disrupt quorum sensing
- Disrupt the functions triggered by quorum sensing
- *In humans,* they may also stimulate local host resistance or circulation

Hydrastis leaf

- Contains all the *Hydrastis* alkaloids but in lower concentration than the root
- Contains at least 2 MDRi which **effectively double the potency of berberine**
- Also contains anti-quorum and anti-biofilm properties unrelated to its alkaloids.
- Sustainably grown Hydrastis leaf may be added in formula to almost any topical antimicrobial to improve results

Cech NB, Junio HA, Ackermann LW, Kavanaugh JS, Horswill AR. Quorum quenching and antimicrobial activity of goldenseal (Hydrastis canadensis) against methicillin-resistant Staphylococcus aureus (MRSA). Planta Med. 2012 Sep;78(14):1556-61.

Host defense against biofilms

Non-inflammatory defense

- Mechanisms which "self-clean" the body, especially in the skin, respiratory, and urinary tracts.
- Impaired action of cilia
- Impaired or obstructed urinary flow
- Impaired Eustachian tube function
- Impaired circulation to skin.

Immune responses

In the host response to chronic biofilms, the cellular components normally present only during the acute phase of the innate immune system are chronically activated, especially **Polymorphal nuclear leukocytes (PMN).** This *chronic activation of an acute response* can result in tissue inflammation and damage.

PMN: Neutrophils, Eosinophils, Basophils, Mast Cells

Polymorphal nuclear leukocytes (PMN)

The biofilm protects bacteria from otherwise bactericidal PMNs.

Oxidative bursts from the PMN *damage the tissues* around the biofilm and produce inflammation.

Endobronchial Michrography from Infected CF Lung

PMN stained in blue surround the biofilm.
Their oxidative bursts can damage tissues.

Damage-response model of infection

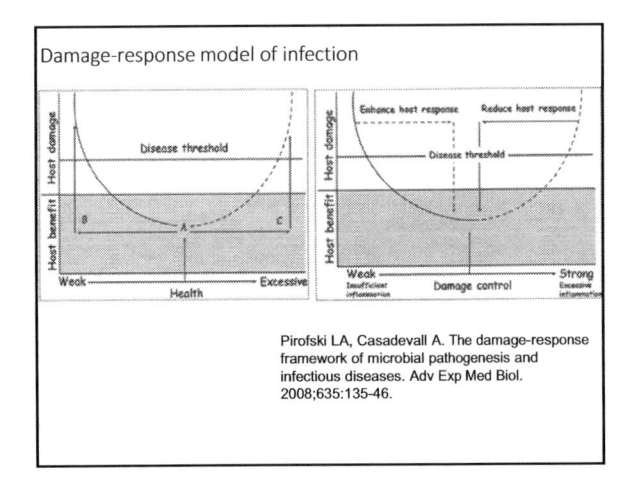

Pirofski LA, Casadevall A. The damage-response framework of microbial pathogenesis and infectious diseases. Adv Exp Med Biol. 2008;635:135-46.

Examples of host damage

- Non-healing wounds and ulcers. Immune response damages tissues.
- Tuberculosis. Damage to lung by immune response.
- Chronic viral hepatitis. Damage to liver by immune response.
- HIV infection triggering autoimmune response
- Chronic Lyme infection. Damage to connective tissues by response.
- Possible chronic-infection triggered autoimmunity
- Permanent presence of high volumes of antigenic food substances produce systemic inflammation.

The "Biofilm Complex"

- Planktonic microorganisms
- Microorganisms in a biofilm matrix
- Microorganisms actively resisting antimicrobial substances through efflux pumps.
- A continuous and ongoing evolution of resistance to host and antimicrobials.
- Damage to the tissues through invasion or toxins
- An ineffective active immune response which may further damage the tissues
- Non-resolving inflammation

A Plant Constituent-Synergy model of therapeutics for the chronic biofilm complex

Damage-response therapeutics

A synergy model for multi-constituent topical applications

Antimicrobial Effects
Direct antimicrobial effects
MDR pump inhibition
Anti-quorum effects

Enhance immunity
Increase local circulation
Enhance local immunity
Support systemic immunity

Reduce damage
Modify local inflammation
Repair local tissue damage

These properties are all possessed by some single plants, and with some simple plant combinations

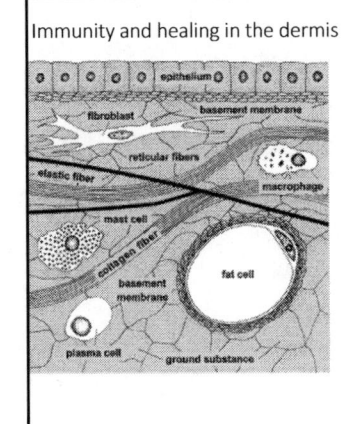

Immunity and healing in the dermis

- Circulation can increase or decrease from external or internal (or herbal) stimuli
- The immune-cell-rich dermis is semi-independent of the larger immune system, and can be regulated or stimulated by local factors, including herbal applications.
- Collagen and elastin forming fibrocytes circulate in the system in the same manner as white blood cells, and can migrate into an injured or inflamed dermis to produce healing and **scarring.**

Direct applications

- The plant material or its extract comes in direct contact with the cell and its environment.
- *All* of the plant constituents can come directly into contact with tissue in high concentration, and can act synergistically. Significance for large molecules, essential oils.
- Plants may be combined for multiple effects
- Plants may be delivered in media with anti-biofilm effects
- May apply to external skin, throat, ear, sinus, stomach, vagina, and some constituents may be delivered through the urinary tract.

Potential synergistic actions against the biofilm complex

	Anti-inflammatory	Vulnerary	Antiseptic	Anti-biofilm	MRDi	Local Immunity
Calendula	x	x	x		x	x
Plantago	x	x	x	x	x	x
Hypericum	x	x	x	x	x	x
Echinacea	x	x	x		x	x
Althaea	x	x	x	x	x	x

Infused oils: Olive oil also has wound healing and anti-inflammatory effects
Echinacea wash from decoction of 1 ounce per liter for 40 minutes.
Echinacea wash from tincture 1 part Echinacea to 3-6 parts water.

Some cautions

- Caution in applying herbs with strong wound healing effects to suppurating wounds. Potential to "seal in" a biofilm and produce septicemia.
- Case: A man applied comfrey poultices to an extensive burn on his hand. This resulted in severe infection of the hands, swollen nodes in the armpit, and fever from septicemia.
- Caution in applying topical herbs in salve form (with wax) to an infection, even if the herbs may be antimicrobial. May create anaerobic environment.
- Case: A young man with fungal infection in pubic hair region shaved the hair and applied a salve. The bacteria flourished in the anaerobic environment and entered the body through the micro-tears. Result: nearly a week in the hospital on IV antibiotics. Systemic infection with both staph and

Herbs with synergistic effects against biofilms

	Anti septic	Immune	Anti Biofilm	MRDi
Larrea	x	x	trad	
Thuja	x	x	trad	
Anemopsis	x		trad	
Baptisia	x	x	trad	x
Hypericum	x	x	science	x
Althaea	x	x	science	x

	Antiseptic	Immune	Biofilm	MRDi
Aloe	x		science	(-)
Commiphora	x	x	science	x
Boswellia	x	x	science	x
Allium	x	x	science	x
Hydrastis	x		science	x
Achillea	x		science	x

Stimulate local circulation

	Stimulant	Antiseptic	Immunity	Biofilm	MDRi
Thuja	x	x	x	trad	
Anemopsis	x	x		trad	
Myrica	x	x	x	trad	
Baptisia	x	x	x	trad	x
Commiphora	x	x	x	yes	x
Achillea	x	x		yes	x
Capsicum	x	x			
Arnica	x				

Some historical combinations

Garden variety infused topical oil

	cool	Anti-inflammatory	Vulnerary	Antiseptic	Anti biofilm	MRDi	Local Immunity
Calendula	x	x	x	x		x	x
Plantago	x	x	x	x	x	x	x
Hypericum	x	x	x	x	x	x	x

Samuel Thomson's Number Six

	Stimulant	Anti inflammatory	Antiseptic	Immunity	Biofilm	MDRi	Vulnerary
Commiphora	x	X	x	x	x	x	
Capsicum	xxx		x				
Echinacea		X	x	x		x	x

- "Rheumatic drops" taken internally, topical antiseptic, throat spray
- Externally: "The most powerful antiseptic known, and is on that account highly serviceable in all putrid affections whatever"
- Used as surgical disinfectant with simultaneous internal immune stimulation by the later Physiomedicalists (post germ-theory)
- RS Clymer later recommended substitution of Echinacea for Capsicum in the formula. Can use all three in suitable proportions

A classical pair

	Stimulant	Anti-inflammatory	Antiseptic	Immune	Biofilm	MDRi
Hydrastis			x		x	x
Myrrh	x	x	x	x	x	x

Traditionally used for oral infections and non-healing wounds

Hydrastis and Myrrh

- Topical wash for infection
- Antibacterial, antiviral, antifungal
- Spray for sore throat
- Gum disease
- Topical for gastric mucosa
- Powerful systemic effects (mucous membrane tonic, general alterative and tonic, antimicrobial through separate mechanisms, in low dose is balanced warm, cold, moist and dry.

Sinusitis spray

- Get a 2 ounce sinus spray bottle
- Add 1 teaspoon of glycerine. Not more.
- Add 15 drops each of *Hydrastis* and *Myrrh**. Not more.
- Fill to 2 oz with water.
- Spray into sinuses up to 4 times per day.
- Frequently will clear chronic sinusitis within 4 days.

*Original recipe called for 30 drops of *Anemopsis*

Possible combination

		Stimulant	Anti inflammatory	Antiseptic	Immune	biofilm	MDRi
Commiphora (sub: Bursera?)	warm	x	x	x	x	science	x
Larrea	cool		x	x	x	trad	

Esberitox

		Stimulant	Anti inflammatory	Vulnerary	Antiseptic	Immune	Biofilm	MDRi
Echinacea	cool		x	x	x	x	x	x
Baptisia	cold	x			x	x	trad	x
Thuja	warm	x	x		x	x	trad	

- Developed in Europe for internal use as an immune stimulant.
- A very potent potential topical treatment. Prepare as decoction.
- Note traditional use of Baptisia was primarily external application of the tea

Roberts formula for ulcers

- *Helicobacter pylori* is a normal component of the gastric microbiome. In some cases it is the dominant species.
- It normally grows in a biofilm separated from the mucosa by a mucous layer. Pathology may be due to loss of the mucous layer.
- For a complete discussion of H Pylori, the history of its discovery, and subsequent discovery of systemic harms that can result from it eradication, see *Missing Microbes* by Glaser.
- Roberts formula for ulcers was developed mid 20th century, long before the possible infectious basis of gastric ulcers was known, and before the discovery of H pylori. Most of the herbs are those that would traditionally be used on topical ulcers or poorly healing wounds. Later in the 20th century, J. Bastyr added Baptisia and several other components to the formula.

Roberts Formula for Ulcers

		Antiseptic	Anti biofilm	MRDi	Local Immunity	Anti-inflammatory	Vulnerary
Althaea	cool	x	x	x	x	x	x
Geranium maculatum	cool	X*	x	x			
Hydrastis (leaf)	cold	X*	(x)	(x)			
Echinacea	cool	x		x	x	x	x
Phytolacca	cold	x			x		
(Baptisia)	cold	x	x	x	x		

*Specific strong activity against *H. pylori* in vitro

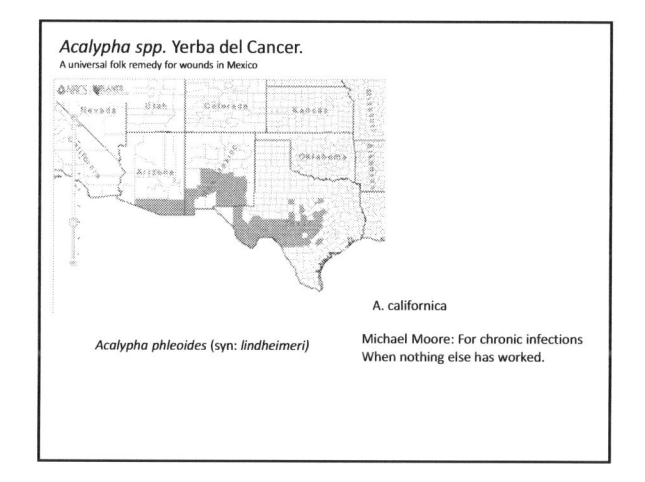

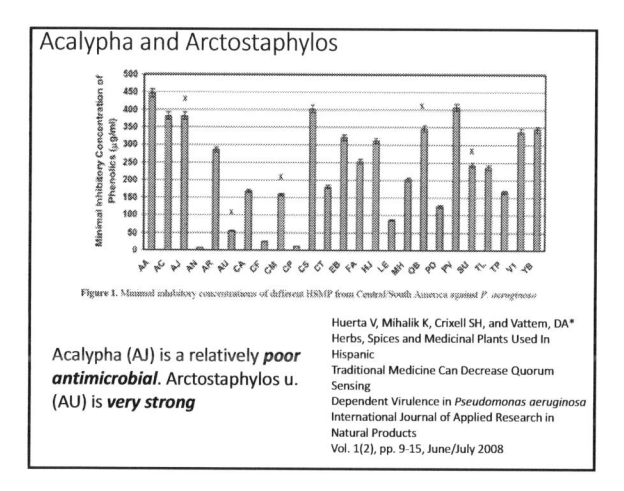

Acalypha spp. Yerba del Cancer.
A universal folk remedy for wounds in Mexico

A. californica

Acalypha phleoides (syn: *lindheimeri*)

Michael Moore: For chronic infections
When nothing else has worked.

Acalypha and Arctostaphylos

Figure 1. Minimal inhibitory concentrations of different HSMP from Central/South America against *P. aeruginosa*

Acalypha (AJ) is a relatively **poor antimicrobial**. Arctostaphylos u. (AU) is **very strong**

Huerta V, Mihalik K, Crixell SH, and Vattem, DA*
Herbs, Spices and Medicinal Plants Used In Hispanic
Traditional Medicine Can Decrease Quorum Sensing
Dependent Virulence in *Pseudomonas aeruginosa*
International Journal of Applied Research in Natural Products
Vol. 1(2), pp. 9-15, June/July 2008

Of 25 Mexican plants tested, Acalypha and Uva ursi were #1 and #2 in one measurement of anti-quorum activity Most had no activity

In another measure of quorum sensing activity, Acalypha was #1 of the 25.

Quercus species
Constituent synergy for anti-quorum properties

- Dried then rehydrated *Quercus* bark
- The whole plant had mild anti-microbial but very strong anti-quorum sensing activity.
- Ten constituents tested individually
- Two of ten showed anti-microbial and anti-quorum activity
- Five more showed anti-quorum activity without anti-microbial activity
- Only a recombination of all constituents together showed activity equal to the whole plant.

Deryabin DG, Tolmacheva AA. Antibacterial and Anti-Quorum Sensing Molecular Composition Derived from Quercus cortex (Oak bark) Extract. Molecules. 2015 Sep 17;20(9):17093-108.

Allium sativum

- Raw fresh cut garlic contains high amounts of allicin, which has broad spectrum antimicrobial and anti-biofilm effects
- Allicin breaks down rapidly once garlic is cut or crushed. Breakdown products have anti-biofilm and antimicrobial effects.
- The constituent *ajoene*, which is abundant in oil-infused garlic preparations, has a potent anti-biofilm effect.
- Some of these non-allicin constituents may be delivered to a biofilm after oral ingestion.
- **Fresh garlic can produce second and third degree in burns.**

Allium sativum applications

- Two cloves (not whole bulbs) in liter of water, blended and strained through cheesecloth.
- Poultice
- Foot bath or handbath.
- Mouthwash for thrush
- Douche
- Infused oil to ear

Chronic otitis media

- Dysfunction of the Eustachian tube may allow normal oral flora to form chronic biofilms in the middle ear.
- Biofilms can readily be detected in the exudate after eardrum rupture.
- Traditional treatment with warm infused oil of garlic.
- Antimicrobial and anti-biofilm constituents including oil-soluble *ajoene*.
- The eardrum is permeable to medications and plant constituents.
- Administration in outer ear results in expectoration in the sinuses with garlic flavor to the exudate.

May add the astringent *Verbascum* and antimicrobial *Phytolacca* to the formula.

Ancient formula from *Balds Leechbook**

- The recipe instructs the reader to crush garlic and a second *Allium* species (whose translation into modern English is ambiguous), combine these with wine and oxgall (bovine bile), and leave the mixture to stand in a brass or bronze vessel for 9 days and nights
- The researchers made two versions of the formula, exactly as described, with allium cepa (onion) in one and Allium ampeloprasum (leek) in the other.
- These were tested against *Staphylococcus aureus* in both planktonic and established biofilm form in synthetic wound fluid

* Cockayne O. 1864–1866. Leechdoms, wortcunning and starcraft: being a collection of documents, for the most part never before printed, illustrating the history of science before the Norman conquest. Rolls series 35th, 3 Vols. Longman, Green, Longman, Roberts, and Green, London, United Kingdom

---

- Both formulas were 100% bactericidal against planktonic bacteria.
- Both also significantly reduced the biofilm (see chart)
- *None of the elements individually had any effect on the biofilm.*
- The combination of wine, garlic, and leek demonstrated the full effect of the formula
- If onion was used instead of leek, then the bile was necessary also for the full effect of the formula.
- Brass had no effect, but because it is sterile, it was probably valuable in medieval times
- Take-home: **Addition of leek or possibly onion to a topical antimicrobial garlic preparation has strong synergistic activity.**

Harrison F, Roberts AE, Gabrilska R, Rumbaugh KP, Lee C, Diggle SP. A 1,000-Year-Old Antimicrobial Remedy with Antistaphylococcal Activity. MBio. 2015 Aug 11;6(4):e01129.

Media

Vinegar and biofilms

- Acetic acid has an anti-microbial effect against established biofilms both in-vitro and in open wounds.
- It is effective at 100% eradication of established *P. aeruginosa* and *S. aureus* at a concentration of 1% acetic acid.
- The anti-biofilm effect is not due to pH value of the bacteria, because HCl at the same pH has no effect.
- The effect is due to the acetic acid molecule itself.
- Application six times a day for twenty minutes on non-healing diabetic ulcers. (See following slides)

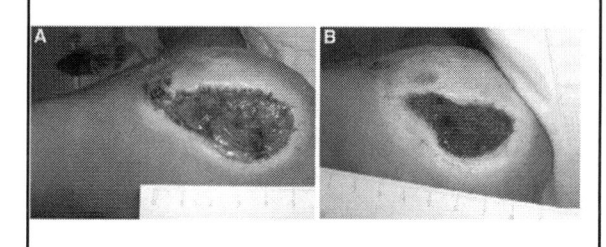

Day 0 vs Day 11 of antibiotic resistant diabetic foot ulcer treated with vinegar. Note complete lack of suppuration.

Days 0, 3, and 6 of vinegar treated antibiotic resistant diabetic foot ulcers. Note disappearance of suppuration and appearance of circulation by day 3.

Treatment of a year-long antibiotic resistance diabetic foot ulcer with vinegar. Days 0 and 6. See method of application in middle slide.

Stages of chronic ulcers

Antibiotic treatment results in resistance, evolution of the biofilm, and ultimately to co-infection by additional species and yeasts (purple circles) in multispecies biofilms

Honey

- Honey in a dilution of ½ was tested against planktonic and biofilm forms of antibiotic resistant *P. aeruginosa* and *S. aureus*
- Tested honey was Manuka honey, which may contain antimicrobial volatile substances. Some Canadian honey samples were ineffective.
- The honey completely eradicated planktonic forms and reduced biofilm forms of both bacteria by 63-91%

Alandejani T, Marsan J, Ferris W, Slinger R, Chan F. Effectiveness of honey on Staphylococcus aureus and Pseudomonas aeruginosa biofilms. Otolaryngol Head Neck Surg. 2009 Jul;141(1):114-8.

Oral biofilms

- A healthy microbiome may exist in the biofilm on the teeth.
- Sugars drive evolution of the biofilm on the teeth toward acid producing bacteria and caries.
- Poor hygiene results in evolution of the a multispecies biofilm of anaerobes which can live under the gum line. Subsequent inflammation is destructive to the tissues.
- An entirely new biofilm of anaerobes evolves in a tooth abscess.
- Anaerobes in severely infected gum pockets or abscesses may spread through virulent planktonic bacteria to other areas of the body, to medical implants, kidney stones, atherosclerotic plaque, etc.

Treatments for oral infection

- Combinations of *Hydrastis* and Myrrh, applied generously, diligently, and persistently have saved teeth that were due to be pulled because of severe gum disease. Consider Hydrastis leaf.
- May also work with powdered Myrrh and sea salt.
- Will not work without first mechanical cleaning of the teeth.
- Abscesses or infected root canals cannot be addressed with herbs.
- Strong *Echinacea* teas internally, and also held as a mouth wash, have effectively prevented or treated oral infections following gum surgery when antibiotics were refused.
- Also effective internally in a case study of facial cellulitis following root canal, when antibiotics were refused.

Tooth powder
For treatment or maintenance after cleaning

	Parts	Stimulant	Anti-inflammatory	Antiseptic	Immune	Biofilm	MDRi
Quercus alba	4		x	x		x	
Myrrh	4	x	x	x	x	x	x
Myrica	2	x		x		x	
Hydrastis	1			x		x	x
Cinnamomum cassia	1	x	x	x			
Eugenia	1	x		x			

This is a formula from Candis Cantin Kiriagis

Bacterial vaginosis

- The normal biome of the vagina is dominated by one of several vagina-specific *Lactobacillus* species.
- BV is characterized by strongly tissue-adherent multi species biofilms constructed on a dominant *Gardnerella* matrix.
- Antibiotics are ineffective because of the biofilm, and because restoration of the vaginal specific Lactobacillus is necessary.
- The general pattern of therapy is:
- Keep the environment acidic
- Apply probiotics of vaginal-specific lactobacillus.
- Apply topical therapeutics with antimicrobial and anti-biofilm effects

Some traditional treatments

- Vinegar douches. May have anti biofilm effects independent of pH effects
- Boric acid capsules. BID. Boron may have anti-biofilm effects independent of pH.
- Boric acid mixed with powder of *Hydrastis, Mahonia*, or *Berberis*. Might be enhanced by the use of leaf of *Hydrastis* or *Mahonia*.
- Douche of *Hydrastis* tea. Consider adding the leaf, with the entire Berberine compound formula.
- Douche of *Allium sativum*. Must strain the blended preparation through cheesecloth (*allicin* from cut garlic can cause burns)

Boric acid and biofilm formation

Beneficial effects in BV may be due to the effect of the Boron molecule on biofilm formation rather than to the acidity.

Sayin Z, Ucan US, Sakmanoglu A. Antibacterial and Antibiofilm Effects of Boron on Different Bacteria. Biol Trace Elem Res. 2016 Feb 11.

Garlic vs Flagyl for Bacterial Vaginosis

- 500 mg powder of *Allium sativum*
- 250 mg Metronidazole
- Two tablets with meals orally each 12 hrs.
- Successful oral application with reduction of the biofilm implies that the anti-microbial and possibly the anti-biofilm constituents are delivered systemically to the vaginal mucosa

Mohammadzadeh F, Dolatian M, Jorjani M, Alavi Majd H, Borumandnia N. Comparing the therapeutic effects of garlic tablet and oral metronidazole on bacterial vaginosis: a randomized controlled clinical trial. Iran Red Crescent Med J. 2014 Jul;16(7):e19118.

Internal biofilms

- These usually require mechanical assistance to remove.
- High doses of single antibiotics are ineffective
- High dose antibiotic combinations *may* be effective.
- Tooth abscess
- Medical devices and implants
- Tissue fillers
- Chronic tissue infection (Borrelia)

Find supplemental notes and readings at http://naimh.com/scbm

Paul Bergner
Director, North American Institute of Medical Herbalism
Editor, *Medical Herbalism* Journal

http://naimh.com

All material copyright Paul Bergner 2/1/2016. All Rights Reserved

---

Note: The text and illustrations on many of the slides in this presentation are quite small. A more consistently legible digital version of this power point presentation is available for purchase and download at www.botanicalmedicine.org under "Past Conferences/2016 Southwest Conference on Botanical Medicine pdf"

Herbal Galactagogues

Plants which increase the production and secretion of breast milk

Mary Bove ND
marybove.com
herbaldocmb@gmail.com

Herbal Preparations in Lactation

- Alcohol enters breastmilk by passive diffusion
- Alcohol enters breastmilk 30-60 min post ingestion
- Takes 2 hours to clear one drink from breastmilk
- 5mls of a 50% ethanol tincture gives about 2.5 gr ethanol
- Ethanol is slow to metabolism in neonate and may accumulate
- Ethanol may inhibit milk enjection reflex and decrease breastmilk

Role of Galactagogues

- Low Milk Supply
  - Delayed lactation
  - Return to work
  - Stress-induced
  - Pump-dependency
  - Relactation or Adoptive lactation

Herbal Galactagogues

- Increase prolactin
  - Dopamine receptor antagonist
  - Blocks inhibitory effect of dopamine
- Diaphoretic reflex
  - Mammary is modified sweat gland
- Hormone Modulation
  - Estrogen, progesterone,
  - Increases insulin sensitivity
- Nervine, Thymoleptic Actions
  - Promotes prolactin response, let down reflex
- Increase mammary blood flow
- Carminative action for baby

Botanical Galactogues

- Alfalfa
- Ashwaganda
- Blessed Thistle similar to milk thistle
- Borage Seed/ GLA high plants
- Hops – milk ejection refex
- Holy Basil
- Shatavari
- Marshmallow
- Oatstraw
- Raspberry
- Red Clover
- Saw Palmetto
- Vervain
- Vitex

Herbal Galactagogues

- Anise, Fennel, Coriander, Dill seed
  - Trans-anethole
  - Dopa receptor antagonist
  - 15 -40 g/day dried seed infused
  - 3-5 mls TID 1:5 tincture
  - 3-6 g/day dry seed powder
- Galega officinalis/ Goats Rue
  - Traditional use as galactagogue
  - Diaphoretic
  - Increases insulin sensitivity
  - 2-3mls 1:5 tincture TID

Goat's Rue

Herbal Galactagogues

- Trigonella foenum-graecum/ Fenugreek seed

  - Most commonly utilized galactagogue in the published literature
  - May have estogenic like affects
  - Increases sweat production
  - 2 grams powdered seed TID
  - 2-3 grams decocted as a tea TID
  - Effective in 24-72 hrs
  - Increases pump volume overall in one week
  - Can reduce need for intervention to increase milk supply

Urtica diocea/ Nettle

- Traditional food for breastfeeding
- High mineral, enzyme, and vitamin green
- Tea, tincture, food, juice

Herbal Galactagogues

- Silybum marianum/ Milk Thistle

Virgin Mary's Milk dropped on the leaves

Traditionally the whole plant was boiled as a food to support breatfeeding.

Clinical Studies show;
  - 420 mg/day is effective dose
  - Increases volume 60-80%
  - Effects seen in 30 to 63 days
  - Possible dopamine receptor antagonist

Milk Thistle
(Silybum Marianum)

50 healthy women with borderline lactation (700 ml/day)
- 2600 kcal diet for placebo and test group
- 25 women 420 mg of micronized silymarin; 25 women placebo
- Silymarin group increased supply by 64.4% in 30 days and 89.95% in 63 days
- placebo 22.5% in 30 days and 32.09% in 63 days
- (? breast pump factor)
- No difference in milk composition
- No drop outs/good compliance and tolerability

Acta Biomed Dec 2008; 79(3): 205-210

Vitex Agnus-Castus

- Two clinical studies showed that vitex is effective in increasing the mild production of lactating women with poor milk production.
- One study found favorable effect in 80% of the 125 participants.
- In the second controlled trial with 817 patients, those taking Vitex produced and average of three times as much milk as that of the controls after 20 days of treatment.
- Pharmacological studies with animals have also demonstrated increase in lactation and enlargement of the mammary gland. No hazards to nursing infants has been noted in any of these studies.

Lawrence Review of Natural Products

Holy Basil
Ocimum sanctum

- Mental cloudiness
- Uplifting
- Enhancing mental clarity and meditation
- Tones CNS
- Sleep restorative

Holy Basil

- Adaptogen, antiviral, galactogogue, radioprotective, hypoglycemic, anti-inflammatory, cortisol regulator
- Enhancing metabolic functions and natural resistance
- Cortisol reducing compounds
- Ursolic acid, a constituent in Holy Basil, reveals it's activity as an anti-inflammatory and COX-2 inhibitor.
- Enhances the activity of glutathione S-transferase, a key enzyme in detoxification.

Holy Basil

Preparations:

- Fresh leaf
- Herbal tea
- Dried powder-250-1000mg/d
- Tincture-4-10mls/day 1:5 LE
- Mixed powdered herb with ghee

Aspargus Racemosus

- **Common name**: Shatavari
- **Active Constituents**: steriodal saponins with estrogen modulating activities
- **Actions:**
  - "She who has a hundred husbands"
  - Toning to pituitary gland; HPA axis
  - Demulcent
    - Urinary
    - Respiratory
    - Gastric (ulcers)

Aspargus Racemosus

- Common uses:
  - Reproductive tonic
    - Increase fertility, libido
    - Menopause: vaginal dryness/dry skin
  - Galactogogue – increases prolactin levels
  - Nutritive & immune system tonic
  - Anemia
  - Chronic fatigue
  - Cystitis, gastric ulcers,
  - Irritable coughs (difficult to expectorate & sticky mucus)

Culinary Herbal Galactogogues

- Aromatic Seeds - Anise, dill, fennel, caraway, cardamom, fenugreek, coriander
- 2 tsp of seeds
- 12 oz of water
- Simmer seeds in water for 10 minutes covered
- Strain and drink 1 cup three time per day

Herbal Galactagogues

Herbal Seed Tea to Enhance Breastmilk
  Fennel
  Fenugreek
  Milk Thistle

Mix 2 ounces of @ with 1 ounce
  Cardamom- coarsely chop
  Anise

Use 2 tsp to 12 ounces boiling

Water steep covered 5-10 min

Herbal Tea to Support Lactation

- Foeniculum vulgare/Fennel- seed
- Silybum marianum/ Milk Thistle-seed
- Urtica dioca/ Nettle leaf
- Blessed Thistle-whole herb
- Rose petals

Use equal parts of each herb, mix well in a large glass jar and use 2-3 teaspoons per 8 ounces boiling water, steep 5-10 minutes, strain and drink 1-3 times daily

Herbal Galactagogue Tincture

- Foeniculum vulgare/Fennel- seed
- Silybum marianum/ Milk Thistle-seed
- Urtica dioca/ Nettle leaf
- Galega officinalis/ Goat's Rue-leaf
- Verbena spp/ Blue Vervain
- Aspargus Racemosus/Shatavari

Mix equal parts and use ½ to 1 tsp BID to TID before meals

Herbal Galactagogues

- Infusions, tablets or capsules
- Tinctures if necessary (dose post feed)
- Effects start to be observed in 3-4 days
- Use higher doses initially
- Adjust dose after 2-3 weeks
- Include herbal nervines & relaxants if indicated

Foods to Enrich Milk Supply

- Oats, barley
- Peas, legumes
- Walnuts, almonds
- Sunflower, sesame, flax seed, pumpkin
- Hemp seed and oil

Avoid coffee and black tea as decreases supply as does pineapple and sage

Herbal Salve used for Tender Cracked Nipples

- Althea root or Slippery elm
- Chickweed or witch hazel
- Calendula, Chamomile or Yarrow flowers
- Make an oil or salve from a combination of the above herbs, use several times a day after nursing baby. Wipe gently with a dry cloth before nursing baby again

Mastitis

Systemic Therapies

- Hydrate and take electrolytes
- Buffered Vitamin C, dose 3-6 grams/day
- Herbal Formula
  - 30 mls Echinacea
  - 20 mls @ Calendula, Baptisa, Fucus, Tumeric
  - 10 mls @ phytolacca

  Use ½ to 1tsp TID/QID

Mastitis

Topical Preparations:

- Grated Potato Poultice
- Chamomile & scored Cabbage Leaf Poultice
- SWS- Seaweed Slim (fomentation)
- Castor Oil Pack; cold or warm

Grated Potato and Slippery Elm Poultice

- 1 medium potato grated
- 2-3 tsp slippery elm powder

- Mix well, form into small patty and place on area for 10-15 minutes, 1-3 times a day
- *This may be used on sore or cracked nipples as well*

References

Journal of Human Lactation 29(2) 154 –162© The Author(s) 2013
Reprints and permission: sagepub.com/journalsPermissions.navDOI: 10.1177/0890334413477243jhl.sagepub.com

Luteal Phase Deficiency
What is it all about?

Mary Bove ND
herbaldocmb@gmail.com
SW Herbal Conference 4/2106

Luteal Phase Deficiency (LPD)

- A condition in which endogenous progesterone is not sufficient to maintain a functional secretory endometrium and allow normal embryo implantation and growth

- Controversy regarding the clinical significance of LPD is due in part to the lack of a reliable test to diagnose this disorder

---

The Ovarian Cycle

- The ovarian cycle consists of the follicular phase, ovulation and the luteal phase.
- During the follicular phase, day 1 to ovulation, FSH causes the growth of the ovarian follicle readying it for ovulation.
- Post-ovulation the ovary enters the luteal phase, which lasts until menstruation.

The Luteal Phase

- Ovulation occurs 10-12 hrs post LH peak and 36-48 hrs post estradiol peak
- With LH rising there is a rapid drop in estrogen, followed by a drop in LH
- Progesterone production increasing by the luteinized cells in the follicle
- 8-9days post ovulation peak vasculation of the follicle is reached. This is crucial in the delivery of LDLs to the corpus luteum, as progesterone is made from the LDLs
- Corpus luteum production of progesterone, peaks 6-8 days post ovulation. Small amounts of estrogens are produced and also peaks at day 6-8.
- 9-11 days post ovulation if conception does not occur the corpus luteum degenerates causing estrogen ad progesterone to drop and menses to occur.
- The endometrium enters the secretory phase, becoming thick with blood
- Luteal phase is the most predictable in length, as the life span of the corpus luteum is relatively constant at 14 days +/- 2 days.

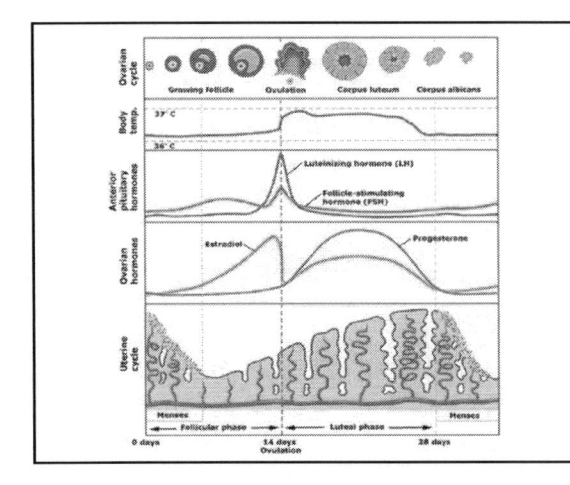

LPD

- Given the importance of the luteal phase in the establishment of a normal pregnancy, LPD has a strong association with fertility issues
- Although there appears to be an association with infertility, it has not been established that persistent LPD is a cause of infertility

LPD has been associated with

- Fertility issues
- First trimester pregnancy loss
- Short cycles
- premenstrual spotting
- anorexia, starvation, and eating disorders
- excessive exercise
- Stress
- obesity and polycystic ovary syndrome (PCOS)
- Endometriosis
- Aging
- Thyroid dysfunction and hyperprolactinemia

Fertility and Sterility® Vol. 103, No. 4, April 2015 0015-0282/$36.00
Copyright ©2015 American Society for Reproductive Medicine, Published by Elsevier Inc.
http://dx.doi.org/10.1016/j.fertnstert.2014.12.128

Luteal Phase Deficiency

- Occurs during the postpartum period
- With significant weight loss or exercise
- In random cycles of normally menstruating women
- LPD is only clinically relevant if it is consistently present in most cycles

Infertility and LPD

- Due to the fact that the endometrium is not adequately developed, it is then not prepared for implantation of a fertilized ovum.
- Multiple miscarriages in the first trimester can be due to lack of progesterone caused by LPD.
- Progesterone is needed not only to prepare the uterine wall for implantation; it also helps the implanted ovum to remain in place during the delicate first trimester.

PMS and LPD

- Relates to the physical and emotional events occurring during the luteal phase of the cycle that resolve once bleeding begins
- Mood: anger, anxiety, tearfulness
- Altered cognition "fog brain"
- Physical: breast pain, swelling, headaches, palpitations
- Most common in early puberty and perimenopause
- Worsened by stress

Botanical Medicines for LPD

- Alchemilla vulgaris – Ladies Mantle
- Angelica sinensis – Dong Quai
- Eleutherococcus senticosis – Siberian ginseng
- Glycyrrhiza glabra - Licorice
- Medicago sativa – Alfalfa
- Trifolium pratense - Red Clover
- Viburnum opulus – Cramp bark, Highbush Cranberry
- Vitex agnus castus – Chaste tree
- Withania somnifera - Ashwaganda

Botanical Approaches for LPD

- Anti-spasmodic and nervine herbs
- Uterine tonics
- Hormone normalizers
- Pelvic decongestants
- General and local nervines
- Adaptogens

Anti-spasmodic & Nervine Herbs

- Included in this group of herbs are those plants which not only relax the muscular tissues, but also those which act to relax the whole body, so as to bring a generalized relaxed state. The different botanicals in this group do that to differing degrees. These medicines can be important in the treatment of various gynecological conditions, ranging for dysmenorrhea to infertility.
  - Artemisa vulgaris - Mugwort
  - Avena sativa - Wild oats
  - Cimicfuga racemosa - Black Cohosh
  - Hypericum perfoliatum - St John's wort
  - Piscidia erythrina - Jamaican Dogwood
  - Verbena spp - Blue vervain
  - Viburnum opulus - Cramp Bark, Highbush Cranberry

Wild Oats
Avena sativa

Wild Oats

- Nervine (for "nervous exhaustion")
- Stabilizes blood glucose

- Eur J Clin Nutr. 2013 Apr; 67(4):310-7

Uterine Tonics

- These are the plants that feed and support the normal function of the reproductive organs. They act more slowly and are usually given over a period of time to bring about a long lasting and regulating effect. Some of the plants work due to their nutrient content, others by increasing blood and lymph flow to and from the organs and others due to secondary hormonal effects.
  - Alchemilla vulgaris - Lady's Mantle
  - Leonurus cardiaca – Motherwort
  - Mitchella repens - Squaw Vine
  - Rubus ideaus - Red Raspberry
  - Verbena spp – Blue vervain

Rubus Idaeus

Hormone Normalizers

- This is an important group of plants in the treatment of reproductive disorders as they tend to normalize and optimize the function of the endocrine glands. These plants should always be considered in the treatment of menstrual irregularities, fibroids, fertility issues, hormonal imbalance and breast disorders.
  - Medicago sativa - Alfalfa
  - Cimicfuga racemosa - Black Cohosh
  - Salvia officinalis – Sage leaf
  - Taraxacum officinalis – Dandelion
  - Trifolium pratenses – Red clover
  - Verbena spp – Blue vervain
  - Vitex agnus-castus – Chaste tree

Red Clover
Trifolium pratense

Red Clover

- Improves follicular steroidogenesis and upregulates estrogen receptors (animal study)
  - Theriogenology. 2013 Oct 15;80(7):821-8
- Activates progesterone receptor signaling
  - Steroids. 2012 Jun;77(7):765-73
- PPAR agonist; helps glucose/insulin control
  - J Steroid Biochem Mol Biol. 2014 Jan;139:277-89
- Clinically helpful for vasomotor symptoms, though not supported by research

Chaste tree berry
Vitex agnus-castus

Chaste tree berry

- Dopaminergic (lowers prolactin)
- Action likely via FSH/ LH and subsequent effect on estradiol/progesterone ratio
- Principal constituents include diterpenoids, flavonoids, iridoids, fatty oils

  » Pharmacogn Rev. 2013 Jul-Dec; 7(14): 188–198.

Pelvic Congestion

- A dysfunctional state of the pelvic circulation and movement which can manifest as many symptoms, syndromes and disease states of the female reproductive system.
- As the term implies the pelvic region of the body becomes congested, engorged, and stagnant be it with lymph fluids, blood, inflammation, emotions, traumas, and energy.
- The normal movement of the pelvic region becomes compromised and lack of vitality sets in, leading to dysfunction and disease.

Pelvic Decongestants

- This group of plants acts to:
  - decrease congestion in the pelvic region
  - increase circulation of fluids to and from pelvic region
  - balance tissue, muscle, and vascular tension
  - increase vitality of the organs and tissues
- Used in formulas for fibroids, painful menses, heavy menses, prolapsed uterus, prolapsed vaginal walls, endometriosis, PMS, labial varicosities, painful intercourse, vaginal discharge, abdominal water retention, low back pain, infertility, irregular menses, bladder issues, and constipation.

Botanical Pelvic Decongestants

- Angelica sinensis – Dong Quai
- Cimicfuga racemosa - Black Cohosh
- Leonurus cardiaca - Motherwort
- Mitchella repens - Squaw Vine
- Taraxacum officinalis – Dandelion
- Trifolium pratenses – Red clover
- Viburnum opulus - Cramp Bark

Dandelion
Taraxacum officinale

Dandelion

- Supports liver function (estrogen breakdown?)
- Upregulates estrogen receptors, progesterone receptors and FSH receptors
    – Int J Mol Med 2007 Sep;20(3):287-92
- Decreases CRF, ACTH and corticosterone in animal models
    – Pharm Biol 2014 Aug;52(8):1028-32

Combine pelvic decongestants with

- Circulatory stimulates such as: capsicum, ginger, cinnamon, xanthoxyllum, rosemary.
- Anti-spasmodic and nervine herbs to relax the muscular tissues in the pelvis region, but also to relax the whole body, so as to bring a generalized relaxed state to the whole person.
- Consider aromatic herbs with pleasant flavors such as melissa, rose petals, lavender flowers, holy basil, hops, or linden flowers.

Botanical Adaptogens

- Asparagus racemosus - Shatavari
- Eleutherococcus senticosus – Eleuthero root
- Medicinal Mushroom Species
    - Reishi, Shiitake, Maitake
- Ocimum sanctum – Holy Basil
- Rhodiola rosea
- Withania somnifera - Ashwagandha

Holy Basil
Ocimum sanctum

Holy Basil

- Complex adaptogen
- Anti-inflammatory, antihistaminic
- Hypotensive, immunomodulatory, anticoagulant
- Diuretic

– Indian J Exp Biol. 2007 May;45(5):403-12

Mood Changes
(Hormonally-mediated)

- Present in both PMS and Perimenopause
- Anxiety
  - Often from higher estrogen / lower progesterone
  - Potentially from elevated cortisol
- Depression
  - Low cortisol, low DHEA affects neurotransmitters

Treatment of Mood Issues

- Anxiolytics
- Nervines
  - Wild oats
- Adaptogens
  - ashwagandha, holy basil
- Hormone modulators
  - Chaste tree berry

Herbal Tea for Depression

- Mix in a large jar 1 oz of each
  - Avena
  - Lemon Balm
  - Linden Flowers
  - Rose Petals
  - Vervain

Use 1 tsp herbal mix to 1 cup boiling water steep covered 1-3 minutes. Drink several times daily.
A stronger tea may be made and added to the bath

Case Study #1
31 yr old woman with PMS

- Thirty one year old woman who presents with PMS symptoms including tender breasts, constipation, mood swings, and headaches.
- Reports one miscarriage in the first trimester of pregnancy 2 yrs ago, allergies, migraine headaches, and low back pain.
- History of oral birth control use for 10 years, ceasing 5 years prior to visit.
- She has suffered much emotional trauma related to her miscarriage and feels apprehensive about getting pregnant, yet that is what she wants most.

Case Study
31yr old woman

- Menstrual cycle were 30 –39 days, with 5-6 days of moderate to mild bleeding, PMS symptoms from 12 weeks of her cycle.
- P.E. shows a chronic bacterial vaginosis with secondary yeast flare
- Lab values show low progesterone in the second half of her cycle, normal thyroid, mild iron deficiency anemia, and normal LH surge at her mid-cycle.

Botanical Formula
31 yr old woman

- Chaste Tree berry
- Elderberry
- Mitchella repens
- Cramp bark/ Viburnum opulus
- Blue Vervain
- Raspberry leaf
- Dandelion leaf and root
- Prickly Ash bark

Take 5 mls 2 times a day for several months

CASE STUDY #2
36 y/o Female Multiple Miscarriage

- History of 4 previous miscarriages in past 2 years
- Emotionally distraught and fearful of the stress of future miscarriages
- Referred by ND colleague
- Librarian at high school, main $ for couple
- Generally healthy, seasonal allergies, constipation and bloating, often cold

---

36 y/o Female

- Nml menstrual hx; 26 days, heavy for 1st day w/cramps, hypotensive, dizziness, 5-6 days total, midcycle discomfort
- Miscarriage hx – 10 to 14 weeks gestation
- No issues conceiving
- Low Progesterone, saliva & serum, Using 50 mg bio-identical progesterone

---

36 y/o Female

- Labs; CBC ESR, ferritin, metabolic panel, Vt D
- Rule out Anti-Phospholipid Syndrome (APS)
- Functional labs; IGg Food Allergy-90, BBT for 1 month, Urine Iodine spot & load
- Prior labs – serum progesterone 3.7 luteal, TAP saliva cortisol - nml levels, abnml curve, low saliva progesterone, TSH - nml

---

36 y/o Female

- Uterus retroverted position
  - Pelvic uterine massage, cat pose, hoola hoop
- Lab Outcomes
  - Low ferritin, Vt D,
  - Iodine low and poor saturation,
  - BBT average 97.6 w/ little variation
  - Food Allergy + for almonds, dairy, egg white

Treatment Plan

- Address food/ GI issues, improve thyroid function, improve blood sugar function, reduce system inflammation, improve uterine tissue, tone, and circulation
- No active conception for 4 months
- Supplement iodine, Vt D, Vt E, probiotics, magnesium, EFAs, Pancreatic enzymes

Herbal Medicines

- Vitex, Rhodiola & Shatavari blend 5mls BID
- Ashwagandha capsules, 1cap BID
- Holy Basil Tea 1-2 cups daily
- Turmeric, Licorice and Ginger blend
- Cramp Bark and Blue Vervain blend used during menses for cramps

Progress

- After 4 months; iodine nml, progesterone improved in luteal phase, digestion better with good bowel habits, wgt lose, hair growth, ok to try for pregnancy, BBT-98.2
- Off iodine, enzymes, Turmeric, Licorice and Ginger blend
- Switch Vitex, Rhodiola & Shatavari blend to Rhodiola/Ashwagandha Phytocaps

Outcome

- No pregnancy after 2 month, got severe cold with fever, dizziness, lymph swelling and tenderness
- Tx - Cleaver, Burdock Rt, and Calendula
- Continue conception plan
- Switch 50 mg oral Progesterone to vaginal suppository, day 12- 26

Outcome

- No pregnancy after 4 month
- Visit to support her and continue plan
- Pregnancy 5th month
- Early progesterone and HcG levels good with increase in levels one week later - nml
- Continue Rhodiola/Ashwagandha/ progesterone until week 10-12
- Ruby born healthy and happy at 40 weeks

Exploring Botanicals Impacting Thyroid Function and Female Endocrine Health

Mary Bove ND
herbaldocmb@gmail.com
marybove.com

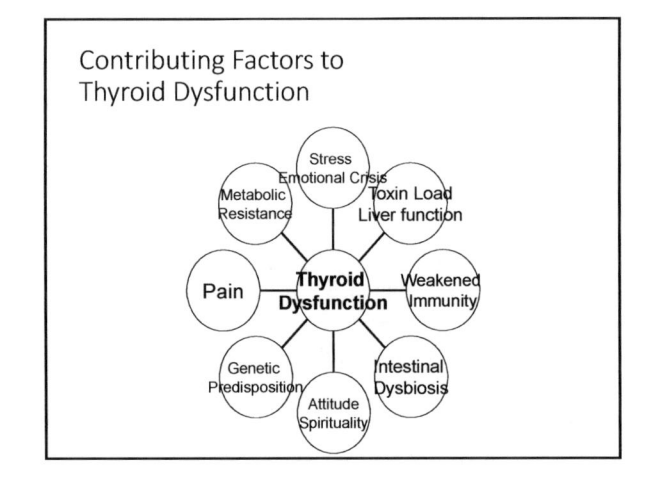

Contributing Factors to Thyroid Dysfunction

- Stress/Emotional Crisis
- Toxin Load/Liver function
- Weakened Immunity
- Intestinal Dysbiosis
- Attitude/Spirituality
- Genetic Predisposition
- Pain
- Metabolic Resistance

Endocrine Stressors

- Substances capable of disrupting normal function of the endocrine system
- Impacts male & female reproductive system leading to fertility issues
- Disrupts thyroid hormone metabolism & increases anti-thyroid antibodies
- CNS-chronic stress, mood disorders

Chemicals and Xenobiotics

- Hormones, PCBs, phenolic compounds
- Disrupt thyroid hormone metabolism
- Production of antithyroidal antibodies
- Inhibition of thyroid hormone activity
- Inhibits iodine metabolism
- Increased risk for infants and children

Environmental Toxins

- HALIDES: Bromine, Chlorine, Flourine May Interfere With Iodine Uptake
- HEAVY METALS: Cadmium, Lead, Mercury May Interfere with T3-T4 Conversion, and ultimately lower T3 levels
- CHEMICALS: Organochlorides, PCBs. PBDEs May agonize, antagonize TH Receptors, and other with other endocrine disruption
- LOW ANTIOXIDANT LEVELS: Vitamins E, C, Selenium May Reduce Protective Mechanisms against the above heavy metals and chemicals

Environmental Hazards

Heavy Metals
Electromagnetic radiation
- Computers and electrical devices
  - Immune and endocrine suppression
  - Altered red and white blood counts
  - Hair loss in a uniform pattern

Insights from Medical Anthropology

- Indigenous peoples of northern latitudes have higher BMRs than tropical peoples as an adaptation to colder climates.
- Medical anthropologist have found that thyroid function is strongly shaped by environmental factors such as changes in temperature and nutrition.

Insights from Medical Anthropology

- The presence of a supportive and tactile community is vital for optimal thyroid function.
- Feeling of alienation and loneliness

Exposure to Sunlight

Morning light starts;
- Physical activity
- Hormone secretions
- Urine output
- Body temperature
- Stimulates the thyroid to burn fat

Stress is a silent factor

- Immune dysregulation due to the increased levels of immune complexes
- Stress effects thyroid hormone function
- Decreased production via HPT axis
- Impacts the peripheral conversion of thyroid hormone via inhibition of 5'-deiodinase

Stress is a silent factor

Excessive cortisol associated with:

- Depressed levels of active T3
- Reduced peripheral hormone metabolism
- Increased risk for autoimmune disorders

Autoimmune Thyroid Disease

- **Hyperthyroidism – Grave's Disease**
  - female to male ratio of 8:1
  - ages 20 to 40years old
  - common etiology of hyperthyroidism
- **Hypothyroidism – Hashimoto's Disease**
  - most common cause of hypothyroidism in US
  - 10-20% of women over the age of fifty
  - female to male ratio of 10:1[1]

Factors linked to thyroid autoimmune processes

- Epstien-Barr virus, intestinal tract parasite or yeast infection, bacterial infections
- Pregnancy and the postpartum period
- Allergies-foods, chemicals, plastics, environmental pollutants
- Genetics
- Stress

Hypothyroidism

- Condition of deficient thyroid secretion or conversion of T4 to T3
- Subclinical: minimal or no symptoms in the present of normal serum free T4 and T3 with elevated TSH.

Hypothyroidism: Etiology

- Primary
- Secondary
- Tertiary
- Autoimmune (Hashimoto's disease)
- Conversion disorder (Wilson's Temperature Syndrome)
- Postpartum

Hypothyroidism

In hypothyroidism, levels of thyroid hormone are low. The thyroid gland can be small or large (goiter), depending on the cause of the disorder

Atrophied thyroid

*ADAM.

Hypothyroidism

- • Hypothyroidism affects a significant % of the population, and may occur in tandem with Metabolic Syndrome, both being associated with:
- – Hyperlipidemia
- – Dysglycemia
- – Reproductive Issues

Hypothyroid Symptoms

- Fatigue, weight gain, cold intolerance, muscle weakness
- Depression, insomnia, memory loss, poor concentration, headaches
- Dry skin, brittle hair constipation
- Irregular menstruation, loss of libido, infertility, miscarriage, premature delivery
- Hyperlipidemia
- Recurring infections

Hashimoto's Disease

- Antibodies are formed against thyroid peroxidase enzyme, thyroglobulin, and TSH receptors preventing the manufacture of sufficient levels of thyroid hormone.

- These antibodies may also bind to the adrenal glands, pancreas, and acid-producing cells of the stomach (parietal cells).

Hypothyroidism: Laboratory Evaluation

- Serum TSH
- Serum free T4 or Free Thyroxine Index
- Serum free T3
- Anti-thyroid antibodies
- Thyroid urine or saliva profiles

Drug →	Thyroid Tablets, USP (Armour® Thyroid)	Liotrix Tablets, USP (Thyrolar™®)	Liothronine Tablets, USP (Cytomel®)	Levothyroxine Tablets, USP (Unithroid® ⁵, Levoxyl® ᵈ, Levothroid® ⁵, Synthroid® ᶠ)
Approx. Dose Equivalent	1/4 grain (15 mg)	1/4		25 mcg (.025 mg)
Approx. Dose Equivalent	1/2 grain (30 mg)	1/2	12.5 mcg	50 mcg (.05 mg)
Approx. Dose Equivalent	1 grain (60 mg)	1	25 mcg	100 mcg (.1 mg)
Approx. Dose Equivalent	1 1/2 grains (90 mg)	1 1/2	37.5 mcg	150 mcg (.15 mg)
Approx. Dose Equivalent	2 grains (120 mg)	2	50 mcg	200 mcg (.2 mg)
Approx. Dose Equivalent	3 grains (180 mg)	3	75 mcg	300 mcg (.3 mg)

Nature-Throid was formulated with the following ingredients:

Active Ingredient:
Thyroid USP (desiccated porcine thyroid)
*Lactose Monohydrate (Lactose is not added to our formula but it is already present in Thyroid USP raw material as a diluent per USP (United States Pharmacopeia). Lactose is not contraindicated for individuals with allergies to dairy, as lactose is a milk sugar (vs. dairy allergies, which are caused by proteins in milk). It is, however, contraindicated for individuals with lactose intolerance. We have had many physicians reporting no side effects while using Nature-Throid with lactose intolerant patients. The amount is very small – less than 5 mg. per 1 Grain vs. 12,000 – 15,000 mg. in a typical 8 fl. oz. glass of milk.)
Inactive Ingredients:
Colloidal Silicon Dioxide
Dicalcium Phosphate
Magnesium Stearate
Microcrystalline Cellulose
Croscarmellose Sodium
Stearic Acid
Opadry II 85F19316 Clear – tablet coating

Possible Drug Interaction with Armour Thyroid

- Asthma medications such as Theo-Dur
  Blood thinners such as Coumadin
  Cholestyramine (Questran)
  Colestipol (Colestid)
  Estrogen preparations (including some birth control pills such as Ortho-Novum and Premarin)
  Insulin
  Oral diabetes drugs such as Diabinese and Glucotrol)

The Armour® Thyroid by Forest Pharmaceuticals contains:

- 1. Thyroid Powder, USP
  2. Dextrose, Anhydrous
  3. Microcrystalline Cellulose, NF
  4. Sodium Starch Glycolate, NF
  5. Calcium Stearate, NF
  6. Opadry White (titanium dioxide used as a whitening agent)

- *Armour Thyroid does not contain gluten or lactose*

Treatment Goals for Thyroid Disease

- Support the thyroid gland and function
- Eliminate microorganism infections and allergies
- Reduce inflammation, balance immune function

Treatment Goals for Thyroid Disease

- Repair the gut function, permeability of gastrointestinal mucus membranes, improve gut dysbiosis and absorption
- Correct nutritional deficiencies
- Reduce toxic load improve detox pathways
- Stress reduction both internal and external sources.

Hypothyroidism: Evidence Based Botanical Therapy

- Coleus forskohli
- Commiphora mukul
- Fucus spp.
- Laminaria spp.
- Withania somnifera

Coleus forskohlii

- Essential oil and diterpenes
- Increases thyroid hormone production
- Increases thyroid hormone secretion
- Activates cAMP production
- Activates hormone sensitive lipase
- Acts synergistically with Crataegus to inhibit phosphodiestrase

Withania somnifera Ashwagandha

- Alkaloids, steroidal lactones, saponins
- increases T4 hormone production
- increases conversion to T4 to T3
- Anti-inflammatory, sedative nervine, tonic
- Adaptogen

Comminphora mukul Guggul

- lipid-soluble steroids found in resin
- thyroid stimulating activity, but not via pituitary – TSH mechanism, direct action on gland
- peripheral conversion of T4 to T3 increasing T3 levels
- reduces LDL cholesterol in individuals with functional hypothyroidism, may be related to the stimulation of T3 by guggulsterones
- Increases weight lose

Fucus and Laminaria spp

- provide iodine in its natural state

- seaweeds acts to support thyroid hormone synthesis by providing one of the precursors used in thyroid hormone synthesis

- polysaccharides that bind to heavy metals, such lead, mercury, and cadmium which can interfere with thyroid function

---

Sea Vegetables

- • Seaweeds are high in numerous minerals and halides including iodine.
- • The bioavailability of the iodine in seaweed has been shown to be quite good, though slightly less than direct KI supplementation.

Cell Mol Biol 2002 Jul;48(5):563-9. Bioavailability of seaweed iodine in human beings.

Sea Vegetables

- Not only do seaweeds such as Fucus provide iodine, seaweeds are reported to contain di-iodotyrosine or DIT.
- Seaweeds, containing DIT may promote thyroid function by making it easier for the thyroid gland to make active thyroid hormones.

Eur. J. Biochem. 51 (2): 329–36; February 1975

Seaweed provides DIT

- The presence of di-iodothyronine (DIT) within the colloid of the thyroid gland may stimulate the gland to produce thyroxine.
- Of various seaweeds tested, iodine content is highest in young freshly cut blades and lowest in sun dried seaweeds.

Bladderwrack

- Fucus vesiculosus contains the flavonoid flucoxanthin reported to have the greatest antioxidant activity of all the edible seaweeds tested.
- This may contribute to stabilizing effects in thyroiditis

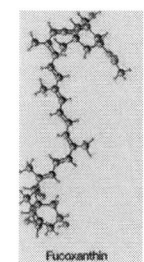

Fucoxanthin

Hypothyroidism: Botanical Therapy

- Adjunctive Botanicals
  - Glycyrrhiza glabra
  - Astragalus membranaceous
  - Eleutherococcus senticosus
  - Panax quinqefolium
  - Rhodiola rosea
  - Scutellaria baicalensis

Hypothyroid Botanical Formula

- Coleus forsika 1:3: 45% 20mls
- Withania somnifera 1:2 50% 20mls
- Fucus 1.2 55% 20mls
- Licorice 1:1 20% 15mls
- Guggul 1:3 55% 15mls
- Urtica 1:1 45% 15mls
- Rieshi mushroom 1:2 50% 10mls
- Ginger 1:5 60% 5mls
- Take 5mls am and noon.

Hypothyroidism: Additional Therapies

- Identify and eliminate food allergies
  - Gluten & endocrine autoantibodies
- Adequate iodine consumption
- Exercise: increases thyroid function and tissue sensitivity to thyroid hormone.
- Stress reduction and management
- Exposure to morning light

Hypothyroidism: Nutrient Therapy

- Selenium: necessary for conversion of T4 to T3
- Zinc: involved in synthesis of TRH, cofactor for 5'-deiodinase, delta desaturases
- Copper: cofactor for iodothyronine iodinse

Selenium Cofactor

- All the iodinase, deiodinase and peroxidase enzymes are selenium dependent.
- Selenium and iodine work synergistically.
- Selenium can affect iodine metabolism, homeostasis, and bioavailability, and thereby also play a role in thyroid function

Hypothyroidism: Nutrient Therapy

- Tyrosine: 500-1500 mg qd
- Essential fatty acids: decreased delta 6- and delta-5 desaturease activity in hypothyroidism.

Dietary goitrogens

- broccoli, cauliflower, brussels sprouts, cabbage, kohlrabi
- sweet potatoes
- almonds, pine nuts, peanuts
- millet
- peaches
- soy

Case--53 y.o. woman

- Menopausal complaints – severe hot flashes, insomnia, forgetfulness
- Hypercholesterolemia - 238 total, 144LDL, 52 HDL
- Hypertension -146/90
- Overweight by 40 pounds
- Anxiety

53 y.o. woman

- Complains of being cold most of the time
- Exercises recreationally, yoga
- Eats a whole foods diets, craves chocolate, avoids caffeinated drinks
- Hx of severe dysmenorhea, mennorhagia, and PMS, 2 children
- No family history of thyroid disease

53 y.o. woman

- Complains of being cold most of the time
- Exercises recreationally, yoga
- Eats a whole foods diets, craves chocolate, avoids caffeinated drinks
- Hx of severe dysmenorhea, mennorhagia, and PMS, 2 children
- No family history of thyroid disease

Treatment Plan for 6 months

- Exercise 20 minutes daily in the morning outside. Yoga evenings 3x/wk
- Gluten free diet
- Pancreatic digestive enzymes with HCL
- Astragalus, Althea offinalis & Ulmus falva (2-1-1) Powder 1Tbsp daily ac

Hypothyroidism: Nutrient Therapy

- Selenium: necessary for conversion of T4 to T3
- Zinc: involved in synthesis of TRH, cofactor for 5'-deiodinase, delta desaturase
- Copper: cofactor for iodothyronine iodinase
- Tyrosine: 500-1500 mg qd
- Essential fatty acids: decreased delta 6- and delta-5 desaturase activity in hypothyroidism.

Hypothyroid Botanical Formula

- Coleus forskohlii 1:3: 45%   20mls
- Withania somnifera 1:2 50%   20mls
- Fucus 1.2 55%   20mls
- Rehmannia 1:5 45%   15mls
- Guggul 1:3 55%   15mls
- Urtica 1:1 45%   15mls
- Reishi mushroom 1:2 50%   10mls
- Ginger 1:5 60%   5mls
- Take 5mls TID cc.

Outcomes 6 month later

- TSH– 2.10, T4 – 1.2, T3 - 133
- Antibodies
- Adrenal Stress DHEA low, cortisol – slightly low am, low SIgA
- Cholesterol 218, LDL 124, HDL 54
- BBT 97.8
- BP 136/80
- Weight lose 13 lbs

Hyperthyroidism

- Autoimmune: Graves disease
- stimulatory anti-TSH receptor antibodies
- comprises the majority of hyperthyroid cases
- increase growth, size, and function of gland
- several common features including: thyrotoxicosis, goiter, ophthalmopathy, and pretibial myxedema.

Thyrotoxicosis symptoms

- Heat intolerance, diaphoresis, fatigue, weakness, weight loss
- Hair loss, nail and skin changes
- Diarrhea, increased appetite
- Palpitations, tachycardia
- Personality changes, nervousness, tremor

Hyperthyroidism: Laboratory Evaluation

- Increase total T4, free T4, free T4 index
- Increased total T3, free T3, T3 resin uptake (T3 can be elevated out of proportion to T4)
- decreased TSH
- Anti-TSH receptor antibodies (Grave's)

- Basal metabolic rate is increased in the hyperthyroid state, which is physiologically similar to a chronic reaction to stress with catabolic consequences including impaired glucose tolerance, impaired liver function and increases calcium needs

Excessive thyroxine

- potentates the actions of catecholamines, using up glucose, accelerating degradation of insulin and further increasing the work load of the pancreas to secret more insulin

- burns large amounts of glucose and the liver stores of glycogen become depleted, increasing the susceptibility to liver damage.

Treatment Goals

- Support thyroid function
- Eliminate infection and allergies
- Reduce inflammation/balance immune function
- Treat underlying gut permeability, dysbiosis
- Correct nutrient deficiencies
- Reduce toxic load/ improve detoxification
- Stress reduction

Hyperthyroidism
Evidence Based Botanical Therapy

- Lycopus spp.
- Lithospermum officinale
- Melissa officinalis
- Leonurus cardiaca

Botanicals

- Aqueous, freeze-dried extracts of Lycopus spp., Lithospermum officinale and Melissa officinalis have been studied in vivo and in vitro[5,6,7,8]
- preliminary results support their use in Graves' disease.
- inhibit TSH effects on TSH receptor sites on thyroid cell membranes,
- block effects of antithyroid immunoglobulins on TSH receptors
- inhibit peripheral deiodination of T4 to T3.

Lycopus spp
Bugleweed

- blocks the TSH receptors
- inhibits peripheral conversion of T4 to T3
- contains caffeic acid, rosmarinic acid and chlorogenic acid which were found to exert antithyroid activity

Lithospermum offcinale

- blocks TSH receptors,
- influence the hypothalamic-pituitary-thyroid axis
- inhibits peripheral T4-deiodination

Leonurus cardiac
Motherwort

- contains the flavonoid, quercetin
- anti-inflammatory activity
- Inhibits the enzyme 5-deiodanase
- Traditionally used in the treatment of tachycardia and palpitations

Melissa officinalis
Lemon Balm

- caffeic acid, rosmarinic acid, chlorogenic acid, which exert antithyroid activity
- acts to block TSH receptors acting to inhibit stimulation of the receptor and thus thyroid gland function
- Traditional nervine and visceral relaxant

Melissa Extract and TSH

- • One study on whole Melissa extract showed that binding of TSH to the TSH receptor was interfered with by direct effects on TSH.

- • And stimulation of cells was interfered with by direct effects on the TSH receptor.

J Endocrinol Invest. 2003 Oct;26(10):950-5. vitro assay of thyroid disruptors affecting TSH-stimulated adenylate cyclase activity Santini F, Vitti P, Ceccarini G

Rosmarinic Acid for Hyperthyroidism

- Rosmarinic acid is a phenolic compound derived from caffeic acid and is most common in Lamiaceae and Boraginacea family plants including:
- Melissa officianalis (Lemon Balm)
- Lycopus europeas (Gypsywort)
- Lycopus virginia (Bugleweed)
- Lithospermum officianalis (Stoneseed or Gromwell)

All have been traditionally used for hyperthyroid symptoms

Rosmarinic Acid

- Rosmarinic Acid Also Shows a Binding Affinity for Graves Autoantibodies
- Grave's antibodies mimic TSH and bind to TSH receptors leading to excessive stimulation of the thyroid.
- Melissa has been shown to inhibit the ability of a TSH receptor antibody t promote intracellular cyclic AMP responses

---

RA in Autoimmune Inflammatory States

- Rosmarinic acid appears to reduce:
- • Autoimmune responses,
- • Auto antibody production
- • And Autoimmune processes contributing to Graves Dz
- Rosmarinic acid appears useful in other immune and autoimmune diseases including:
- • Asthma
- • Allergies

ROSMARINIC ACID
Avoid in Hypothyroidism

- NO.
- Even though Rosmarinic acid has the ability to reduce thyroid activity in cases of hyperthyroidism, ...
- It may also have the polar effect of enhancing thyroxine output or having a thyroxine-like effect within the hypofunctioning thyroid.

Hyperthyroidism: Botanical therapy

- Adjunctive Botanicals
    - Scutellaria laterifloria
    - Valeriana officinalis
    - Iris versicolor
    - Fucus spp
    - Eleutherococcus senticossus
    - Crataegus spp.
    - Silybum marianum

Hyperthyroid Botanical Formula

- Lycopus 1:1 45%   20mls
- Lithospermum 1:3 45%   20mls
- Melissa 1:1 45%   20mls
- Leonurus 1:3 45%   15mls
- Scutellaria laterfloria 1:3 50%   10mls
- Valerian 1:5 45%   10mls
- Elethrococcus 1:3 65%   15mls
- Take 5mls TID with meals
- Astragalus Capsules 500mgs BID

Hyperthyroidism: Nutrient Therapy

- Vitamin C offsets oxidative damage due to higher metabolic rate.
- Flavonoids: decrease serum T4, inhibit 5'-diodinase activity.[9]
- Calcium metabolism is altered increasing the risk for osteoporosis
- Selenium: alters conversion of T4 to T3, decreases anti-TPO-ab
- Zinc increased urinary excretion

L-carnitine

- Inhibits thyroid hormone uptake by the cell nucleus
- Treatment of hyperthyroidism
- 2-4 grams daily

Hyperthyroidism: Additional Therapies

- Hydrotherapy: cold application over thyroid gland for 5-15 min, bid inhibits thyroid activity[9]
- Yoga, tai chi, mediation
- Exposure to light
  - 2 hours of bright light in the morning reduces nocturnal restlessness by increasing serotonin levels.

Botanical Adaptogens

- The nature of thyroid dysfunction is often due to hyper or hypo function.
- Adaptogenic herbs have a role as supportive agents for normalizing thyroid function.
- Thyroid dysfunction results in metabolic dysfunction.

Adaptagenic Herbs for Thyroid Deregulation

- Rehmannia glutinosa
- Withania somnifera (Ashwagandha)

Rehmannia (R. glutinosa)

- Root, Scrophulariaceae
- Uncured- sweet, slightly bitter, cold, clear heat, cools blood
- Cured- sweet, warming, nourishes, blood
- 3-10ml/day 1:3 liquid extract
- 10-20 g/day dry uncured root

Rehmannia

- Adrenal trophorestorative, HPA axis
- Inhibits cortisol breakdown in liver
- Non hypertensive
- Buffer suppressive effects of corticosteroid drugs on endogenous levels of corticosteroids
- RA, asthma and urticaria
- Immune modulation
- With Astragalus m. for chronic nephritis

Ashwagandha Withania somnifera

- Root, Solanaceae
- Alkaloids, steroidal lactones, saponins
- Improves and conserves adaptive energy
- 5-15 mls/day 1:3 liquid extract
- 3-6g/day dry root

Withania somnifera (Ashwagandha)

- Increases T4 hormone production
- Increases conversion to T4 to T3
- Immune modulator, anti-inflammatory, anti-anemic
- Promoter of learning and memory retrieval; cognitive enhancer
- Enhances conception
- Increases stamina
- Tonic- debility, chronic exhaustion, low WBC, convalescence

Hypothyroidism with PCOS, Infertility, and Amenorrhea

- PCOS with amenorrhea and Infertility may involve sob-optimal thyroid function.

Formula
- Commiphora mukul
- Fucus
- Vitex
- Serenoa
- Glycyrrhiza

Formulated by Dr J Stansbury

Hyperthyroidism with Anxiety and Insomnia

- Hyperthyroidism may present as an anxiety disorder with racing thoughts, agitation, and poor sleep. Treat the nervous system and Adrenals as well as the thyroid.

Formula
- Melissa
- Leonurus
- Glycyrrhiza
- Hypericum
- Withania

Formulated by Dr J Stansbury

The Diamond of the Forest
Chaga Mushroom
Inonotus obliquus
Phyllis Hogan

Often times we search for something that ends up being just under our noses. Other times, the thing we are looking for is actually thousands of miles away, and it does the work in finding us. Allow me to take you on a journey that exemplifies a time when the perfect medicine did the work in finding me. I am a Southwest herbalist. I was taught the virtues of desert and mountain plants by legendary indigenous healers. One of the important lessons I received from the indigenous people is: The plants will find you when you are in need of healing. There are many ways this can occur. Sometimes they will come to you in the form of a dream. A teacher may introduce them to you. Or the ancient divine intelligence that governs the universe will flow through the plant and telepathically teach you what you need to know. Plants can even appear in a human form, and it is believed they themselves birthed us into existence, and we are their children. Plants should never be picked without prayer and with some type of an offering such as cornmeal, corn pollen, or tobacco. After collection, a symbolic gesture of cornmeal is given to feed the spirit of the plant. These ceremonious methods of harvesting provided me a life-long spiritual connection to the plants, but I had yet to experience what was to come next.

In the late winter of 2015, I realized I wasn't feeling my energetic self. My sleep wasn't deep, and at times I felt grouchy, tired, and depressed. I had been experiencing adrenal stress, gastrointestinal upset and generally felt rundown. These were all low-grade symptoms, but I felt like the natural order of my life was not quite in balance. It was about that time that a mycologist friend and an acupuncturist friend inquired if I had any experience with Chaga mushroom, or if I sold it in my herb store. I hadn't had any experience with Chaga, but listened intently about what they had to say. In my herb store, I focused on plants within my bioregion that we picked ourselves or were brought in by Native American collectors. I hadn't considered using or selling this fungus that grows in a bioregion so different from the one I am used to. Then, I realized what the elders said would happen, was happening to me. Chaga mushroom found me. It came to me from across the continents, just when I needed it most.

Chaga intrigued me because of its use by the Siberian shamans to increase longevity. It is known in Japan as the "Diamond of the Forest", and in China as "The King of Mushrooms". Chaga, a polypore fungus, grows as a wood conk on Birch in the form of a black, cankerous mass (sclerotium) on the living tree. Mycologists believe that many of the gilled mushrooms have evolved from polypores, which have pores instead of gills in their fruiting bodies. My quest to find the perfect Chaga began. I knew I had to find a supplier who gathered with respect and intent, the way I was taught 40 years ago. Oddly enough, it did not take me long to find an individual in Maine, an individual in Quebec, and a company in Siberia that had similar politics, and a spiritual connection to this life form. In hindsight, I believe this all came together so easily because Chaga knew I needed it.

When the first package of raw, wild-crafted Chaga finally arrived at Winter Sun, I was surprised to see how interesting it looked, not at all like what I expected. It was dense, hard, black and deeply cracked on the surface and beautiful yellow-brown in the interior. I was excited to try it, so on July 4th 2015; I began my love affair with the King of Mushrooms. When I cooked it up, it had a dark, rich, robust color, and looked intriguing. I was not prepared for what was about to happen next. After ingesting the preparation I had made, I felt a profound effect on my body that was almost instantaneous. After drinking 3 cups throughout the day, I went home that night with far more stamina than usual. I felt a re-birth that evening, a feeling that things were about to look up for me. That night I nestled into a deep sleep, and awoke feeling that same spark of optimism. During the next 6 weeks my symptoms of gastric distress improved, the depression vanished, and my patience was restored. Zest for life had returned. Since that initial experience, Chaga has continued to greatly enhance my vitality and health, helping me to counteract the effects of stress.

Chaga is consistently teaching me new lesson, and is furthering my trust in the time-honored traditions passed on by the elders of the southwest. At times we find our medicines, at other times they find us, and in both instances the results can be unexpected, mysterious, and exciting. I write about my experience to touch on the spiritual union that exists between plants and people. Along with my personal spiritual truth, there is also much scientific backing to the beneficial effects of Chaga on the human body. I believe plants are more than the sum of their chemical constituents, but learning the constituents helps to increase our understanding of their effects.

What is Chaga Mushroom?

Chaga is a highly prized tonic mushroom, and has many beneficial health effects. It has long been used in folk medicine, and was well researched in the 20th century by Russian and Scandinavian scientists. Current contributions to the growing body of research come from Japan, Korea, and China. Chaga contains a multitude of active constituents and cofactors, many of which are being investigated for their potential health benefits.

Chaga presents a complex living pharmacy, and some of the benefits are:

- Anti-bacterial
- Anti-inflammatory
- Anti-tumor
- Anti-viral
- Blood sugar regulation
- Liver protection
- Immune modulation
- Adaptogen
- Anti-oxidant
- Gastrointestinal tonifier

Important constituents in Chaga include:

- Polysaccharides (Beta glucans) - Immune enhancement, cell communication
- Melanin - Energizer, gene protection, DNA repair
- Inotidol- Lanosterolterpine; an apoptosis agent
- Betalinic Acid- Terpine - fights viruses and tumors
- Polyphenols- Antioxidants and free radical quenchers

~How To Use and Store~

Store Chaga in a glass container with holes in the lid to allow the Chaga to "breath". Avoid storing or preparing in plastic or metallic items.

To Prepare:

Crock Pot: Place 4-5 pieces in 1 quart of cold "alive" water (spring water or non-chlorinated). Turn on high for 2 hours, reduce heat to medium for another 2 hours, and keep on a warm setting until enjoyed. This batch can be re-used for up to 2 weeks, adding a couple fresh chunks of chaga each time you add the fresh water.

Stove top: Using the above ratios, bring to ALMOST boiling then reduce to a simmer for 3 hours - overnight.

Enjoy hot or cold. Chaga is great alone or brewed with cinnamon, cardamom, ginger, or any of you favorite herbs to enhance flavor. Due to its detoxing effects, be sure to drink extra water. Always compost your chaga, and give thanks to the sacred mushroom!

References and Further reading:

McDow, Ron, M.D. Wild Chaga: The Miraculous Medicinal Mushroom.

Pubmed. http://www.ncbi.nlm.nih.gov/pubmed.

Staments, Paul. Mycelium Running: How Mushrooms Can Help Save the World. Ten Speed Press, Berkley: 1987.

Staments, Paul. MycroMedicinals: An Informational Treatise on Mushrooms. Olympia: MycoMedia Productions, 2002 3rd edtion.

Wolfe, David. Chaga: King of the Medicinal Mushrooms. Berkeley: 2012.

Breast Cancer: Prevention, Breast Health Essentials
Botanical/Nutritional Influences
SW Conference April 2016

Tori Hudson, N.D.
Professor, NCNM/Bastyr U
Medical Director, A Woman's Time
Program Director, Institute of Women's Health and Integrative Medicine
Education/Research Director, Vitanica

Disclosures

- Co-Owner; Director Research and Education for Vitanica

- Scientific Advisory Boards
  - Nordic Naturals
  - Gaia Professional Solutions
  - Integrative Therapeutics
  - Natural Health International
  - Nutritional Fundamentals for Health
  - Pharmaca Integrative Pharmacies

Cancer in Women

Site	incidence	deaths
Breast	192,370	40,170
Lung	103,350	70.490
Colorectal	71,380	24,680
Endometrial	42,160	7,780
Ovarian	21,550	14,600
Skin	29,640	3,100
Cervical	11,270	4,070

Leading Cancers Worldwide

MEN	WOMEN
Lung	Breast
Stomach	Cervix
Colon/Rectum	Colon/Rectum
Mouth/Pharynx	Stomach
Prostate	Uterus

Breast Cancer, Worldwide

- 1 in 33 women will die from breast cancer
- Less than 5 percent of women diagnosed with breast cancer are younger than 40
- By 2020, 70% of all breast cancer cases will be in developing countries

Breast Cancer 2012 U.S.

- About 1 in 8 U.S. women will develop invasive breast cancer over the course of her lifetime - chance of dying 1 in 35
- In 2011, an estimated 230,480 new cases of invasive breast cancer were expected to be diagnosed in women in the U.S.
- Right now there are more than 2½ million breast cancer survivors in the United States.
- White women are slightly more likely to develop breast cancer than African-American women.
- Overall, African-American women are more likely to die of breast cancer. Asian, Hispanic, and Native-American women have a lower risk of developing and dying from breast cancer.

Breast Cancer Etiology

- Multiple factors--- some inherited and some acquired
- Genetic mutations, alterations in gene expression or damage to genes.
- No one single exposure or event is responsible for this affect on genes but rather the timing, duration and pattern of exposure, as well as the dose of a damaging agent.
- Small doses of a carcinogenic agent potentially damaging if in critical window of opportunity

Chemicals in our Environment

- More than 100,000 synthetic chemical are in use in the U.S. today
- 1,000 or so added each year
- More than 90% have never been tested for their effects on human health.

[i] National Cancer Institute. Cancer and the Environment: What you need to know, what you can do. National Institutes of Health. 2003
[ii] Bennett M, Davis B. The identification of mammary carcinogens in rodent bioassays. Environmental and Molecular Mutagenesis. 2002;39(2-3):150-157.

Breast Cancer Risk
What about our Environment?

- **Lack of evidence:** Long Island Breast Cancer Study Report
- **Evidence:** multiple laboratory, animal and human studies covering a wide array of implications including ionizing radiation, xenoestrogens, hormone replacement therapy, oral contraceptives, polycyclic aromatic hydrocarbons, DDT, solvents, polyvinyl chloride, bisphenol-A, polychlorinated biphenyls, dioxin, flame retardants, ethylene oxide, insecticides, phthalates, food additives, methyl mercury, nicotine, hormones used in cattle feed and more items each year

[i] The Long Island Breast Cancer Study Project. Nature Reviews Cancer 2005 Dec;5(12):986-94.
[ii] Gray, J. Breast Cancer Fund; State of the Evidence- The connection between the environment and breast cancer. 2010, 6th edition.

Environmental Health
What Can We Do

- Reduce chemical exposures-- cumulative, timing, multiple and low-dose chronic
- Reduce workplace exposures- chemists, laboratory technicians, dental hygienists, paper mill workers, microelectronic workers, dry cleaners, industrial pollution, roadside workers and more
- Reduce home exposures--cosmetics,cleaning supplies
- Reduce non-ionizing radiation exposures- homes, schools and work place environments
- Reduce exposures based on poverty-- ex/substandard housing, low-income dangerous jobs, housing next to industrial pollution
- Less invasive as well as more effective breast cancer screening methods

Environmental Health 10 point plan for reducing risk of Breast Cancer

The "Breast Cancer Fund" and "Breast Cancer Action"
- Establish **environmental health tracking programs** at state and federal levels
- Practice healthy purchasing by adopting **precautionary purchasing laws** at local, state and federal lands.
- **Protect workers** from hazardous exposures
- Educate the public about the **health effects of radiation** and how to reduce exposure to both ionizing and non-ionizing radiation
- Hold **corporations accountable** for hazardous practices
- Offer local, state and federal **incentives for clean green** practices
- Strengthen **right-to-know legislation** and public participation in decisions about toxic exposures
- Enforce existing **environmental protection laws**
- Require greater **transparency in funding** of scientific and medical training, research and publications
- Create a **comprehensive chemicals policy** based on the precautionary principle

American Cancer Society Guidelines

- Maintain a Healthy Weight Throughout Life
  - Balance caloric intake with physical activity
  - Avoid excessive weight gain throughout the life cycle
  - Achieve and maintain a healthy weight if currently overweight or obese
- Adopt a Physically Active Lifestyle
  - Engage in 30 minutes of moderate to vigorous physical activity, above usual activities, 5 or more days a week
  - Children need 60 minutes or more a day

American Cancer Society Guidelines

- Consume a Healthy Diet, with an Emphasis on Plant Sources
  - Eat 5 or more servings of vegetables and fruit each day
  - Choose whole grains in preference to processed (refined) grains
  - Limit processed and red meats
- Limit Alcohol Consumption, if you drink
  - 1 drink daily for women

    CA Cancer J Clin 2006;56:323–353

"Diet Doesn't Matter ?..."

- Most 'Low Fat' studies for breast cancer and heart disease have not shown significant benefit

  Nurses Health Study, Womens Health Initiative JAMA 2006;295:629-42

- But there is powerful evidence that some dietary patterns, and exercise, DO make a difference

Diet and Cancer: Research Studies

Lyon Study: Mediterranean diet

- 60% less cancer, 4 years

  Arch Intern Med 1998;158:1181-87

- Greek EPIC: 24% less cancer deaths for every 2 points increased adherence to a Med Diet.
  - a 10 point scale, over 4 years

    NEJM 2003;348:2599–608

- Mediterranean Diet: More vegetables, fruit, legumes, grains, fish, nuts, olive & canola oil. Less meat (particularly preserved or cured meats), cream, butter. Moderate alcohol OK

DIANA Research Studies

DIANA 1 & 2

- Mediterranean diet emphasizing whole food lowers weight, cholesterol and insulin resistance, improves hormones linked to breast cancer risk

  Berrino Cancer Epid Bio Prev 2001;10:25–33

- Lower testosterone associated with lower breast cancer recurrence

  Berrino Int J Ca 2005;113:499–502

Breast Cancer Prevention Dietary Fat

Protective

- Fish fat (fish high in omega-3 oils esp.)
- olive oil
- Prospective studies: + and –

  for low fat diets

Non Protective

- Lower risk in some studies but seemed to be unrelated to cancer risk in many studies
- High fat correlates with increased risk
- Breast cancer patients may have reduced chances of survival by eating high saturated fat

Fat and Breast Cancer

Low fat diets:

- Benefit of low fat may be due to a better diet overall and weight loss
- Mortality data for breast/colorectal cancer for 24 European countries show inverse relationship with fish and fish oil
- Seemed to be unrelated to cancer risk in many studies

Omega-3/Omega-6 and Breast Cancer Risk with Obesity

- Overall, there was no significant association between omega-3 PUFA intake and breast cancer risk.
- But...increased risk of breast cancer associated with increasing omega-6 PUFA intake in premenopausal women.
- And...a decreased risk of breast cancer increasing omega-3 PUFA intake in obese women.

Cancer Epid Biomarkers Prev 2011;21(2):319–326

PUFA intake and breast cancer risk –Shanghai Women's Health Study

- No association of breast cancer risk to dietary intake of linoleic acid, arachidonic acid, ALA or fish oils.
- However…
  – Women with lower intake of omega-3 PUFA and higher intake of omega-6 PUFA had an increased risk for breast cancer compared to women with higher intake of omega-3 PUFAs and lower intake of omega-6 PUFAs.
- **The message:** relative amounts of omega-6 PUFA to omega-3 PUFAs may be more important for breast cancer risk than individual dietary amounts of these fatty acids

Murff H, et al. IJC 2011;128:1434–1441

WINS Research Study: Lower recurrence rate in women treated for breast cancer

- WINS: Low fat diet vs. usual care. Low fat diet (20% of calories as fat) associated with significant (6lb) weight loss and various changes in food and nutrient intake. After 3 years, 24% less recurrence overall, 40% less ER- tumor recurrence rate for breast cancer p=0.034

Chlebowski JNCI 2006;98:1767–76

WHEL study

Patients with early breast cancer did not have fewer recurrences of cancer or improved mortality after eating a diet rich in vegetables and fruit and low in fat.

Pierce J, et al. JAMA 2007;298(3)

Life After Cancer Epidemiology Study

- Two dietary patterns were identified:
  – Prudent diet vs Western diet
- Increasing consumption of a Western diet was related to an increasing risk of overall death and death from non-breast cancer causes.
- Neither dietary pattern was assoc with risk of breast cancer recurrence or death from breast cancer.
- Conclusion:
  – women diagnosed with early-stage breast cancer might improve overall prognosis and survival by adopting healthier dietary patterns.

J Clin Oncol 2008;27:919–926.

Mediterranean Diet-PREDIMED

- A benefit of the MeDiet supplemented with extra-virgin olive oil provides primary prevention of breast cancer. This is the first randomized trial to see the effect of a long-term dietary regimen on breast cancer incidence.
- 4282 postmenopausal women; follow-up of 4.8 years; rates for breast cancer were 1.1. for those on the MeDiet supplemented with extra virgin olive oil (1 liter per week for the woman and her family), 1.8 for MeDiet with supplemented nuts (mixed nuts=walnuts 15 g, hazelnuts 7.5 g, and almonds 7.5 g), and 2.9 for those women on a low-fat diet.
- The risk for a malignant breast cancer was 62% lower in women randomized to the MeDiet supplemented with extra-virgin olive oil compared to those randomized to the low-fat diet. The MeDiet supplemented with nuts was also associated with a lower risk, but it was not statistically significant, as was the diet with the extra virgin olive oil.

Toledo E, et al. JAMA Intern Med 2015 Nov;175(11):1752-60

Omega-3 F.A. and Breast Cancer Prognosis

- **Purpose:** whether intake of EPA and DHA were associated with prognosis in a cohort of women who had been diagnosed and treated for early stage breast cancer.
- **Results:** women with higher intakes of EPA and DHA from food (fish) has an approximate 25% reduced risk of additional breast cancer events compared with the lowest tertile of intake. Women with higher intakes of EPA and DHA from food had a dose-dependent reduced risk of all-cause mortality.

Patterson R, *et al*. J Nutr 2011;141:201–206

Laboratory Evidence for EPA+DHA from Fish

- Inhibit proliferation of breast cancer cells
- Reduce initiation and progression of breast tumors
- Anti-inflammatory
- Proapoptotic
- Antiangiogenic effects
- Down regulation of estrogen synthesis
- Modulation of insulin sensitivity
- Lower levels of CRP, TNFalpha and IL-6

Fish oils and Breast Cancer Risk Reduction (VITAL study)

- 35,016 postmenopausal women who did not have a history of breast cancer: Vitamins and Lifestyle (VITAL) cohort study.
- Regular use of fish oil supplements was linked with a 32 percent reduced risk of breast cancer. The reduction in risk appeared to be restricted to invasive ductal breast cancer
- Mechanism??? omega-3 fatty acids, impede nuclear factor kappa-B, a major inflammatory molecule

Cancer *Epidemiol Biomarkers Prev* 2010 Jul;19(7):1696–708

Alcohol and Breast Cancer Overview

- Several meta-analyses and major reviews: dose response effect at 1-2 drinks per day.
- Higher if $\geq$ 3 drinks/day compared with abstainers
- A significant dose-response relationship as low as 1 drink/day
- 2% of U.S. cases attributed to alcohol
- 15% of Italian cases attributed to alcohol

Breast Cancer and Alcohol

- Observation regardless of kind of alcohol
- Assoc with both pre and postmenopausal breast cancer risk
- breast cancer risk shows a dose response relationship with recent alcohol intake
- Age at drinking initiation and lifetime consumption = ???
- Possible: reduction in breast cancer risk if age of drinking is delayed (30 y.o.) (Colditz)

Lifetime Alcohol Consumption and Postmenopausal Breast Cancer Rate

Postmenopausal women; recent intake of alcohol is a more important predictor of breast cancer risk than either earlier lifetime exposure, or cumulative lifetime intake.

J Nutr 2004;134:173-178

Breast Cancer and Alcohol
New Research

- 1,898 women; early-stage invasive breast cancer
- After 8 years of f/u, 275 women had had a recurrence of breast cancer, and 232 had died of cancer or other causes.
- women who drank three to four standard servings of alcohol a week- the equivalent of 3-4 glasses of wine =34 % more likely to have experienced a recurrence of their cancer than those who drank very little or not at all
- greater risk among post-menopausal, ER negative tumors and overweight women.
- The most elevated risk was in women who drank 2 or more servings per day compared to none.

BJ Kaiser Permanente, Oakland, CA

NIH-AARP Diet and Health Study
Fiber

- Dietary fiber intake was inversely associated with breast cancer risk.
- The inverse association was stronger for ER-/PR- tumors than for ER+/PR+ tumors
- Stronger for lobular than for ductal
- Dietary fiber associated with a 13% lower risk of breast cancer in postmenopausal women in the highest quintile of total dietary fiber as opposed the lowest quintile.
- Soluble, not insoluble fiber
- Low fiber 11 g/day; high fiber 26 g/day

Am J Clin Nutr 2009;90:664-671

Other fiber studies

- Most studies
  No relation between dietary fiber and breast cancer in postmenopausal women
- Swedish Mammography Cohort Study
  fiber from fruit was significantly inversely associated
- 2 Swedish studies
  inverse association
- Nurses' Heath Study
  fiber from fruits was also weakly associated
- Pectin- inhibitory effect on mammary tumor growth, angiogenesis, metastasis

Other fiber studies

- Melbourne Collaborative Cohort Study= positive assoc with ER+/PR+ tumors and an inverse assoc with ER-/PR- tumors

Fruits, Vegetables & Breast Cancer

- **Benefit may be greatest in those with family history**
  - High blood levels of carotenoids associated with 40% lower recurrence. Rock. J Clin Onc 2005;23:6631-6638

Family *Cruciferae*, genus *Brassica* (cabbage family)

- Associated with lower human breast, prostate, colon cancer incidence
  Nutrition and Cancer. 2001;41:17-28
- Suppresses breast cancer cell growth
  Tseng Exp Biol Med 2004;229:835-42
- Targets breast cancer susceptibility gene
  Br J Ca 2006;94:407-26
- Reduces breast tumor incidence or delays onset in animal models
  J Ag Food Chem 200;49:2679-83

Breast Cancer and Flaxseed

- RCT: Women fed 25gm (4 TBS) ground flaxseed in a muffin =reduced tumor growth at 39days.
  Significant reduction in Ki67 and Cerb-B2 labeling index, increased apoptosis N=47 Thompson, Goss, Clin Cancer Res 2005;11:3828-3835

- Flaxseed lignans reduce breast cancer cell adhesion, invasion and migration *in vitro*
  Br Ca Res Treatment 2003;80:163-170

Soy and Breast Cancer

- Weakly estrogenic
- Selective hormone modulator
- Antagonist-inhibits binding of estrogen
- Antioxidant
- Antiangiogenesis
- Inhibits aromatase, tyrosine kinase
- Increases SHBG
- Lowers serum estradiol
- Decreased breast density

Soy and Small Reduction in Breast Cancer Risk

- Evaluation of epidemiologic data= 18 studies
- 10 of the studies: inverse assoc between soy exposure and breast cancer risk stronger in premenopausal women

Trock B.J NCI 2006;98

Soy and Breast Cancer Review 2008

- Overall: Little clinical evidence to suggest that isoflavones will increase breast cancer risk in healthy women or worsen the prognosis of breast cancer patients.
- No evidence that isoflavone intake increases breast tissue density in pre or postmenopausal women
- No evidence that isoflavones increase breast cell proliferation in postmenopausal women with or without a history of breast cancer

Nutrition J 2008;7:17

Soy food intake and Breast Cancer Survival

Shanghai Breast Cancer Survival Study

- Among women with breast cancer, soy food consumption was significantly associated with decreased risk of death and recurrence

- Women who had the highest level of soy food intake and who did not take tamoxifen had a lower risk of mortality and a lower recurrence rate than women who had the lowest level of soy food intake.

JAMA 2009;302(22): 2437-2443

Soy and Risk of Breast Cancer Recurrence

LACE study

- Suggested trends for a reduced risk of cancer recurrence were observed with increasing quintiles of daidzein and glycetin intake compared to no intake among postmenopaual women and tamoxifen users.

- Postmenopausal and tamoxifen use: 60% reduction in breast cancer recurrence comparing the highest to the lowest daidzein intakes (> 1,453 vs < 7.7 mcg/day).
- No interference with the efficacy of tamoxifen

Breast Cancer Res Treat 2009;118:395-405

SOY AND BREAST CANCER
Prognosis- 2011

- As soy isoflavone intake increased, the risk of death decreased. Women at the highest levels of soy isoflavone intake (> 16.3 mg isoflavones/day) had a 54% reduction in risk of death.

Cancer Epidemiol Biomarkers Prev 2011;20(5):854-858.

Body Mass and Weight

- BMI correlates inversely with cancer incidence in premenopausal women
- BMI in postmenopausal women-positive but weak association
- BMI < 22.8 – 72% reduction in breast risk compared to sedentary counterparts

---

Breast Cancer Risk and Obesity

- **Postmenopausal women who are obese have a breast cancer risk 60 -100% higher compared to thin women.** Nurses Health study, in McTiernan, A. McPherson et al, BMJ 2000;321:624-28.
- **>50lb weight gain after 18 years old doubles risk.** McTeirnan, 'Breast Fitness' St. Martins 2000
- **In postmenopausal women with breast cancer, survival appears to be better in those who are not obese.** Am J Epid 2003;158:963-68
- **Higher mortality** Jain, Int.J Obesity, 2005; 29:792-797

Breast Cancer and Insulin Resistance

- **Postmenopausal breast cancer associated with insulin resistance** Furberg JNCI 2004;96:1152-60
- **Diet and exercise approaches that reduce insulin resistance are related to lower breast cancer risk**

Weight Gain and Chemotherapy

- **Weight gain common during chemotherapy, and this is associated with:**
  - reduced survival
  - loss of muscle
- **There is a likely benefit in maintaining physical activity during chemo if possible, and keeping energy intake appropriate to needs.**

Harvie B Ca Res Treatment 2004;83:201-210

Exercise

- More exercise- lowered cancer incidence
- Sedentary to walking to heavy manual labor risk of breast cancer decreases proportionately
  pre-menopausal: 1 to .82 to .48
  postmenopausal: 1 to .87 to .78
- Breast cancer risk
    52% reduction for premenopausal
    22% reduction for postmenopausal

Lifestyle summary plan (research/opinion)

- Low saturated and polyunsaturated fats
- Increase fish= 2+/week
- Increase olive oil 1-2 tbsp/day
- Soy- one serving/day
- Increase-cruciferous; flax seeds; fiber
- Low alcohol
- Manage weight
- Exercise 4+/week; more if needed to lose weight

Nutraceuticals and Breast Health

Breast pain/FBD

Vitamin E
EPO
Vitex
Vitamin A
Iodine

Nutraceuticals and Breast Health
Breast Cancer

11 categories of targeted nutrients
1. DNA damage prevention-ex/Turmeric, green tea, NAC
2. Control regulatory genes-ex/ fish oil, soy, resveratrol
3. Anti-inflammatories-Turmeric, fish oils, CLA, ASA
4. Inhibit cell proliferation-ex/I3C, melatonin, Se, ASA
5. Cell differentiation-ex/ CLA, NAC, D
6. Apoptosis promoters-ex/CLA, turmeric, Quercitin, soy, D
7. Receptor restoration-ex/Turmeric, green tea, metformin
8. Aromatase inhibition-ex/grape seed, lignans, D
9. Growth factor inhibitors-ex/Turmeric, green tea, fish oil
10. Antiangiogenics-Apigenin, Turmeric, Soy, green tea
11. MMP inhibitors –ex/CLA, soy, green tea, turmeric

Mastalgia and EPO

- N=291 women
- 3 grams per day EPO x 3–4 mo
- almost half of the 92 women with cyclic breast pain experienced improvement vs one-fifth of the patients on placebo.
- For those women who experienced breast pain throughout the month, 27 % (just over one-fourth of the 33 women) responded positively to the EPO vs 9% placebo

•Lancet 1985; 2:373–77

Mastalgia and EPO

- N=73 women with breast pain with or without lumpiness
- 3 gm/day of EPO or placebo.
- After three months, pain and tenderness were significantly reduced in both cyclical and noncyclical groups; the women who took placebo did not significantly improve.

•Br J Surg 1981; 68:801–24.

Vitex and Mastalgia

- 1. 80% of patients rated their response as a good and 81% rates it as a very good treatment for their mastalgia.
- 2. Cyclical mastalgia decreased significantly along with a smaller degree of improvement even 3 months after stopping the plant. Thirty-eight women rated the effectiveness as moderate to excellent, with 5 reporting no effect.
- 3. Cyclical mastalgia= twice the decrease in intensity of pain after one or two treatment cycles as compared to placebo The duration of pain also improved in the chaste tree group. In the chaste tree group, half the women did not have severe pain at all during any time of the menstrual cycle and only 25% had severe pain for 4% of the days compared with severe mastalgia one fifth of the time before their use of chaste tree began.
- 4. 58% of patients being treated with chaste tree had an improvement in their cyclical mastalgia and 68% of patients had improvements in their psychological symptoms.
- 5. The improvement in breast pain was greater in the chaste tree group (52%) compared with the placebo group (24%).

- Loch E, et al. J Womens Health Gend Based Med 2000;9:315-320.)
- Berger D, et al. Arch Gynecol Obstet 2000;264:150-153.)
- Halaska M, et al. Breast 2000; 8:175-181.)
- Atmaca M, et al. Hum Psychopharmacol 2003;18:191-195.)
- Schellenberg R, et al. Br Med J 2001;322:134-137.)

Vitamin E-Mastalgia

- DBCT; n=150; 2 groups of 75 women each
- Chewable tablets of either vitamin E 200 mg tablets or a placebo; bidx 4 mo.; severity and duration of breast pain was evaluated at the end of the second and fourth month.
- Results: results at two months for vitamin E was dramatically better than placebo in severity and duration; achievable in about 70% of the women.

Parsay S, The Breast Journal 2009;15(5):510-514.

NAC- Breast Density

- 25 postmenopausal women; 1 – 1.5 g metformin or 400 – 600 mg of NAC over a median of ten months.
- Mammographic breast density was measured before and after completion of the study. Both groups exhibited reductions in mammographic breast density with the metformin group eliciting reduction in 28.5% of women and the NAC group exhibiting reduction in 27.3% of cases.

Bershtein, LM, et al. *Vopr Onkol.* 2012;58(1):45-49.

LECITHIN AND BREAST CANCER RISK

- **Ontario Women's Diet and Health Study. 3101 breast cancer cases in women ages 25-74 and 3471 age matched controls**
- **Ever-use of lecithin supplements was associated with reduced breast cancer risk (age-adjusted OR = 0.77 [95% CI = 0.62–0.97]) and was stronger in postmenopausal women (age-adjusted OR = 0.71 [0.55–0.92]) than premenopausal women (0.96 [0.62–1.49])**

Epidemiology, May 2001, 22(3): 444-446

MULTIPLE VITAMIN USE AND BREAST CANCER OUTCOMES
THE LACE STUDY

- The use of MVM after diagnosis was not associated with any outcome when compared to women who never used MVMs.
- For women who used MVMs persistently from pre- to post-diagnosis, there was a decreased risk or recurrence, although not statistically significant, when compared to never users.
- There was a protective association in women who had been treated with radiation only and both radiation and chemotherapy.
- Women who consistently used MVMs before and after their diagnosis ate more fruits and vegetables, were more physically active and had better overall survival.
- In essence, those women who have a habit of MVM use before and after diagnosis and have overall healthier diet and exercise habits may improve their survival outcome after a breast cancer diagnosis.

Breast Cancer Res Treat 2011;130:195-205.

Nutraceuticals and Breast Cancer
DIM

- DIM= Diindolylmethane
  - a natural compound found in cruciferous vegetables
  - extracellular antioxidant
  - promotes beneficial metabolism of estrogen
  - Higher 2-OH and lower 16-OH= lowers risk of breast cancer
  - promotes programmed cell death
  - reduces level and activity of estrogen receptor alpha
  - reduces 4-OH estrogen

DIM

- Nutritional support to inhibit aromatase enzyme for beneficial metabolism of estrogen

- Beneficial in hormone mediated oncological conditions: Breast, Ovary, Uterus and Prostate

Vitamin D and Cancer

- Higher serum vitamin D- lower cancer risk: prospective and retrospective studies below 20 ng/ml = 30% to 50% increased risk of breast cancer (also colon, prostate) and increased mortality
- higher latitudes and lower cancer risk
  - colon and colorectal
  - breast
  - prostate
- 1,25(OH)2D3 is extremely potent in inhibiting cancer cell growth.
- Colon cancer, breast cancer and lung cancer cells all have the ability to make 1,25 (OH)2D

Vitamin D, Breast Cancer

- Women who were in the top quintile of reported outdoor activities between 10 and 19 y.o. had a 35% reduced risk compared with those in the bottom quintile

Knight et al. Cancer Epid Biomarkers Preve 2007;16

Vitamin D and Breast Cancer

- average follow-up of 10 years, the overall incidence of invasive breast cancer was 2.6% among premenopausal women and 3.6% among postmenopausal women.
- Among premenopausal women, the hazard ratio for developing breast cancer was 0.61 for women in the highest versus lowest quintiles of calcium use and 0.65 for vitamin D intake.
- No benefit was seen in postmenopausal women.

Lin J et al. Arch Intern Med 2007, May 28; 167:1050-1059.

More on Vitamin D, Bone Health and Cancer Prevention

- The risk for cancer in the calcium-plus vitamin-D group was less than half that in the placebo group (RR 0.4; P=0.013). The calcium only group had no statistically significant risk reduction.
- Women in the calcium plus vitamin D group had higher serum vitamin D levels that correlated with lower cancer risk, both at baseline and at one year.

Am J Clin Nut 2007; Jun;85(6):1586-1591

Vitamin D and Breast Cancer

- **Patients with highest Vit D associated with one fifth of the risk of breast cancer as lowest quartile**

- **High self-reported Vit D intake with supplements or sun associated with less risk of breast cancer**

Holick Mayo Clin Proc 2006;81:353-73

Vitamin D and Breast Cancer

- **Blood levels of 25-OH Vitamin D at upper end of normal (>52ng/ml) associated with 50% lower risk of breast cancer**
  JAMA 2006;295:2128-29
  - May require over 2000IU Vitamin D daily
  - If being tested, make sure the request is for 25-OH Vitamin D

Prognostic Effects of serum D in Early Breast Cancer

- 75 nmol/L = 30 ng/mL
- Prospective cohort of 512 women with early breast cancer. Mean age = 50.4 years
- Mean vitamin D was 58 nmol/L.
- 37.5% of women had vitamin D deficiency (< 50 nmol/L 38.5% were insufficient (50-72 nmol/L)
- 24% were sufficient (> 72 nmol/L)
- 116 women had distant recurrences, 106 women died.
- Women with deficient vitamin D levels had an increased risk of distant recurrence (HR = 1.94) and death (HR= 1.73) compared with those with sufficient levels.

J Clinic Oncology 2009;27(23):3757-3763

Botanicals- Green Tea

Camellia sinensis – rich in epigallocatechin gallate
Potential properties----
- Antioxidant and free radical scavenging
  Antiatherogenic and anticarcinogenic
- Chelating properties
- Inhibition of tumor initiation and promotion
  inhibits cell-to-cell communication and angiogenesis
- Prevention of mutagenicity and genotoxicity
- Arresting abnormal cell growth or inducing apoptosis
- Excretion of detoxified metabolites of cancer cells
- Inhibits metastasis by inhibiting collagenase effects

Green Tea & Cancer

- Green tea extract and EGCG affected angiogenic factor vascular endothelial growth factor (VEGF) expression.
- The extract or the EGCG significantly decreased the levels of the VEGF peptidesecreted into the medium of human breast cancer cells. The green tea was also able to suppress the expression of protein kinase C, a VEGF transcription modulator, and decrease the RNA levels of VEGF.

N Nutr 2002;132:2307-2311

- EGCG inhibited mouse mammary tumor HER-2 neu cell growth in vitro and dose of green tea polyphenols slowed the growth of estrogen receptor-negative breast cancer cell lines.

Cancer Res 2002;62:652-655

- Green tea polyphenols slowed the growth of estrogen receptor-negative breast cancer cell lines.

Japan J Cancer Res 1998;89:254-261

Botanicals-Green Tea

- 472 women with stage I,II, III breast cancer
- 7 year follow-up
  Increased consumption of green tea correlated with a decreased recurrence of stage I, II breast cancer (P<0.05) for crude disease-free survival
- Recurrence rate 16.7% 5 or more cups 24.3% for 4 or less cups.

Japan J Cancer Res 1998;89:254-261

Green tea and Detoxification

- Green tea polyphenols: catechins, EC, ECG, EGCG
- Catechins, ECG, and EGCG have demonstrated antimutagenic effects against bacterial mutagens (in vivo)
- EGCG counters the carcinogenic effects of chemical carcinogens (ex/ benzenes)

Kuroda and Hara, Mutation Res 1999;436-469

Green Tea Benefits Chemotherapy

- Counteracts the modification of fatty acid composition induced by Adriamycin in cultured cardiomyocytes
- Enhances the effects on Adriamycin induced antitumor activity by increasing the drug concentration in the tumor, reverses multidrug resistance and improves the metastasis-suppressive efficacy of Adriamycin and improves the quality of life in cancer chemotherapy.

Hrelia S, Bordoni A, et al. *Prostagl Leukot Essent Fatty Acids.* 2002 May-Jun;66(5-6):519-24.
Sadzuka Y, Sugiyama T, et al. *Toxicol Lett.* 2000 Apr 3,114(1-3):155-62.
Sugiyama T, Sadzuka Y. *Clin Canc Res.* 1999 Feb;5(2):413-6.
Sugiyama T, et al.. *Clin Canc Res.* 1998 Jan;4(1):153-6.
Stammler G, Volm M. *Anticancer Drugs.* 1997 Mar;8(3):265-8.

Green tea: the Ohsaki study

- Green tea consumption….
  - inversely associated with mortality due to all causes
  - inversely associated with cardiovascular disease

  This inverse association for all-cause mortality association and for cardiovascular disease was stronger in women and even a greater association with cardiovascular disease

- No beneficial effect of green tea consumption and reducing the hazard ratio of cancer mortality.

  JAMA 2006 Sept 13; 296 (10): 1255-1265

Fish Oils: Clinical Importance

Fish oil supplementation
- Competitive inhibition limits release of AA and pro-inflammatory prostaglandins
- Outcome: manage inflammatory and chronic disease

Inflammation and F.A. intake in Breast Cancer survivors

N=633; Stage 1-3 breast cancer survivors

CRP levels and diet questionnaire 30 months after diagnosis and a fatigue and vitality questionnaire 39 months after diagnosis

Conclusion: higher intake of omega 3 PUFAs, decreased inflammation and decreased physical aspects of fatigue

Alfano C, et al. J Clin Onc 2012;12(30):1280-1287

Fish Oils Supplements as Adjunct to Conventional Treatment

- Surgery---- in doses of 1-4 gm/day

  Lack of significant bleeding with omega-3 f.a. supplementation in CVD studies, pregnant women and in dialysis patient

  omega-3 f.a. supplements do not increase risk for clinically significant bleeding, even in patients being treated with antiplatelet or antithrombotic medications.

  Anecdotal reports: increased bruising tendency- not tested in a controlled setting

Fish Oils Supplements as Adjunct to Conventional Treatment

Chemotherapy-positive study
- Supplementation with fish oil may increase chemotherapy efficacy
- Study: Patients in the FO group had an increased response rate and greater clinical benefit compared with the SOC group.
- The one year survival tended to be greater in the FO group.

Murphy R, et al. Cancer 2011;117:3774-80

Fish Oils Supplements as Adjunct to Conventional Treatment

Chemotherapy- negative study
- In animal experiments: stem cells in the blood of mice responded to cisplatin, by producing, two fatty acids. These fatty acids referred to as PIFAs (platinum-induced fatty acids)

The two PIFAs make cancerous cells resistant to a broad spectrum of chemotherapies.

Fish oil supplements as well as some algae extracts containing omega-3 and omega-6 fatty acids would stop chemotherapy's effects on some tumors in mice.

When they gave fatty acids to the mice, the tumors were unaffected by the chemotherapy and continued to thrive.

When medications which block the production of these fatty acids were used, the tumors' resistance to chemotherapy went down

Roodhart J, et al. Cancer Cell, Volume 20, Issue 3, 370-383

Fish Oils Supplements as Adjunct to Conventional Treatment

- Chemotherapy-weight loss
- Sixteen took 2.2 grams of fish oil per day, while the remaining 24 received standard care; 10 weeks
- The majority of patients (69%) in the study who supplemented their diet with fish oil, either maintained or gained weight.
- Less than a third of the patients in the other group kept their weight up- they lost an average of 5#
- Most of the patients taking fish oil also maintained muscle mass for the duration of the study, while the majority of those receiving standard care lost a significant amount of muscle mass.

Murphy, R, et al. *Cancer* 2011; DOI: 10.1002/cncr.25709.

Fish Oils Supplements as Adjunct to Conventional Treatment

Radiation- theoretical issues---
- Potential benefits:
  radiosensitivity enhancer
  reducing inflammation
  reducing weight loss from treatment
- Potential harm:
  enhance side effects due to enhancement of radiosensitivity
  free radical interference

Fish Oil Quality & Potency Matters

- Choosing the right fish oil product for your patients is key
- Burping/Fish repeat due to rancid, poorly manufactured oil
- Rancid oils are a source of harmful free radicals
- Effective distillation is critical to removing impurities
- Desired results cannot be achieved without sufficient levels of EPA & DHA
- Learn about quality: freshness, purity, concentration, sustainability

Lifestyle summary plan (research/opinion)

- Low saturated and polyunsaturated fats
- Increase fish= 2+/week
- Increase olive oil 1-2 tbsp/day
- Soy- one serving/day
- Drink Green tea daily
- Increase-cruciferous; flax seeds; fiber
- Low alcohol
- Manage weight
- Exercise 4+/week; more if needed to lose weight
- Daily sunshine or take Vitamin D

Dr Hudson Resources

- Women's Encyclopedia of Natural Medicine;2nd Edition 2008; Hudson; McGraw-Hill

- www.drtorihudson.com
- www.vitanica.com
- www.instituteofwomenshealth.com
- www.awomanstime.com

- womanstime@aol.com
- vitanica@aol.com

Abnormal Uterine Bleeding

SW Botanical Conference
April 2016

Tori Hudson, N.D.
Medical Director, A Woman's Time
Clinical Professor, NCNM/Bastyr/SCNM
Program Director, IWHIM
Director Education/Research, Vitanica

Characteristics of Normal Menstruation

TABLE 1: CHARACTERISTICS OF NORMAL MENSTRUATION[12]

	NORMAL	ABNORMAL
Duration of flow	4-6 days	<2 days or >7 days
Volume of flow	30 mL	>80 mL
Length of cycle	24-35 days	

Usual Causes of AUB Throughout a Woman's Lifetime

(diagram of causes across lifespan)

Usual Causes of AUB Throughout a Woman's Lifetime

- Complications from pregnancy
- Infection
- Trauma
- Cancer
- Pelvic pathology (benign)
- Systemic disease
- Medications/iatrogenic causes

Differential diagnosis in the adolescent girl

- Anovulation
- Pregnancy
- Infection
- Vaginal lacerations
- Blood dyscrasia
  - Thrombocytopenia
  - Clotting disorders
  - Liver disease
- Ovarian problems
  - Cyst or neoplasm
- Endocrine disorders
  - Thyroid disease
  - Adrenal disorders
  - Hyperprolactinemia
  - Polycystic ovary syndrome

Ovulation Failure/Problems---Perimenopause

irregular timing, and skipped cycles compared with your Patient's 'usual' bleeding history

unpredictable ovulation usually due to:
- ---short luteal phase
- ---follicle depletion

AND, Other Causes are common in Perimenopausal Women:

Structural Problems
-endometrial polyps, uterine fibroids, ovarian cysts/tumors, adenomyosis/endometriosis, endometrial hyperplasia,

Age Related
-Molar pregnancies, cancers

Other
-pregnancy (especially ectopic), thyroid disorders, coagulopathies, chemotherapy, radiation therapy, end-stage liver and renal disease.

Regulation of Normal Menstruation

ovulatory dysfunction evaluation

Blood/Lab Tests
* Pregnancy test
* FSH (should be <12)
* Thyroid (TSH, Free T4 or more)
* Chem Screen
* possibly LH (for PCOS), karyotype (for high FSH in patients age <35)
* no clinical use presently for Anti-Mullerian Hormone (AMH) except infertility evaluation (AMH decreases with follicle depletion— Low in perimenopause)

And, as applicable:
* Pap smear, pelvic exam
* Pelvic Sonogram (transvaginal best.."TVUS")
  —saline sonogram if irregular endometrial echoes
* Hysteroscopy?
* Endometrial sampling/biopsy: sample women over age 40 even if endometrium measures < 5 mm. Use curette for 5mm +, use Gynecore Tao Brush if < 5mm (unlikely to get tissue with curette if < 5mm)

Ovulatory dysfunction treatments

OCs

Lysteda (tranexamic acid) for heavy flow, start PRN, use TID for 3-5 days
** the menstrual endometrium arterioles form fibrin plugs to stem the bleeding. The fibrin is degraded by plasmin, which allows the plugs to be resorbed/break down.

Women who have heavy menstrual bleeding have higher than normal levels of the enzymes that produce plasmin in the endometrium. Tranexamic acid stops the production of plasmin by blocking the action of the enzymes that produce it. This reduces the breakdown of fibrin and stops the plug degredation, which in turn reduces bleeding.

Tranexamic acid can reduce menstrual blood loss by up to 58 per cent.

Progesterone IUD.... extremely popular
Cyclic progestins – Provera 10 mg or Prometrium 100-200 mg daily cycle days 14-28
Endometrial Ablation

There are no Western Medicine therapies to treat the underlying ovulation defects... we offer control of bleeding

Ovulatory Dysfunction Conventional Treatments

- OCPs
- Lysteda (tranexamic acid) for heavy flow, start PRN, use TID for 3-5 days
- Progestin IUD.... extremely popular
- Cyclic progestins – Provera 10 mg or Prometrium 100-200 mg daily cycle days 14-28
- Endometrial Ablation
- There are no Western Medicine therapies to treat the underlying ovulation defects... they offer control of bleeding

OCPs for Chronic Use

- Use continuous or long cyclic:
  - After 4 days off OCs, ovarian follicles begin to grow, so there is loss of suppression with 7 days off. More BTB and pregnancy risk on cyclic OCs
  - warn patient to expect some light flow and keep on OC. 75% will make 3 months without break thru... hence the 3 month packaging
  - if intolerable, take 3-4 days off and begin again. average 30-40 days spotting in the first year... tell them to stay on OC and live with light flow and it will end
- Start with lowest Estrogen products and increase as needed
- ? add 50 mg Doxycycline for chronic spotting (ongoing study at OHSU)

Acute Bleeding, stable Conventional Treatment

- Lysteda (tranexamic acid) 650 mg, 2 tabs BID for 3-5 days
- OCs (30-35 microgram dose)
  - QID for 7 days (nausea), so: BID for 7 days, or TID 3 days then BID 3 days then daily til end of pack (stay at same dose until flow slows significantly)
  - then, continuous OCs, or Mirena IUD or ablation or watch
- Estrogen, oral
  - oral Premarin 2.5 mg or Estradiol 2 mg QID until bleeding slows dramatically, then TID for 3 days, BID for 3 days, and daily for a total of 20-21 days
  - Add Progesterone 100-200 mg (or Provera 5-10 mg) for last 7 days (15-21) Progestins only won't work... need endometrial estrogen which is low or absent in perimenopause
- NSAIDs
  - Mefenamic acid 500 mg TID for 3 days can reduce flow 30%, Aleve 2 tabs TID, Ibuprofen less effective

Hypotensive, nauseated, dizzy, e.g.

Acute Bleeding, unstable

- Transfer patient to hospital
- CBC, bHCG, PT, PTT
- IV Premarin 12.5 mg - 25 mg q 4 hour up to 24 hours until bleeding has stopped
- If bleeding does not stop after 24 hours, perform a hysteroscopy, D & C
- If bleeding continues consider Uterine Artery Embolization, Hysterectomy, or Ablation
- After patient's bleeding is under control
  - Transfusion or oral iron
  - Any of the regimens used for stable patients, probably using oral estrogen or OCs and at least a 21-28 day regimen to eliminate another bleeding episode soon
- Consider concomitant antibiotic if patient is very anemic and bleeding has been present > 7 days

Oral Contraceptives

- There are many doses of estrogen, and many types of progestins and doses
- *** Get familiar with a few in each progestin and estrogen dose category
- *** Familiarize yourself with common symptoms of progestins
- ————so you don't change the patient to an identical formulation :)
- 2 estrogens... 1 used in 99%, ethinyl estradiol, and estradiol valerate (in Natazia)
- Progestins : levonorgestrel, norethindrone, norgestimate, desogestrel, drospirinone, norgestrel, ethnodiol, dienogest.
- Several doses in each category
  - Estrogen... 10, 20, 25, 30, 35, 50 micrograms
  - Progestins... 0.1, 0.2, 0.3, 0.35, 0.5, 0.75, 1.0, 1.5 milligrams
- Monophasic
- Multiphasic... originally designed to rest break-thru bleeding, useless if using continuous or long cyclic
- Progestin only or 'mini-pill' uses norethindrone 0.35
- and TRANSDERMAL... the vaginal ring,"Femring" and the patch "OrthoEvra"

Endometrial Ablation Types

- **Electrical or electrocautery.** An electric current travels through a wire loop or rollerball that is applied to the endometrial lining to cauterize the tissue
  - first method, uneven therapy (rows)
- **Hydrothermal.** Heated fluid is pumped into the uterus and destroys the endometrial lining with high temperature
  - possible vaginal burns
- **Balloon therapy.** A balloon at the end of a catheter is inserted into the uterus and filled with fluid, which is then heated to the point that the endometrial tissues are eroded away
  - popular, works on many uterine sizes
- **Radiofrequency ablation.** A triangular mesh electrode is expanded to fill the uterine cavity. The electrode delivers electrical current and destroys the endometrial lining.
  - most popular, highest amenorrhea and lowest immediate post procedure pain.
- **Cryoablation (freezing).** A probe uses extremely low temperatures to freeze and destroy the endometrial tissues
- **Microwave ablation.** Microwave energy is delivered through a slender probe that has been inserted into the uterus and destroys the endometrial lining.

Balloon Ablation

TVUS

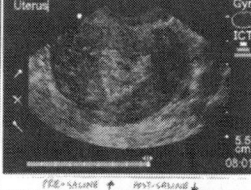

Saline Sonogram

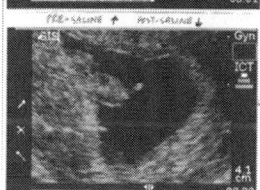

Endometrial Polyps

- Benign localized overgrowth of endometrium
- Peak incidence in 40 - 49 age group but can occur in all ages
- Only 0.5-1 % will have malignant transformation
- Diagnosed on Ultrasound or hysteroscopy
- Treated with hysteroscopic resection

Fibroids

Leiomyomas

Benign smooth muscle tumors unique to the uterus, composed of smooth muscle cells and varying amounts of fibrous tissue and collagen matrix. They vary in consistency.
They are true neoplasms, composed of clonal cells, not hypertrophied cells.
---Present in 20-50% of women (or more)
---Clinically affects 25% of women
---200,000-300,000 hysterectomies/ year due to fibroids...
  # 1 cause of hysterectomy
---Increase with age

Typical fibroid locations and terminology

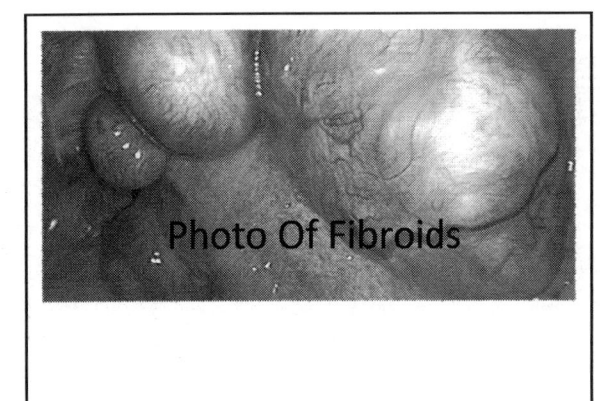

Photo Of Fibroids

Fibroid Treatments
Conventional Treatments

Treatment depends on location and size
Submucous leiomyomas can be resected hysteroscopically
Intramural fibroids require abdominal or laparoscopic myomectomy or hysterectomy
Uterine Artery Embolization results in significant shrinkage of the majority of fibroids
Medical treatment of fibroids includes progesterone or oral contraceptives to reduce menorrhagia by shrinking and stabilizing the endometrium
GnRH agonists will shrink leiomyomas and may be used preoperatively treat anemia or simplify the surgical approach, but are temporary.
Endometrial ablation controls bleeding
MRI guided focused ultrasound in a few centers in the US heat/destroy fibroids selectively under direct visualization without invasive procedures (just starting up)
Under study...
  SERMs selective estrogen receptor modulators to decrease local estrogen effect on tumors
  SPRMs selective progesterone receptor modulators, RU-486, decrease local progesterone effect on tumors
  Anti-angiogenic agents to reduce tumor blood supply/growth
  Tumor genetics... abnormal genes found in fibroids and not in normal uterine cells may lead to targeted therapies.

Adenomyosis---- Endometriosis

Endometriosis

*Endometrial tissue found outside the interior of the uterus... bleeding/pain/infertility
*Especially associated with metrorrhagia
*Laparoscopic diagnosis
*Treated with surgery, OCs, GNRH meds, Danazol, progestins, progestin IUDs.

Adenomyosis

*Endometrial gland invasion of myometrium
*Diffusely enlarged and sometimes tender uterus mistaken for fibroids
*Dysmenorrhea, PMS, exaggerated cyclic symptoms can clinically suggest that it is not fibroids
*Diagnosis by ultrasound, MRI, or pathology after hysterectomy
*Treatment is hysterectomy, possibly progestin IUDs

Endometrial Hyperplasia Treatments

Megace 20-80 mg/day for 3-6 mo
Provera 20-40 mg/day   "
Progesterone 200 mg/day   "
Need to repeat EMBx to assess therapy

Hysterectomy if atypia present and no need to preserve fertility

Endometrial Adenocarcinoma

- Occurs in women over age 45 and peaks between 55 and 69
- Diagnosed on pap 50% of the time
- Presents with postmenopausal or perimenopausal abnormal bleeding
- Risk factors include unopposed estrogen, menopause after age 52, obesity, nulliparity, diabetes, PCOS, granulosa cell tumors, tamoxifen therapy

Cervical Cancer...
glandular or adeno is on the rise....

Molar Pregnancy Ultrasound

- like swiss cheese

Bleeding Disorders

Disorders include: Van Willebrand's disease, Thrombocytopenias, Leukemias, Factors II, V, VII, X, and XI deficiencies

Rarely present in mid-life... usually found in adolescents

Von Willebrand's is quite variable in severity, so may be missed until a pregnancy-related bleed, or in perimenopause because of synergistic factors (ovulatory dysfunction or fibroids + VonW)

Chronic Liver disease:
Alcoholism Cirrhosis Hepatitis

Decreases the ability to metabolize estrogen and decreases fibrinogen and clotting factors

Chronic Renal disease:
Chronic renal failure
Renal transplant patients

Interferes with normal secretion of estrogen and progesterone

---

Thyroid Disorders

* Up to 45% of patient's with hypothyroidism will have menorrhagia
  -- In one study, 15 of 67 patients with menorrhagia were found to have subclinical hypothyroidism which was measured with sensitive TSH
* 10% of patients with hyperthyroidism will have metrorrhagia
* TSH very important test in women with change in bleeding patterns at any age.

Overview of Natural Treatments

- Goals
  determine cause
  control bleeding
  prevent anemia
  treat anemia
  restore menstrual pattern
  prevent additional complications

Overview of Natural Treatments

- Initiate ovulation
- Anti-inflammatory
- Astringent
- Tonification
- Stress

Principles

- Healing Power of Nature
- First, Do No Harm
- Identify and Treat the Cause
- Treat the Whole Person
- Physician as Teacher
- Prevention is the Best Cure
- Establish Health and Wellness
- Resonance
- Choice

Nutrition

- Soy
- Flax
- Fish
- Iron foods
- General whole foods diet

Nutrition
Soy

- Soy protein
  n=6 premenopausal women
  60 grams of soy protein (45 mg isoflavones) daily for 1 month
  - Increased follicular phase length and/or delayed menstruation by 1-5 days

  Cassidy, et al. Am J Clin Nutr 1994

Nutrition
Flax Seeds

- N=18 normally cycling women
- Low fiber diet x 3 months
- Low fiber diet plus flax seeds (10 grams) x 3 months

Results: 3 anovulatory cycles in control
no anovulatory cycles during flax

Nutrition
Fish

- Cold water fish=salmon, tuna, halibut, swordfish, mackerel, herring, sardines
- High in omega 3 oils
- Goal: increase EPA=eicosapentaenoic acid
- Therapeutic dose: 1.8 grams EPA/day

(consider flax oil=13 grams; 1.5 tbsp/day)

Nutrition
Iron Content of Foods per 3 ½ oz (100 g)

- Kelp   100.0 mg
- Yeast, brewer's 17.3
- Molasses   16.1
- Wheat bran   14.9
- Pumpkin seeds   11.2
- Wheat germ   9.4
- Beef liver   8.8
- Sunflower seeds   7.1
- Millet   6.8
- Parsley   6.2
- Clams   6.1
- Almonds   4.7
- Prunes, dried   3.9
- Cashews   3.8
- Raisins   3.5
- J Artichoke   3.4

Nutrition
Whole Foods Diet "Anti-inflammatory Diet"

- Whole grains
- Legumes
- Vegetables, Fruits
- Nuts, Seeds
- Fish
- Reduce saturated fats

Nutrition
Vegetarians vs Non-vegetarians

- Nonvegetarians = 4.9% menstrual irregularity
  - greater intakes of saturated f.a., protein, cholesterol, caffeine and alcohol
- Vegetarians = 26.5%
  - greater amounts of PUFAs, carbohydrates, B-6, fiber, magnesium

Am J Clin Nutr 1991

Nutrition
Influences on menstrual regularity

- High fiber or magnesium assoc with increased likelihood menstrual irregularity
- High cholesterol or high protein assoc with increased likelihood of menstrual regularity

WHY?

- High cholesterol- role as estrogen precursor
- High protein-changes in steroid concentrations; lower SHBG
- High fiber-lower circulating estrogens
- Lower concentrations of estrogens in vegetarians

Exercise
Menstrual Irregularity

- Average = 2-5%
- Swimmers = 37%
- Sprinters = 42%
- Athletes who began training before menarche = 43%

Nutritional Supplements

- Vitamin A
- B complex
- Vitamin K
- Bioflavonoids
- Vitamin C

Nutritional Supplements
Vitamin A

- Deficiency of vitamin A
- Intervention
  n=40 women with menorrhagia
  Vit A 60,000/d for 35 days.
  Results: normal menses in 23 women
           decrease in 14 women
           ineffective in 3
      overall: 92.5% cases were cured or ameliorated.
  Lithgow, Politzer S A M J 1977

Nutritional Supplements
B-Complex

- May be correlation between B deficiency and menorrhagia and metrorrhagia.
- Liver loses ability to inactivate estrogen in B complex deficiency
- Old study (1940s): B complex (3-9mg thiamin, 4.5-9mg riboflavin, 60 mg niacin)
  Improvement in menorrhagia/metrorrhagia

Nutritional Supplements
Vitamin K

- Vitamin K deficiency, rare
- Role in manufacture of clotting factors (prothrombin and clogging factors VKK, IX, X)
- Sources: Fat-soluble chlorophyll; fresh green juices, green leafy vegetables
- Doses: 150-500 mcg per day

Nutritional Supplements
Vitamin C

- Vitamin C
  Strengthens capillaries
- Reduce heavy bleeding in 87% women
- Increases absorption of iron
- Sources: Red chili peppers, Guavas, Red sweet peppers, Kale, Parlsey, Collards, Turnip greens, Green sweet peppers, broccoli, brussels sprouts, red cabbage, strawberries, papayas, oranges
- Dose: 2,000mg – 6,000 mg per day

Nutritional Supplements
Bioflavonoids

- Citrus Bioflavonoids
  -Strengthens capillaries
  -May have anti-estrogenic effect on endometrium
  -Anti-inflammatory
Sources: grape skins, cherries, blackberries, blueberries, pulp and white rind of citrus fruits
Dose: 1,000mg – 2,000 mg chronic

Botanicals

- Vitex
- Ginger
- Turmeric
- Astringents
- Uterine tonics

Botanicals
Vitex agnus castus (chaste tree)

- N=126 women with menstrual disorders
- 33 women had polymenorrhea
  Results: Cycle lengthened from 20.1 days to 26.3 days
- 58 women with menorrhagia
  Results: shortening of menses

Bleir. Zentralblatt Gynakol 1959

Botanicals
Zingiber officinalis (Ginger)

- Shown to inhibit prostaglandin synthetase
- Shown to inhibit leukotriene formation

Both mechanisms=anti-inflammatory agent

Gingerol-most potent constituent
Dose: Dry powder 1-5 grams
Ginger root st extract (5%) gingerols 100 mg 1 tid

Botanicals
Curcuma longa (Turmeric)

- Ginger family
- Turmeric contains 0.3-5.4% curcumin
- Chinese and Ayurvedic medicine- antiinflammatory agent
- Mechanisms: inhibits leukotrienes, inflammatory mediators and platelet aggregation; promotion of fibrinolysis (is this a good idea?)
- Dose: 400-600 mg tid
- Toxicity: generally safe; 100mg/kg body weight= ulcerogenic in rats

Botanicals
Astringents

With tannins:
- Yarrow (Achillea millefolium)
- Ladies' mantle (Alchemila vulgaris)
- Cranesbill (Geranium maculatum)
- Beth root (Trillium erectum)
- Greater periwinkle (Vinca major)

Botanicals
Astringents

- Without tannins
  - Horsetail (Equisetum arvense)
  - Goldenseal (Hydrastis canadensis)
  - Shepherd's purse (Capsella bursa pastoris)
    - can coagulate blood
    - best used in combination with other astringent and hemostatic herbs

Botanicals
Uterine Tonics

- Regulate tone-both reduce excess tone and increase tone (amphoteric)
- Dong quai (Angelica sinensis)
- Blue cohosh (Caulophyllum thalictroides)
- Helonias (Chamaelirium luteum)
- Squaw vine (Mitchella repens)
- Squaw vine (Mitchella repens)
- Raspberry leaves (Rubus idaeus)
- Life root (Senecio aureus)

Botanicals
Liferoot

- Aka ragwort
- "female regulator"
- Traditional uses: menstrual cramps, menorrhagia, suppressed menstruation
- Classic uterine tonic
  Tonify soft, boggy uterus

Botanicals
Uterine stimulants/emmenagogues

- Squaw vine (Mitchella repens)
- Yarrow (Achillea millefolium)
- Chaste tree (Vitex agnus castus)
- Penyroyal (Mentha pulegium)
- Mugwort (Artemisia vulgaris)
- Blue cohosh (Caulophyllum thalictroides)

Anovulatory DUB
Natural Treatments

- OMP 100 mg daily for 10-12 days per month
- Consider E3 1mg/E2 .25mg/P50 mg 1 bid 21 days on and 7 off
- Stimulation/regulation of ovulation:
  - Vitex S.E. 1 cap daily
  - Symplex F 1 tid
  - Progest ¼ tsp 1-2 times daily days 7-14
     (or Progonol= 40 mg per ¼ tsp)
- Squawvine, Yarrow, Blue Cohosh, Pennyroyal

Anovulatory bleed
Natural Treatments

Oligomenorrhea

- Squawvine	1 ½ oz	Sig ½-1 tsp 2-3
- Yarrow	1 oz	x/day
- Blue cohosh	1 oz	
- Pennyroyal	½ oz	

- Progesterone cream ¼ tsp 1-2x/d, day 7-14; 1/2 tsp 2x/day, day 15-26
- Vitex 1 cap daily
- Symplex F 1 tid

Anovulatory Bleed
Natural Treatments

Polymenorrhea

Soy, flax seeds
Chaste tree 1 daily
Natural progesterone ¼-1/2 tsp bid 21 on and 7 off
Cons/ higher doses-OMP 200-400 mg 12 days/mo
Consider E3/E2/P
"Slow Flow" 2 caps bid throughout the month
Consider/extra bioflavonoids, vitamin A

Combination
Proprietary formula

- Vitamin A   10,000 iu
- Vitamin C   500 mg
- Vitamin K1   150 mg
- Bioflavonoids   500 mg
- Ginger root   500 mg
- Cranesbill root   200 mg
- Greater periwinkle 200 mg
- Yarrow   200 mg
- Liferoot   200 mg
- Shepard's purse   150 mg

Abnormal Bleeding due to Fibroids

- OMP 100-400 mg per day days 15-26
- Or Progesterone cream ¼ tsp bid 3 week on and 1 week off
- Slow Flow 2 caps 2-3x/day (extra vit A, bioflavs)
- Calc Phox 6x
- Consider conventional tx:
  -OCPs, Myomectomy, Laparoscopic resection, embolization, endometrial ablation, laparoscopic myolysis, GnRH agonists

Abnormal bleeding due to Endometrial Hyperplasia

- If no atypia
  -OMP 100 mg bid for 3 months then repeat biopsy
  No sublingual, transdermal
  -Vitex- improvement in menstrual bleeding
- If atypia
  Conventional=Megace, Provera
      Must monitor closely and cons/Hyst

Endometrial Polyps

- Combination Proprietary formula 2 caps 2-3x/day
- Vitamin A 50,000 i.u. daily
- Extra Bioflavonoids 1,000 mg 1-2 x/day
- Progesterone for bleeding
  -Progesterone cream ¼ tsp bid days 15-26
  -OMP 100-200mg bid days 15-26

Acute Menorrhagia
Integrative Treatment Interventions

Acute Anovulatory bleeding; stable; Natural Treatments

- Botanicals
- Nutrients
- Bio-Identical Hormones

Integrative
- Conventional Hormones
- OCPs

Acute anovulatory bleeding; stable- Botanicals

- Botanicals
  Astringents
  Uterine tonics
  Hemostatics
  Anti-inflammatories
- Nutrients
  Anti-inflammatories
  Vitamin A, C, Bioflavonoids

Acute Anovulatory bleed; stable

- Proprietary Combination formula 3 caps every 3 hours
- Vitamin A 50,000-100,000 iu daily
- Bioflavonoids 1,000 mg tid
- Essential oil of cinnamon 1-5 drops ever 3 hours
- Tincture:

-Erigeron Canadensis(Fleabane)
-Capsella bursa   (Shepard's Purse)   -Secale
-Achillea millefolium (Yarrow)
-Savina officinalis (Savin)
20 drops q 2 hours x 24-48 hours then 1 tsp tid x days of flow

Acute anovulatory bleed; stable

- Consider

-OMP 200 tid until bleeding slows, then bid for 3 days, then once daily for a total of 21 days-

OR

-Estradiol 4 mg qid until bleeding slows dramatically, then 4 mg tid for 3 days, then bid for 3 days then 4 mg daily for a total of 21 days

-Add OMP 200 mg daily for days 15-21

OR OCP regimen options

Acute Anovulatory Bleed-post surgical

- Bromelain
- Vitamin C
- Infection prevention
- "Opti-Recovery" or similar
-

Dr. Tori Hudson Resources

- Women's Encyclopedia of Natural Medicine, 2008, second edition
- www.drtorihudson.com (blog)
- www.awomanstime.com
- www.instituteofwomenshealth.com
- www.vitanica.com or www.vitanicapro.com
- www.naturopathicresidency.org
- Monthly columns:
    Emerson Ecologics
    Townsend Letter for Doctors

Endometriosis
A Comprehensive Approach
SW Botanical Conference April 2016

Tori Hudson, N.D.
Clinical Professor, NCNM/Bastyr
Medical Director, A Woman's Time
Program Director, IWHIM
Education/Research Director, VITANICA

Disclosures

- Director of Education and Research; Co-owner
  - Vitanica
- Scientific Advisory Board
  - Integrative Therapeutics
  - Nordic Naturals
  - Natural Health International
  - Gaia Professional Solutions
  - Nutritional Fundamentals for Health
  - Pharmaca Integrative Pharmacies

Definition

- Common, benign, estrogen dependent associated with pelvic pain and infertility
- The presence of endometrial glands and stroma outside the uterine cavity, mainly on the pelvic peritoneum, but also ovaries, rectovaginal septum (rarely: pericardium, pleura, brain)

Prevalence

- 6-10% general population
- 35-50% in women with pain, infertility or both
- Most commonly diagnosed in women of reproductive age

Endometriosis: Possible Pathogenesis

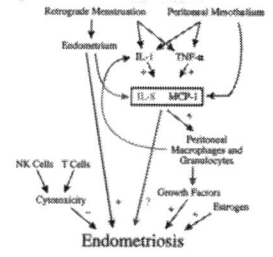

Figure 1. Factors involved in the pathogenesis of endometriosis.

Theories of pathogenesis

- Retrograde menstruation
- Coelomic metaplasia
- Metastasis
- Iatrogenic
- Genetic
- Environmental factors
- Altered cellular immunity

Theories
Retrograde menstruation

- Retrograde menstruation of endometrial tissue sloughed through patent fallopian tubes into the peritoneal cavity
- Endometrial fragments attach to the epithelium of the peritoneum, invasion of the epithelium, establishment of a blood supply and suboptimal immune response that does not adequately clear the implants, resulting in continued growth

Theories
Metaplasia; Metastasis

- Metaplasia of the coelomic epithelium might also contribute to establishment of the disease, perhaps induced by environmental factors, and primarily involving the formation of endometriomas or rectovaginal endometriosis
- Metastasis of lesions could seed other lesions in the pelvis or elsewhere

Theories
Iatrogenic

- Can be iatrogenically induced or disseminated
- Sometimes found after C-section, rarely after an episiotomy scar
- Estrogen dependent disease: can be iatrogenically stimulated postmenopausally by use of exogenous estrogen.

Theories
Genetic

- Risk for first degree relatives of women with severe endometriosis = six times higher
- Familial aggregations observed in clinical, population based studies and in twin studies
- Genetic abnormalities in detoxification enzymes, tumor suppressor genes
- Strong familial tendency reported in non-human primates

Theories
Environmental factors

- Monkeys exposed to whole-body irradiation
- Monkeys exposed to dioxin
- Belgium: highest dioxin pollution in the world, and has the highest incidence of endometriosis and the highest prevalence of severe endometriosis
- No epidemiological study to date, definitively linking one class of chemicals, although estrogen like compounds have been suspected

Theories
Immune system

- Abnormalities in both cell-mediated and humoral components
- Increased cytokine production
- Decreased phagocytic activity
- Increased protein called Endo I(similar to haptoglobin)
- Increased interleukin 6
- Decrease NK cells
- Compromised immune surveillance
- Peritoneal fluid: high concentrations of cytokines, growth factors, and angiogenic factors
- Once endometriosis lesions: secretion of proinflammatory molecules, lipid peroxidation
- Oxidants are proposed to stimulate endometrial cell growth
- Estrogen receptor issues

Theories
Immune system

- Autoimmune etiology?
  -increased polyclonal B-cell activity
  - abnormalities in function of B and T cells
  - Familial inheritance
  - high B-cell and T-cell counts
  - reduced NK cell activity
  - high IgG, IgA, IgM autoantibodies and antibodies to endometrium

Symptoms/Signs

- Chronic pelvic pain (> 6 months)- 78-82% of women with pain >6mo have it
- Dysmenorrhea
- Dyspareunia
- Mid-cycle pain and/or bleeding
- Painful bowel movements
- Endometrioma – found on routine exam or on ER visit for rupture/pain
- Unexplained infertility
- Deep pelvic (culdesac) nodules

Evaluation

- Pelvic exam
  - Tenderness, culdesac pain, deep pain
- Ultrasound to rule out other causes and detection of endometrioma
- Laparoscopy if anti-inflammatories, antibiotics and OCs don't help; (also laparotomy selectively)
- Evaluation of pelvis if having other surgery like a C/section or appendectomy

Conventional Treatment

- Oral contraceptives
- Progestins
  - Depo-Provera – 100 mg IM q 2wks for 4 doses, then 200 mg monthly for 4 months
  - Medroxyprogesterone 30 mg daily
  - Megesterol (Megace) 40 mg daily for 6 mo
- Anti-Progestins RU486 50 mg daily for 6 months (off label, not used much yet)
- Danazol
- Surgery
  - GnRH agonists- Lupron, Synarel, Goserelin
- Counseling
- Anti-inflammatories

Environmental Factors

- Dioxins
- PCBs
- Phthalates
- BPA
- Pesticides
- Formaldehyde
- Solvents
- Cadmium

Sunscreen and Endometriosis

- In this study, the concentrations of five BP derivatives were measured in urine collected from 625 women in Utah and California.
- The association of urinary concentrations of BP derivatives with an increase in the odds of a diagnosis of endometriosis was examined in 600 women who underwent laparoscopy or pelvic magnetic resonance imaging during 2007-2009
- Exposure to elevated 2,4OH-BP levels may be associated with endometriosis.

Environ. Sci. Technol. Publication Date (Web): March 14, 2012

Hormonally Responsive

- Endometriotic lesions contain estrogen, progesterone, and androgen receptors.
- Estrogen receptor (ER)β levels in endometriosis are >100 times higher than those in endometrial tissue
- High levels of ERβ suppress ERα expression.
- A severely high ERβ-to-ERα ratio in endometriotic stromal cells is associated with suppressed progesterone receptor and increased cyclo-oxygenase-2 levels contributing to progesterone resistance and inflammation.

ALTERNATIVE MANAGEMENT

- General considerations
  - Immune modulation
  - Reduce inflammation
  - Decrease influence of estrogen
  - Enhance Liver function; detoxification
  - Pain relief; symptom relief
  - Psychosocial influences and consequences
  - Prevent progression of disease
  - Decrease oxidative damage
  - Inhibition of growth factors
  - Antiangiogenesis agents

Immune modulation

- Decrease cytokines and Increase NK cells
  - Boswellia
  - Omega 3 oils
- Increase phagocytosis
  - Astragalus
  - Coriolus versicolor
  - Withania somnifera
- Antioxidants
  - Flavonoids- especially pine bark
  - E,C,A,Selenium, carotenes, melatonin
- Inhibit growth factors
  - Silymarin
  - Soy
  - Quercetin
- Antiangiogenesis
  - Soy

Alleviate inflammation

- Zingiber officinalis
- Scutellaria baicalensis
- Curcumin
- Flavanoids
- Quercitin
- Hi EPA fish oils

Modulate influence of estrogen

- Estrogen metabolism
  - DIM
  - Soy, flax seeds
  - Fish oils
- Aromatase inhibitors
  - Resveratrol
  - Agaricus
  - Pomegranate
- Lactobacillus
- Liver detoxification
- Colon ecology

Enhance liver function

- Silymarin
- Taraxacum root
- Lipotropic factors
- Liver detoxification programs

Diet and Endometriosis

- In a study of 504 women with laparoscopic confirmed endometriosis compared to 504 women without endometriosis, there was a 40% decrease risk in women who ate high amounts of green vegetables and fresh fruit.
- There was an 80% increase risk in women who ate high amounts of beef, other red meats, and ham
  - Hum reprod 2004;19:1755-1759

Endometriosis Links

- Multiple sclerosis, Sjögren's syndrome, and systemic lupus erythematosus
- Inflammatory bowel disease
  - 37,661 women hospitalized for endometriosis at any time between 1977 and 2007. Of these women, 320 developed IBD (228 women developed ulcerative colitis, 92 developed Crohn's disease).
  - They share a common underlying inflammatory problem, or that treatment for endometriosis (oral contraceptive use) increases the risk for IBD.
- Gut doi:10.1136/gutjnl-2011

Therapeutic Priorities

- Acute pain
- Chronic pain
- Fatigue
- Constipation
- Infertility
- Medications-side effects, risks

Pain relief

- Acute
  Valerian
  Crampbark
  Fennel, Ginger
  Guava
  Essential oils
  Vitamin B3
  Vitamin B6
  Thiamine
  Vitamin C and Rutin
  Calcium, magnesium, manganese
- Chronic
  Curcumin
  Hi EPA fish oils
  Pycnogenol

Endometriosis: Pine bark Extract

- N=58 women with persistent symptoms after endometriosis surgery
- Tx: Pine bark extract 30 mg bid for 48 weeks vs Lupron 6 times every 4 weeks
- Pine bark group: 33% reduction in symptoms
- Lupron= more efficient, but relapse 24 weeks post treatment

  J Reprod Med 2007;52

Botanicals and Endometriosis

- Study on herbal formula consisting of;
  - Frankincense, corydalis, salvia, cinnamon chinese angelica, dahurian angelica, licorice, myrrh, and white peony
- Endometrial biopsies were used to generate cell cultures from subjects with endometriosis and from controls
- The herbal formula was shown to inhibit proliferation, induce apoptosis, and blunt CCL5 gene and protein expression in endometriotic stromal cells
- Biol Reprod. 2009 Aug;81(2):371-7.

Ginger and Dysmenorrhea

- N=150 reproductive aged women with primary dysmenorrheal were divided into three groups, in a double-blind clinical trial. Group 1) ginger rhizome capsules, 250 mg four times a day for three days starting day one of their menses. Group 2) 250 mg mefenamic acid capsules, four times daily days one through three. Group 3) 400 mg ibuprofen capsules four times daily again, days one through three of the menses.
- Severity of dysmenorrhea decreased in all groups and no differences were found between the groups in pain severity, pain relief or satisfaction.
- More women in the ginger group became completely pain free, vs the mefenamic acid and ibuprofen groups. The rate of satisfaction from the treatments was 20/50 women in the mefenamic acid group, 22/50 women in the ibuprofen group and 21/50 women in the ginger group.

J Alternative and Complementary Med 2009; 15(2):129-132.

Ginger and Dysmenorrhea

- 105 Iranian women; moderate-to-severe primary dysmenorrhea
- Ginger capsules were given in one of two methods: 1) 500 mg ginger capsules or placebo 3x/daily starting 2 days before the beginning of menses and continued through day 3 of menses. 2) 500 mg ginger capsules or placebo 3x/daily on days 1,2 and 3 of menses.
- The severity of pain was significantly reduced in the ginger group compared to the placebo group for both dosing methods with better results in the first dosing method.
- A 1.4 to 2.0 point reduction in severity was seen with ginger and with the first dosing method, ginger significantly reduced the duration of pain compared with placebo. There was a 4.6 ± 10.6 hour decrease in the duration of pain versus a 2.3 ± 18.2 hour increase in duration in the placebo group. The second ginger dosing method was not significant in pain duration between ginger and placebo.

BMC Complement Altern Med. July 10, 2012;12(1):92

Fenugreek Seed Powder- Menstrual Cramps

- Ground fenugreek seed capsules at 900 mg three times per day vs P for first 3 days of menses and for 2 consecutive menstrual cycles.
- Outcome: severity of pain significantly decreased in both groups after the second menstrual cycle as compared to baseline (fenugreek group=3.25 vs. 6.4, placebo group=5.96 vs. 6.14).
- After each cycle, pain severity in the fenugreek group was significantly less as compared to placebo (cycle 1=4.32 vs. 6.03, and cycle 2=3.25 vs. 5.96).
- Duration of pain was significantly decreased in the fenugreek group; average use of pain medication in fenugreek group significantly decreased by the end of the study compared to the P group.
- Younesy S, Amiraliakbari S, Esmaeili S, Alavimajd H, Nouraei S. Effects of fenugreek seed on the severity and systemic symptoms of dysmenorrhea. *J Reprod Infertil.* January 2014;15(1):41-48.

Cinnamon- Menstrual Cramps

- Women with moderate menstrual cramps and regular menstrual cycles. Use of hormonal contraception and pain management medications were not allowed during the study.
- 38 women received placebo and 38 received 420 mg capsules of dried cinnamon bark powder
- Dose: two capsules three times daily during the first three days of their menses.
- *Results:* The mean pain severity score and the mean duration of pain were less in the cinnamon group than in the placebo group at all measured times. The amount of bleeding decreased significantly at 24 hours and 48 hours in the cinnamon group but not in the placebo group.
- The mean severity of nausea and the number of vomiting episodes significantly decreased in the cinnamon group at 24, 48 and 72 hours and greater than when compared with placebo.

Jaafarpour M, et al. *Iran Red Crescent Med J.* 2015;17(4):e27032.

Valerian- menstrual cramps

- RDBPCT; n=100; Valerian= 49; placebo=51
- Valerian (dose 255 mg), tid for 3 days beginning at the onset of menstruation, for 2 consecutive menstrual cycles.
- After the intervention, the pain severity was significantly reduced in both groups, but the extent of the reduction was larger in the valerian group.

Int J Gynaecol Obstet. 2011 Dec;115(3):285-8.

Dysmenorrhea and Topical essential oils

- Sixty-seven female college students
- Women were randomized into three groups: the aromatherapy group, a placebo group and a control group. Topically applied aromatherapy was given with abdominal massage using two drops of lavender, one drop of clary sage and one drop of rose in 5 cc of almond oil. The final concentration was 3%. The placebo group received almond oil only and the control group received no treatment.
- In the treatment group, menstrual cramps decreased from 7.40 to 4.26 on day one after the aromatherapy and the trend was the same for day two.
- No side effects were reported.

J Alternative and Complementary Medicine 2006;12(6): 535-541.

Turmeric

- Volatile oil= antiinflammatory activity
  - Inhibition of leukotriene formation
  - Inhibition of platelet aggregation
  - Promotion of fibrinolysis
  - Inhibition of neutrophil response to various inflammatory stimuli
  - stabilization of cell membranes preventing release of inflammatory mediators
  - May also increase and potentiate cortisol action

Dose: 400-600 mg tid for antiinflammatory effect

Green tea

- Epigallocatechin-3-gallate (EGCG) has an antiangiogenesis mechanism in an endometriosis model in vivo.
- Vitamin E had no effect

Fertil Steril. 2011 Oct;96(4):1021-8.

Melatonin and Endometriosis

- N=40 w/endometriosis; randomized to melatonin 10 mg/day (n=20) or placebo (n=20) groups for 8 weeks; moderate-severe chronic pelvic pain
- Melatonin group =significantly lower pain scores vs placebo (=39.3% reduction in melatonin group vs placebo group.
- Melatonin group also had significantly lower pain score during menstruation with mean reduction in analgesic use of 42.2% in the placebo group and 22.9% of patients in the melatonin group.
- Placebo group was 80% more likely to require additional analgesics than the melatonin group. P group =acetaminophen was used by 66.7%, NSAIDS by 60% and codeine or tramadol by 60%. Melatonin group= 33.3% used acetaminophen, 40% used tramadol or codeine and 35% used NSAIDS.
- Schwertner A, Conceicao dos Santos C, Costa G, et al. *Efficacy of melatonin in the treatment of endometriosis: A phase II, randomized, double-blind, placebo controlled trial.* PAIN 2013;154(6):874-881.

N-acetyl Cysteine Endometriosis

- 92 women participated in the study with 47 women receiving NAC, 600 mg three times daily, for three consecutive days a week over three months. 45 women received no treatment.
- NAC treated patient cyst mean diameter slightly reduced (-1.5 mm) vs. a significant increase (+6.6 mm) in untreated patients. NAC treatment: more cysts reduced and fewer cysts increased in size.
- 24 NAC patients (vs. 1 patient within control) cancelled scheduled laparoscopy due to cyst decrease or disappearance and/or relevant pain reduction (21 cases).
- The NAC treatment group resulted in 8 pregnancies with only 6 pregnancies resulting in the controls.
- The study concluded that NAC represents a "simple effective treatment for endometriosis, without side effects, and a suitable approach for women desiring pregnancy".

Porpora, M.G., et al. *Evid Based Complement Alternat Med, vol. 2013*

Fish Oils

- Rats with endometriosis were feed EPA for 6 weeks and compared to rats feed LA
- Endometriotic lesions were morphologically evaluated and their fatty acid composition was examined.
- In the EPA group the thickening of the interstitium, an active site for inflammation in endometriosis, was significantly suppressed

Fertil Steril. 2008 Oct;90(4 Suppl):1496-502.

Nutritional Supplements

Fish Oils
- N=42 adolescent girls with dysmenorrhea
- **Group 1:** 21 = tx fish oil
  - (1,080 mg EPA +720 mg DHA)
  - (+ 1.5 mg vitamin E)
  - daily for 2 months
  - followed by placebo for 2 months
- **Group 2:** 21 = placebo for 2 months
  - Followed by fish oil for 2 months

RESULTS:
- 7 point scale
- (4 = moderately effective)
- (7 = totally effective)
- 73% rated greater ≥ 4

*Harel, et al. Am J Ob/Gyn 1996

Vitamins and Endometriosis

- **Vitamin B** complex and **magnesium** intake, as well as **omega 3** supplements, can exert an anti-inflammatory role in endometriosis.
- Omega 3 and 6 fatty acids were proposed to improve pain symptoms related to endometriosis by modulating the biosynthesis and prostaglandin biochemical activity related to pelvic pain.
- Magnesium and vitamins B are related to anti-inflammatory prostaglandins production and miometrial relaxation.
- Diet based on vegetables, vitamins, omega 3 and magnesium ultimately reduces animal protein intake and therefore reduces the excess of body fat and estrogen peripheral production

Cochrane Database Syst Rev. 2004;3:CD003678.
Fertil Steril. 2007;88(6):1541-7

Bio-IdenticalProgesterone

- Natural Progesterone
  - 1/4 tsp. cream bid 3 weeks on and 1 week off
  - OMP 100-200 mg bid 2-3 weeks per month;
  - (days 15-26)
- Modifies the action of estradiol by decreasing the retention of receptors, causing a fall in serum estradiol levels
- Antispasmodic/Sedative effect

Vitamin D: Caution

- Eighty-seven women with endometriosis and 53 controls were recruited
- Vitamin-D levels measured
- Endometriosis is associated with higher serum levels of vitamin D

Hum Reprod. 2007 Aug;22(8):2273-8.

Caution: L-carnitine

- L-carnitine, when administered to young female mice, has been shown to induce a pathologic condition resembling human endometriosis accompanied by a marked degree of infertility.

Fertil Steril. 2011 Jun 30;95(8):2759-60.

Endometriosis Traditional Options

- **Homeopathics** – colocynth, apis, lyc, lach, bell, bry, sabina, mag phos, plat, rhus tox.
- **Pain botanicals** – piscidia, corydalis, passiflora, valerian, vibernum.
- **Turska's formula** – aconite, gelseminm, bryonia, phytolacca, water – 5 gtt QID
- **Turska's Revised Formula** – (Wise Woman Herbal) – vitex, arctium, ceonanthus, false unicorn, serenoa repens, yellow jasmine, iris versicolor, phytolacca, prickly ash bark, ginger, aconite

Endometriosis Chronic Sample Tx Plan

- Diet:
  -- Garlic, onions, curries, Cold water fish, fruits, veggies, nuts/seeds
  -- Decrease saturated fats, sugar, salt, caffeine
- EPA 1,080 mg/DHA 720 mg
- Anti-oxidant combinations= robust dosing
- NAC 600 mg tid
- Melatonin 10 mg h.s./day
- Pycnogenol 30 mg bid
- Turmeric 1,000 mg bid
- OMP 200 mg daily, days 15-26
- Consider/ MPA cyclic; OCPs/Nuvaring/contraceptive patch

Acute Dysmenorrhea
Sample Treatment Plan

- Acute Pain:
  - Niacin 100 mg every 2-3 hours
  - B 6 100 mg + Mg 100 mg every 2 hours during pain (x 6 mo.)
  - Tincture
    Valerian 2 Oz + Crampbark 2 oz + wild yam 2 oz + Ginger 2 oz
    1 tsp. every 3 hours
  - Ginger caps 250 mg qid
  - (Combination product 2 caps every 2-4 hours)
  - Relaxation techniques; Heat

Dr. Tori Hudson Resources

- Women's Encyclopedia of Natural Medicine, 2008, second edition
- www.drtorihudson.com
- www.awomanstime.com
- www.instituteofwomenshealth.com
- www.naturopathicresidency.org
- Monthly columns:
    Emerson Ecologics
    Townsend Letter for Doctors

Infertility

Dr. Marianne Marchese
www.drmarchese.com

Female factor

- **Ovulation disorders** (40 percent)
- Aging=Diminished ovarian reserve
- Endocrine disorder (hypothalamic amenorrhea, hyperprolactinemia, thyroid disease, adrenal disease)
- Polycystic ovary syndrome
- Premature ovarian failure
- Tobacco use
- **Tubal factors** (30 percent)
- Obstruction (history of pelvic inflammatory disease, tubal surgery)
- **Endometriosis** (15 percent)
- **Other** (about 10 percent)
- Uterine/cervical factors (more than 3 percent)
- Congenital uterine anomaly
- Fibroids/ Polyps
- Poor cervical mucus quantity/quality (caused by smoking, infection)

Pelvic Factors

- Infection: PID, STI, septic abortion, endometritis, pelvic TB
- Prior Surgery: D & C, appendicitis, fibroids, endometriosis, adnexal surgery
- Contraception and Pregnancy History: IUD, DEPO, OCP, ectopics, SAB, abortions
- Menstrual Cycle Issues: oligo- or amenorrhea, long/short cycles, menorrhagia, endometriosis, cyclic abdominal/pelvic pain

---

Ovulatory Factors

- Secondary amenorrhea
- Abnormal uterine bleeding
- Luteal phase defect (short cycle)
- Premature ovarian failure (early menopause)
- Polycystic ovarian syndrome (high androgen)
- Elevated prolactin (assoc. w/ endometriosis, lactation)
- Hypothyroidism
- Prior use of anti-estrogens (lupron, depo-prov)

Other female factors

- Delayed childbearing
- Over- (BMI>25) or underweight (BMI<18)
- Insulin resistance
- Depression, anxiety, stress
- Substance use (alcohol, marijuana, caffeine, tobacco)
- Malabsorption (celiac, IBD)
- **Unexplained 15%**

Male factor

- **Unknown** (40 to 50 percent)
- Primary hypogonadism (30 to 40 percent)
- Androgen insensitivity/ Congenital or developmental testicular disorder
- Cryptorchidism
- Medication s
- Orchitis, including mumps orchitis
- Systemic disorder- **thyroid**
- Testicular trauma/radiation
- Varicocele
- chromosome defect
- Altered sperm transport (10 to 20 percent)
- Absent vas deferens or obstruction/ Epididymal absence or obstruction
- Erectile dysfunction/ Retrograde ejaculation
- Secondary hypogonadism (1 to 2 percent)
- Androgen excess state (e.g., tumor, exogenous administration)
- Congenital idiopathic hypogonadotropic hypogonadism

Toxicants
Mechanism of Action

Endocrine disruptors can act through;
1. Classical nuclear receptors
2. Estrogen-related receptors
   1. (ERR) are a subfamily of orphan nuclear receptors closely related to ERα and ERβ.
3. Cross talk with estrogen receptors after binding on other receptors –Dioxin as an example
4. Nonsteroid receptors- such as the serotonin, dopamine, and norepinephrine receptor

De Coster S, J Environ Public Health. 2012

Toxicants
Mechanism of Action

Endocrine disruptors can act through;
1. Changes in metabolism of endogenous hormones
2. Cross-talk between genomic and nongenomic pathways
3. Interference with hormonal feedback regulation and neuroendocrine cells- GNRH
4. Changes in DNA methylation

De Coster S, J Environ Public Health. 2012

Environmental Factors and Fertility
Women

- Adult exposure in women to **cigarette smoke** results in decreased fecundity, decreased success rates of in vitro fertilization (IVF), decreased ovarian reserve, earlier menopause by 1–4 years, and an increased miscarriage rate.
  - Genius SJ, Hum Reprod. 2006 Sep;21(9):2201-8.

Environmental Factors and Fertility
Women

Increasing levels of urinary bisphenol-A, **BPA** reduced viable oocyte harvesting in IVF patients, possibly through estradiol suppression.

Int J Androl. 2010 Apr;33(2):385-93. Epub 2009 Nov 30.

Environmental Factors and Fertility
Women

- **Phthalates** and endometriosis- Endometriotic women showed significantly higher plasma DEHP phthalate concentrations than controls.
- In a study in India, 49 infertile women with endometriosis showed significantly higher blood concentrations **phthalates** compared to controls
  - Reddy BS, An International Journal of Obstetrics and Gynaecology. 2006;113(5):515–520.
  - Cobellis L, Hum Reprod., 2003 Jul;18(7):1512-5.

Environmental Factors and Fertility
Women

- Higher **PCB** serum levels in women were associated with increasing menstrual cycle length and a trend towards irregular cycles
  - Cooper GS, Epidemiology. 2005 Mar;16(2):191-200.
- 50 Southeast Asian immigrant women mean luteal phase length was shorter by 1.5 days at the highest quartile of serum **DDT** and progesterone metabolite levels during the luteal phase were decreased with higher **DDE** concentration
  - Windham GC, Epidemiology. 2005 Mar;16(2):182-90.

Environmental Factors and Fertility Women

- Among 1240 women from the Danish National Birth Cohort recruited from 1996 to 2002, longer "time to pregnancy" (TTP) was associated with higher maternal levels of **PFOA and PFOS**
  - Fei C, Hum Reprod. 2009 May;24(5):1200-5.
- 2009 study-women with high blood levels of **PFCs** took over one year to get pregnant or needed IVF compared to controls.
  - Journal of Human reproduction Vol 1(1)2009

Environmental factors and fertility women

- cross-sectional study investigated the association between blood concentrations of Pb, Cd, and As and infertility in women.
- concentrations of Pb and As, but not Cd, were significantly higher in the blood of infertile women than in that of pregnant women.
- A higher percentage of the infertile women consumed more alcohol, used Chinese herbal medicine more frequently, and lacked physical activity compared with the pregnant women.
  - LEI HL, et al. BMC Public Health.. 2015 Dec 9;15(1):1220.

Environmental Factors and Fertility Men and Women

- 157 couples with infertility had higher blood **Mercury** levels than control group which correlated with high fish intake
  - BJOG 2002;109:1121-1125.-157

Environmental Factors and Fertility Men

- Sperm quality and perfluorinated substances; perfluorooctanoic acid and perfluorooctane sulfonate. **PFOS and PFOA**
- Among 105 Danish men from the general population (median age 19 years), men in the highest quartile of combined levels of PFOS and PFOA had a median of 6.2 million normal spermatozoa in their ejaculate in contrast to 15.5 million among men in the lowest quartile.
  - Environmental Health Perspectives, vol. 117, no. 6, pp. 923–927, 2009

Environmental Factors and Fertility Men

- Sperm quality and heavy metals; 149 healthy male industrial workers age 20–43
- **Lead** decreased sperm density, counts, motile, and viable sperm and increased abnormal morphology
- Blood **cadmium** contributed to a decrease in sperm motility and an increase in abnormal sperm morphology
  - Environmental Health Perspectives, vol. 108, no. 1, pp. 45–53, 2000.

Environmental Factors and Fertility Men

- Non-occupational exposure links **lead and cadmium** with reduced sperm count motility, viability, and morphology.
- This study of 300 men included exposure to chemicals and metals when living in areas within 50 m of potential sources of pollution for three months or more and Three-wheeler drivers and those who rode motor bicycles more than 40 km a day
  - Wijesekara GU, et al. Ceylon Med J. 2015 Jun;60(2):52-6.

Environmental Factors and Fertility
Men

- Higher **trihalomethane** levels in drinking water might be associated with a decrease in the fecundity of men
  - Epidemiology, vol. 14, no. 6, pp. 650–658, 2003
- Periods of elevated **air pollution** are associated with decrease in sperm motility, morphology, and proportionately more sperm with abnormal chromatin.
  - Environmental Health Perspectives, vol. 108, no. 9, pp. 887–894, 2000

Environmental Factors and Fertility
Men

- Among 234 young Swedish men, those with the highest **phthalate** levels had fewer motile sperm, and lower luteinizing hormone values.
  - Epidemiology, vol. 16, no. 4, pp. 487–493, 2005
- Among 379 men from an infertility clinic, sperm DNA damage was associated with **phthalates**
  - Human Reproduction, vol. 22, no. 3, pp. 688–695, 2007.

Environmental Factors and Fertility
Men

Decreased sperm quality with increasing serum concentration of Bisphenol-A, **BPA.**

Fertil Steril. 2011 Feb;95(2):625-30.e1-4. Epub 2010 Oct 29.

Environmental Factors and Fertility
Men-Glyphosate

- 1. results show that acute **Roundup** exposure at low doses (36 ppm, 0.036 g/L) for 30 min induces oxidative stress and activates multiple stress-response pathways leading to Sertoli cell death in the testis.
  - de Liz Oliveira Cavalli VL, et al. Free Radic Biol Med.2013 Dec;65:335-46

Environmental Factors and Fertility
Men

- Summary of the effects of more than 15 mostly used pesticides on male reproduction.
- pesticide exposure damages spermatozoa, alter Sertoli or Leydig cell function, both in vitro and in vivo and thus affects semen.

Sengupta P Banerjee . R Hum Exp Toxicol. 2014 Oct;33(10):1017-39.

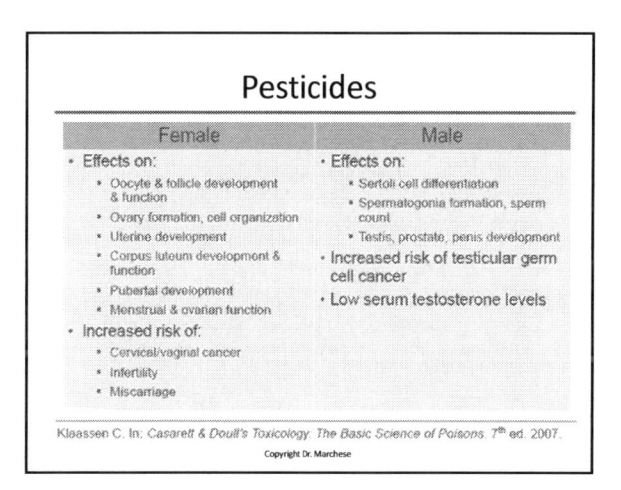

Pesticides

Female	Male
Effects on: • Oocyte & follicle development & function • Ovary formation, cell organization • Uterine development • Corpus luteum development & function • Pubertal development • Menstrual & ovarian function Increased risk of: • Cervical/vaginal cancer • Infertility • Miscarriage	Effects on: • Sertoli cell differentiation • Spermatogonia formation, sperm count • Testis, prostate, penis development • Increased risk of testicular germ cell cancer • Low serum testosterone levels

Klaassen C. In: Casarett & Doull's Toxicology: The Basic Science of Poisons. 7th ed. 2007.

Summary

- Metals- lead, mercury from fish, cadmium, arsenic
- Organochlorine compounds- DDT, PCBs
- Pesticides- roundup
- Phthalates
- BPA
- PFC-Perflourinated chemicals
- Air pollution and trihalomethanes in water

How much fish is too much?

- Consumption of fish and sashimi represented the major source of MeHg exposure in infertile women in 2015 study.
- MeHg levels were elevated in infertile women, and consistent with fish consumption frequency.
  - Compared to the reference level of blood MeHg levels <5.8 µg/L, the elevated blood MeHg levels (⩾5.8 µg/L) in infertile women were 3.35 and 4.42 folds. Frequencies of fish consumption 1-2 meals per week and more than 3 meals per week, respectively.
  - Lei HL, et al. Chemosphere. 2015 Sep;135:411-7.

Environmental Factors and Fertility Smoking

- Smoking
  - Men: Lower sperm count and motility, and more abnormal morphology
  - Women: Higher FSH and Lower AFC

Arch Gynecol Obstet.. 2012 Nov 25

Marijuana

- Men who reported daily marijuana use displayed significant lower sperm concentration and sperm counts compared with nonusers.
- marijuana plays in disrupting the hypothalamus-pituitary-gonadal axis, spermatogenesis, and sperm function such as motility, capacitation
- Am J Epidemiol. 2015 Sep 15;182(6):482-4.
- J Assist Reprod Genet. 2015 Nov;32(11):1575-88.

Alcohol

- two or more drinks per day, or binge drinking (five or more drinks at a time) has been associated with miscarriage and infertility
- large European multi-center study of over 4,000 couples demonstrated that consuming eight or more drinks per week experienced a longer delay to conception compared with non-drinkers.
- A smaller, prospective study also showed a longer delay to pregnancy, even with light consumption of five or fewer drinks per week.
- https://www.scrcivf.com/fertility-and-alcohol/

Autoimmune Infertility

- Celiac, thyroiditis, and lupus are linked to female infertility.
- Celiac not linked to male.
- 5%-10% of infertile women were positive for Transglutimase IgA compared to controls
- Fertility improved with gluten free diet
- Toxicants are linked to autoimmune conditions
- Fertil Steril. 2011 Apr;95(5):1709-13
- Fertil Steril. 2011 Mar 1;95(3):922-7

Lifestyle summary

- Smoking
- Alcohol
- Marijuana
- Gluten
- Fish with mercury

SNPs and infertility

- MTHFR C677T- both male and female factors.
  Zhu X, et al. Ren Fail. 2016 Mar;38(2):185-93., and Stangler Herodez S et al. Balkan J Med Genet. 2013 Jun;16(1):31-40.
- CYP1A1, GSTM1- male factor
  Aydos SE, et al. Fertility and Sterility 2009;92(2):541-547
- CYP1A1, 1B1- female in fertility
  Bankowski BJ, et al. Fertility and Sterility 2004;82(2)s19.
- CYP2D6- male semen abnormalities and failure of clomid in ART in women
  Zalata A, et al. Andrologia.2015 Jun;47(5):525-30

Fertility Work-up
Women

- FSH-Day 3- PMO failure, pituitary fcn
- LH- Day 3-If higher than the FSH, mb PCOS
- E2- Day 3- If elevated, estradiol can lower the FSH, thereby masking elevated FSH levels. If low it could mean low ovarian reserve
- Progesterone- Day 21, if day 14 ovulate
- Cortisol-if elevated affects ovarian fcn
- Testosterone- total and free- mb PCOS
- AMH
- Basic labs- lipids, CMP, CBC, celiac panel, Vit-D, HgA1C, INR/PT

Fertility Work-up
Women

- Prolactin- if elevated affect ovulation
- SHBG- if low mb PCOS or hypothyroidism
- Thyroid and antibodies-
- Ferritin-Levels can be low in patients with infertility. Should be above 50
- Homocysteine- Elevated levels can be found in autoimmune conditions, ovarian aging and endometriosis.
- Anti-sperm AB- Can destroy or damage the sperm Around 5% of infertile women have these antibodies.
- Imaging- Pelvic U/S, HSG

Fertility Work-up
Men

- FSH and LH- for hypogonadism
- Testosterone free and total
- Thyroid and antibodies
- Basic labs- lipids, CMP, CBC, celiac panel, Vit-D, HgA1C, INR
- Prolactin
- Gonorrhea and chlamydia cultures, urinalysis (if genital infection suspected)
- Post ejaculatory urinalysis (if retrograde ejaculation suspected)
- Semen analysis (2 or more samples)
- Post-coital semen test- identifies if there is a sperm/cervical mucus incompatibility
- Imaging- scrotal ultra sound and Transrectal ultrasonography (if ejaculatory duct obstruction suspected)

Fertility Work-up
Men

- Physical examination
  - Genital infection (e.g., discharge, prostate tenderness)
  - Hernia
  - Presence of vas deferens
  - Signs of androgen deficiency (e.g., increased body fat, decreased muscle mass, decreased facial and body hair, small testes, Tanner stage < 5)
  - Testicular mass
  - Varicocele

Environmental work-up

- Exposure history
  - This is how you know what test to run
- Blood and urine tests for chemicals and metals
  - Metals and other toxicants
- Genetic polymorphism testing- SNPs for detoxification and methylation in the cells
  - 23 and Me

Conventional treatments

- **Clomiphene citrate** - 50 mg qd x 5days from day three to seven of the cycle.
- **Follicle Stimulating Hormone,** FSH- stimulates the ovaries to produce more follicles
- **GnRH agonist** (lupron)-stimulate the pituitary gland to release FSH and LH
- **GnRH antagonists-**
- **Gonadotropin**-contains LH and FSH which stimulate the ovaries to produce more follicles
- **IUI and IVF**

Problems with ART

- 2012 study examined **birth defects** in 309,000 Australian children, 6,163 of whom were conceived through ART. Found a 26% increase in risk of birth defects among babies conceived using any form of ART
- A 2005 review showed a 25% or greater increase in risk of **birth defects** in ART infants compared with naturally conceived infants
- 2011 investigators reported a 35% increased risk of **low birth weight** among singletons following fresh-embryo transfer, compared with frozen-embryo transfer.
- Environmental Health Perspectives • volume 120, number 10 .October 2012

Naturopathic treatments

- Treat the cause, both male and female factors
- Treat the whole person
- Treat the toxicant exposure

Find and Treat the cause first not the unexplained first

- Endometriosis/adenomyosis
- PCOS
- Thyroid
- Fibroids
- Oligo or amenorrhea
- PMO- is it really???
- Low AMH
- Smoking, alcohol, marijuana
- Easy to treat cause of abn semen analysis

Mental & Emotional Issues

- Infertility = very stressful, emotionally taxing
- Past/current stress esp. depression may be factor in unexplained infertility (evolutionary)
- Cont'd infertility → vicious cycle of emotional upset & rollercoaster of monthly hopes and let-downs.
- Stress hormones: inhibitory effects on repro system
- Researchers believe addressing fertility issues should begin with stress reduction
- Most agree stress affects fertility in both partners, but data unclear re: effect on IVF

Stress reduction

- Techniques: biofeedback, individual/couple therapy, progressive muscle relaxation, acupuncture, yoga, tai chi, Qi gong, & meditation should be part of the treatment.
- Therapy with mental health practitioner experienced in dealing with infertility best.
- Medications for anxiety & depression that are safe for use in pregnancy are available for women with more severe symptoms.

Treat nutrient deficiencies

- **B12** deficiency can be associated with menstrual cycle dysfunction, recurrent SAB & infertility.
- **Vitamin D3** deficiency reported to have negative impact on fertility that supplementation can reverse
- Preconception **MVM** = higher rates of conception
- Nurses' Health Study indicates decreased risk of ovulatory disorders w/ **MVM**

- Int J Vitam Nutr Res 1996;66:55-58.
- Fertil Steril 2008;89:668–676
- J Reprod Med 2001; 46:209-212

Treat nutrient deficiencies

12pts: h/o unexplained infertility/early SAB all had low magnesium. They were given 600mg qd Mg.
- 6/12 failed to normalize their red cell **Mg** levels after 4 months of 600mg po qd **Mg**
- Added 200mcg po qd **selenomethionine** to the 600mg po qd **magnesium** for both groups fro 2 months
  - All 6 normalized their RBC-Mg and RBC-GSH-Px levels.
  - All 12 previously infertile women produced healthy babies conceiving w/in 8 months of normalizing their RBC-Mg.

Magnes Res. 1994 Mar;7(1):49-57.

Treat nutrient deficiencies

- Forty-five infertile and 30 control women
- Plasma **EPA** and erythrocyte **DHA** levels were reduced in infertile women as compared to controls.
- Levels of MDA, (oxidative stress marker) were increased and **vitamin E** decreased in infertile women.

Hum Fertil ;2009 Mar;12(1):28-33.

Botanicals for fertility
Vitex (chaste tree)

- Re-establishes normal balance of estrogen and progesterone during the menstrual cycle.
- Blocks prolactin secretion in women with excessive levels of this hormone; excessive levels of prolactin can lead failure to ovulate.
- A double-blind trial has confirmed that vitex reduces mildly elevated levels of prolactin before a woman's period.

http://www.uofmhealth.org/health-library/hn-2181002

Botanicals for fertility
Vitex (chaste tree)

- Luteal phase defect
- 48 women (ages 23 to 39) who were diagnosed with infertility took vitex once daily for three months. Seven women became pregnant during the trial, and 25 women experienced normalized progesterone levels

Propping D, Katzorke T. Treatment of corpus luteum insufficiency. Zeitschr Allgemeinmedizin 1987;63:932-3.

Botanicals for fertility
Vitex (chaste tree)

Infertile women 24-42 y.o.
- rFertilityBlend proprietary supplement: **vitex, green tea, L-arginine, vitamins, minerals**
  - After 3m, tx group had increased mid-luteal prog, more days with luteal-phase BBT >98F; both short & long cycles normalized; Placebo group did not show significant changes in these parameters.
  - After 3m, 14/53 pregnancies in tx group (26%) vs 4/40 in placebo group (10%).
  - After 6m, 3 more tx group pregnancies (32%).

Can J Clin Pharmacol Vol 15 (1) Winter 2008:e74- e79
Clin Exp Obstet Gynecol. 2006;33(4):205-8

Botanicals for fertility
Cimicifuga racemosa

- 119 pts w/ unexplained infertility and recurrent Clomid resistant cycles
- 60 pts **Cimicifuga racemosa** 120mg d1-12 with hCG 10000IU IM and clomid 150mg d3-7 plus timed intercourse;
- E2, LH, progesterone, endometrial thickness and pregnancy rate (36% vs. 13%) increased in CR group.

Reprod Biomed Online. 2008 Apr;16(4):580-8.

Botanicals for fertility
Cimicifuga racemosa

- 100 women with PCOS were split into two groups. 50 women received clomid 100mg for 5 days. The other fifty women received a dose of Black Cohosh 20mg for 10 days.
- Black Cohosh group showed significant improvements in LH and LH/FSH ratios. Black Cohosh group had better progesterone levels
- pregnancy rate was also higher in the patients who received Black Cohosh,

Kamel HH. Role of phyto-oestrogens in ovulation induction in women with polycystic ovarian syndrome. Eur J Obstet Gynecol Reprod Biol. 2013;168(1):60-63

Botanicals for fertility
Chinese herbal formula-sperm

- a study on the effects of five herbs on sperm
- *Cornus officinalis, Schizandra chinensis, Rubus coreanus, Cuscuta chinensis,* and *Lycium chinense.* Both in vivo and in vitro in rats
- Sperm count and motility improved compared to controls
- All 5 high in anti-oxidants

World J Mens Health. 2013 Dec; 31(3): 254–261.

Botanicals for fertility
Licorice

- Lowers prolactin in women with elevated prolactin
- Lowers testosterone win women with PCOS
- Mostly used with oligo/anovular in fertility

Arentz S, et al. BMC Complement Altern Med. 2014; 14: 511.

Botanicals for fertility
Tribulus

- Tx for PCOS
- Ovulation induction supported by Increased FSH
- Study of 148 infertile women with oligo/anovular infertility took tribulus and had 60% ovulation rates

Arentz S, et al. BMC Complement Altern Med. 2014; 14: 511.

Botanicals for fertility
Peony and Cinnamon

- Peony combined with Chinese cinnamon
- Study- 157 infertile women aged 17–29 years, including a subgroup of 42 women with hyper-functioning (PCOS) oligo/amenorrhoea.
- Ovulation was confirmed in 30 out of 42 oligo/amenorrheic women.
  - Arentz S, et al. BMC Complement Altern Med. 2014; 14: 511.

Hormones for fertility

- **Progesterone**
  - normalize menstrual cycle
  - improve IVF rates
  - maintain pregnancy in women with hx of repeated SAB
  - d21 <15 may benefit from progesterone after ovulation until menses starts or week 10-12 of pregnancy
- **DHEA**, if deficient may improve ovarian function
  - 73 IVF cases supplemented w/ DHEA; SAB rates decreased for all, but most >35 yo
  - DHEA 50-75mg for at least 4m found to improve natural cycle or IUI/IVF outcome & pregnancy rates in diminished ovarian reserve
  - Increases AMH
  - Curr Opin Obstet Gynecol. 2009 Aug;21(4):306-8. Review
  - Reprod Biol Endocrinol. 2009 Oct 7;7:108.

Curcumin-sperm

- Study examined if curcumin affects sperm function in vitro and fertility in vivo.
- Incubation of sperm with curcumin caused a decrease in sperm motility, capacitation, and murine fertilization in vitro.
- At higher concentrations, there was a complete block of sperm motility and function within 5-15 min.
- Administration of curcumin, especially intravaginally, caused a significant reduction in fertility.
  - Mol Reprod Dev. 2011 Feb;78(2):116-23.

Curcumin-sperm

- Mice were orally administered curcumin (600 mg/kg body weight per day for 56 and 84 days)
- adverse effects on motility, viability, morphology and number of sperm, serum level of testosterone and on fertility and litter size.
- Affects reversible
  - Contraception. 2009 Jun;79(6):479-87

Treatments for sperm

- Antioxidants
  - **Vitamin C & E, glutathione, lycopene, & coQ10** may have beneficial effects in cases of suboptimal sperm
  - l-Carnitine, vitamin C, coenzyme Q10, vitamin E, zinc, vitamin B9, selenium, B12 during a time period of 3 months= increase in concentration, motility, vitality and morphology
    - Andrologia.2012 Sep 3.
    - Curr Drug Metab. 2005 Oct;6(5):495-501.

Treatments for sperm

- **L-Carnitine** was effective in improvement of percentile of motile sperms, grade A sperms, and normal-shaped sperms.
  - J Assist Reprod Genet. 2005 Dec;22(11-12):395-9.
- 60 infertile men with sperm motility problems
  - **L-acetyl-carnitine** (3g po qd) both alone or w/ L-carnitine (LC 2g/d; LAC 1g/d) x 3m
  - Improvement in sperm motility
  - Fertil Steril. 2005 Sep;84(3):662-71.

Summary

- Metals- lead, mercury from fish, cadmium, arsenic
- Organochlorine compounds- DDT, PCBs, dioxin
- Pesticides- roundup
- Phthalates
- BPA
- PFC-Perflourinated chemicals
- Air pollution and trihalomethanes in water

Copyright Dr. Marchese

Cleansing and Chelation

- Remove chemicals to improve fertility
- Remove chemicals to improve the pregnancy
- Remove chemicals to improve health of child

Copyright Dr. Marchese

Panex Ginseng-sperm and toxins

- *Panax ginseng* significantly reduces Dioxin damages in rat testes.[54]
- *Panax ginseng* is found to protect Sertoli cells from the cytotoxic effects of bisphenol A.
- It improves erectile dysfunction and sperm count and motility

- Leung kw, Spermatogenesis. 2013 Jul 1; 3(3): e26391.

Copyright Dr. Marchese

Nutrients and toxicants
Zinc

- Protective role as an antioxidant and antibacterial agent.
- Protective against heavy metal accumulation, specifically lead.
- Low sperm motility is associated with low zinc levels.
- The number of germinal cells and sperm are reduced in the testes of zinc-deficient rats.

- DMAB Dissanayake et. al., J Hum Reprod Sci. 2010 Sep-Dec; 3(3): 124–128.

Copyright Dr. Marianne Marchese

Nutrients and toxicants
Folate

- Aneuploidy may account for over one-third of all spontaneous abortions with a high paternal contribution.
- Chemotherapy, organophosphates, carbaryl and fenvalerate, associated with higher frequency of aneuploidy in human sperm.
- Men with daily total folate intake > 1.8 times the RDA had between 20% and 30% lower chromosomal defects compared with men with lower intake.

- S.S. Young et al, Hum Reprod. 2008 May;23(5):1014-22. Epub 2008 Mar 19.

Copyright Dr. Marianne Marchese

Nutrients and toxicants
Selenium

- Se is an antioxidant and protects cellular membranes and organelles from peroxidative damage.
- The administration of Se to sub-fertile patients induced a statistically significant rise in sperm motility.
- High Se intake (> 500 mcg) has been associated with impaired semen quality.
- Se increases glutathione

- Moslemi and Tavanbakhsh Int J Gen Med. 2011; 4: 99–104

Copyright Dr. Marianne Marchese

Nutrients and toxicants
Vitamin C and E

- Oxidative stress linked to sperm DNA damage.
- Oral antioxidant treatment appears to improve outcomes of assisted fertility tx in those patients with sperm DNA damage.
- Study: 2-month oral treatment with two antioxidants, vitamin C and vitamin E, both at a daily dose of 1 g (500 mg BID).
  - Oxford Journals Medicine Human Reproduction. 2005 Volume 20, 2590-2594.

Nutrients and Toxicants
Oxidative stress

- Study of 40 men treatment with **Carni-Q-Nol** (440mg L-carnitine + 30mg ubiquinol + 75 IU vitamin E + 12mg vitamin C).
- After 3 and 6 months of treatment, improved sperm density and the sperm pathology decreased by 25.8%.
- Concentrations of CoQ10-TOTAL (ubiquinone + ubiquinol) and α-tocopherol were significantly increased and the oxidative stress was decreased.
  - http://www.ncbi.nlm.nih.gov/pmc/articles/PMC4355595/pdf/DM2015-827941.pdf

Nutrients and toxicants
Glutathione

- Glutathione is vital to sperm antioxidant defenses and has demonstrated a positive effect on sperm motility.
- Antioxidant needed for detoxification of toxicants

  - Moslemi and Tavanbakhsh Int J Gen Med. 2011; 4: 99–104

Preconception detoxification

- Increase Fertility
- Reduce Pregnancy Complications
- Improve Health of the Baby
- Decrease the impact of toxicants on pregnancy outcomes

True preventative medicine

- Pregnancy planning and preparation
  - Environmental exposure history
  - Avoidance education
  - Toxin Testing
  - SNP testing
  - Cleansing- maybe with chelation

Removing chemicals from the body

Four steps in a detoxification plan are:
1. Mobilize stored toxins
2. Support liver metabolism
3. Support elimination
4. Avoid re-exposure to toxins

Mobilize stored toxins

- Caloric restriction
- Sauna therapy
- Chelation for mobilizations of heavy metals

Affinities of chelators

DMPS	DMSA	EDTA
Mercury	Lead	Lead
Lead	Cadmium	Copper
Silver	Mercury	Nickel
Cadmium	Silver	Cadmium
Nickel	Nickel	Aluminum
Arsenic	Arsenic	Tin
Antimony	Molybdenum	Antimony
Copper	Copper	Zn, Mn, Fe

- From Dr. David Quig Doctors Data Lab.

Liver metabolism- nutrition

- *Green tea*
  - Catechins increase phase-one and phase-two detoxification and glutathione
- *Pomegranate*
  - Ellagic acid modulates phase-one CYP 450 1A1.
- *Cruciferous family vegetables*
  - Improve liver phase one and two pathways
  - Breakdown estrogen in liver

- Nick, GL. *JANA* 2002;5(4):34-44 [evidence B]
- Liska DJ, Bland J. *Townsend Letter*. 2002 October:42-46 [evidence B]

Liver metabolism- nutrition

- Whey
  - Increases Glutathione
- Psyllium
  - Increases bile acid synthesis

- Balbis E, et al. *Toxicol Ind Health*. 2009;25:325-328. [evidence B]
- Chitapanarux T, et al. *J Gasteroenterol Hepatol*. 2009;24(6):1045-1050. [evidence B]
- Chan MY, Heng CK. *Nutrition*. 2008 Jan;24(1):57-66. [evidence B]

Liver metabolism- supplementation

- Phase one and two enzyme co-factors
- Choloretic and cholagogue
- Estrogen and estrogen mimicking toxin break-down

Polymorphisms

- Liver detox support- example…..preliminary
  - **1A1** Avoid PAHs and amines, charbroiled meats, cigarette smoke, air pollution
  - **1B1** Cruciferous foods, DIM, I3C, Ca-D-glucarate, Rosemary, Fish oil
  - **COMT**-methyl donors
  - **NAT**-see 1A1
  - **GSTs**-glutathione
  - **SOD**-antioxidants

Avoidance at home

- Check for lead paint and pipes, manage dust
- Avoid PVC products; shower curtain liners
- No plastic food storage containers and wrap
- No pesticides in or around home- neighbors
- Air and water filters
- Food- organic, non-gmo, fish low in mercury, no canned food
- Check cleaning, cooking, and cosmetic products

Summary

- Infertility is complicated
- Male and female factors
- Address the cause-the real cause
- Avoid ART
- Incorporate entire tool box including environmental approach
  - Botanicals, nutrition, lifestyle, vitamins, mineral, antioxidants, amino acids, mind-body, acupuncture, homeopathy

Heart Arrhythmias, and Atrial Fibrillation: Balancing the Heart

Presented by Jason Miller LAc, MAcOM

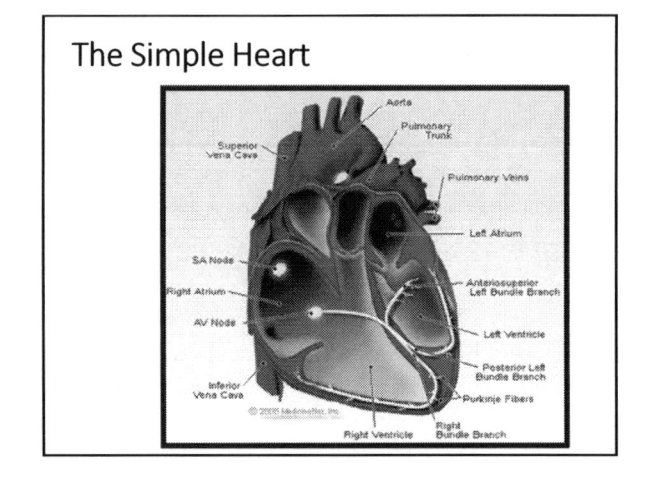

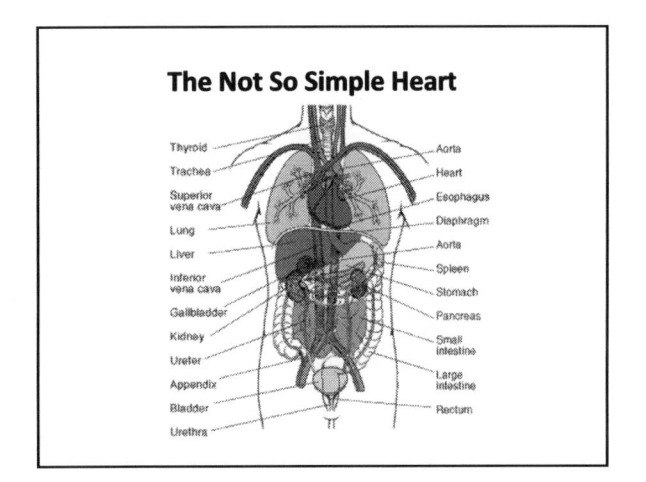

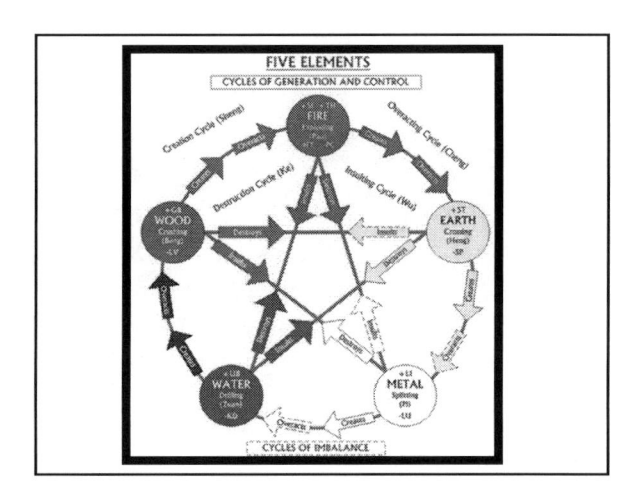

The Simple Heart

The Not So Simple Heart

Arrhythmia

- Abnormal beats.
- A change in the normal sequence of electrical impulses in the heart

Rate or Rhythm
- Too Fast/Too Slow
- Erratic

Types of Arrhythmias

- Atrial Fibrillation
- Ventricular Fibrillation
- Bradycardia/Tachycardia
- Conduction Disorders
- Premature Contractions

Bradycardia

- Abnormally slow heart action
- HR <60
- More common in the elderly
- Atrial, AV, or Ventricular
- Originate in SA or AV nodes

Tachycardia

- Abnormally fast heart action
- HR > 100
- SVT (supraventricular tachycardia)
- Ventricular Tachycardia – "fluttering" of the ventricles – consistent pattern

Ventricular Fibrillation

- Early onset Sx's (an hour before loss of consciousness) - Chest Pain, Rapid heart rate, dizziness, nausea, SOB
- Loss of consciousness or fainting
- AED/CPR

Atrial Fibrillation

- Atrial fibrillation results from quivering, uncoordinated atrial activity
- Most common arrhythmia

Atrial Fibrillation Statistics

- In Europe and North America, as of 2014, it affects about 2% to 3% of the population *Clinical epidemiology* 6: 213–20.
- More than 750,000 hospitalizations per year
- 130,000 deaths each year.
- The death rate from AFib as the primary or a contributing cause of death has been rising for more than two decades.
- $6 billion per year.
- Medical costs for people who have AFib are about $8,705 higher per year than for people who do not have Afib.

Circulation. 2015;131:e29–e322
Journal of the American College of Cardiology. 2014;64(21):2246–80.
HCUP National Inpatient Sample [online]. 2012.
CDC WONDER Online Database. 2014.

Risk Factors for Afib

- Advancing age
- *High blood pressure
- Obesity and sleep apnea
- European ancestry
- Diabetes
- Heart failure
- Ischemic heart disease
- *Heart Valve Disease
- Hyperthyroidism
- Chronic kidney disease
- Heavy alcohol use
- Enlargement of the chambers on the left side of the heart

Circulation. 2015;131:e29–e322

AFib Triggers

- Stress
- Lack of sleep
- Mental/emotional strain
- Physical trauma
- Chemical exposures
- Alcohol
- Caffeine

Alcohol

- Vagal triggers

- Alcohol and vagal triggers often were found in the same patients with PAF, raising the possibility that alcohol may precipitate AF by vagal mechanisms.

  Am J Cardiol. 2012 Aug 1;110(3):364-8

The Importance of Sleep

Sleep-disordered breathing as risk factor – treatment with CPAP has shown to decrease the incidence of AF.

J Thorac Dis. 2015 Dec;7(12):E575-84.

Phenibut

- **Phenibut** - Taurine, 4-amino-3-phenylbutyric acid, B6 – a gabapentinoid
- Lowers stress levels without causing drowsiness.
- Similar to GHB (gamma hydroxy butyric acid) but does not act on the convulsion inducing GHB receptor.
- Dosage 250-1500mg BID
- Can produce sleepiness and hangover-like effects (depression/headaches)
- Alternate with other sleep aids

Caffeine

- Surrounded by controversy in the medical world.
- Recent studies have shown no correlation with caffeine intake and Afib
- Raises heart rate
- Can be a trigger
- SNP - rs762551
  - AA = fast,
  - AC or CC = slowed

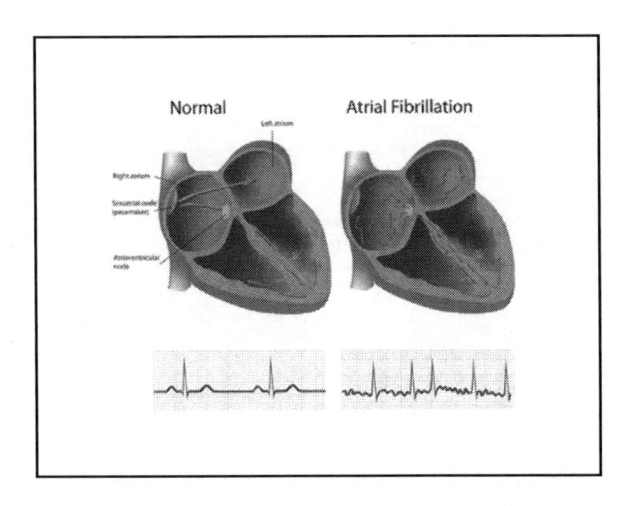

Classes of Afib

- First Detected - one diagnosed episode
- Paroxysmal (PAF) – less than 7 day episodes
- Persistent – more than 7 day long episodes
- Permanent – on going long term
- Lone Atrial Fibrillation (LAF)
- Non-valvular
- Secondary

Afib and Clotting

- *Non-valvular atrial fibrillation is **the most common cardiac source of emboli and cardioembolic stroke.**
- The "eddy effect"
- Can lead to clot formation
- Mobile clots = emboli
- Strokes/TIA's

Evaluating Stroke Risk

- $CHADS_2$ score
- CHA_2DS_2-VASc

Score	Recommendation
0	no anti-coagulant therapy
1	anti-coagulant should be considered
2+	anti-coagulant recommended

Risk factors: Congestive Heart Failure, Hypertension, 75yrs+, Diabetes Mellitus, Prior Stroke, Vascular Disease, Thromboembolism, Age 65+, Female

Warfarin/Coumadin

- Warfarin reduces the risk of stroke in patients with AF by approximately two-thirds.

  Expert Rev Cardiovasc Ther. 2011 Mar;9(3):279-86.

- Bleeding complications, including gastrointestinal bleeding, are a common complication of anticoagulant treatment, and limit their use.

Warfarin/Coumadin Issues

- Warfarin is not a long term solution, especially for Asians, who have more bleeding complications with Vit K inhibitor therapy. Circ J. 2016 Jan 21.

- Bleeding is a real issue with current pharmaceutical anti-coagulation therapy. Cardiol J. 2016 Jan 18

- Patients with Afib and CKD are more difficult to treat due to more bleeding issues and ischemic stroke.

Vitamin K

NOAC's

- Show some improvements over warfarin but have other issues
- The NOAC therapies are associated with an increased risk of major gastrointestinal bleeding compared with warfarin
- **Dabigatran** is also associated with an increased risk of non-bleeding upper GI symptoms such as dyspepsia and heartburn.

Pradaxa/Dabigatran

- Approved for non-valvular Afib   Expert Rev Cardiovasc Ther. 2011 Mar;9(3):279-86.
- Inhibits thrombin
- Does not require routine INR/PTT
- Lower risk of overall mortality, ischemic stroke, and bleeding in the brain than warfarin.
- Gastrointestinal bleeding more common

FDA Drug Safety Communication

Natural Blood Stasis/Clot inhibiting Therapies

- Nattokinase
- Lumbrokinase
- Ginkgo
- EFA's
- Turmeric
- TCM Botanical Formula

Inhibitors of Platelet Aggregation

- **Ginkgo Biloba**
  - Inhibits platelet activation by lowering intracellular Ca^{2+} levels.   Platelets. 1999;10(5):298-305.
  - Redox-cycling, anti-inflammatory, anti-angiogenic, anti-platelet aggregation, and gene-regulatory actions

- **Aspirin**

Fibrin Digesting Enzymes

Lumbrokinase   **Nattokinase**

Nattokinase

- Serine protease extracted exclusively from Natto
- Thrombolytic properties documented in vivo   Acta Haematol. 2014;132(2):247-53.
- Fibrinolytic Enzyme
- Reduces HTN
- Resembles Plasmin
- Dose every 8 hours
- Nattokinase has been the subject of 17 studies, including two small human trials

Health Sciences Institute, March 2002. Maruyama M, Sumi H. Effect of Natto Diet on Blood Pressure. JTTAS, 1995. Sumi H. Healthy Microbe "Bacillus natto". Japan Bio Science Laboratory Co. Ltd

Dr Milner's Dosing

- Low dose = one 100 milligram/2000 FU softgel capsule 2 or 3 times a day
- Medium dose = two capsules 2 or 3 times a day
- High dose = three to four capsules 2 or 3 times a day.
- Capsules are taken on an empty stomach.

Lumbrokinase

- Anti-thrombotic
- Direct effect on fibrin
- Also activates plasminogen
  Chin Med J (Engl) 2007;120:898–904.
- Similar to tissue plasminogen activator (TPA)
- Works only in the presence of fibrin

TCM Botanical Therapeutics for Blood Stagnation

- **Invigorate Blood**
    - Dang Gui (Radix Angelica S.)
    - Chuan Xiong (Radix Ligusticum)
    - Chi Shao (Red Peony)
    - Mu Dan Pi (Radix Moutan)
- **Remove Blood Stasis**
    - *Jiang Huang (Rhizoma Curcumae Longae),
    - Hong hua (Flos Carthamus),
    - Tao Ren (Persica Seed),
    - Dan Shen (Salvia Miltiorrhizome)
- **Break Blood Stagnation**
    - E Zhu (Zedoaria)
    - San Leng (Rhizoma Sparganii)
    - Shui Zhi (Leech)

Hirudo – Leech

At least 14 different anticoagulants have been obtained from leeches.

The therapeutic capacity of the leech is based on secreted anticoagulants that are released while feeding.

Hirudin – a specific inhibitor for thrombin – similar to Heparin

Altern Med Rev 2011;16(1):50-58)

Antiplatelet Properties of Natural Products

- Olive Oil
- Onion and Garlic
- Tomatoes
- Mushrooms
- Wine and Beer
- Cocoa

Vascular Pharmacology 59 (2013) 67-75

Herb/Drug Interactions

- Individuality
- "Currently, there are no reports of bleeding associated with concomitant administration of warfarin and any of these herbs"
    - Coumarin containing
        - angelica root, arnica flower, anise, asafoetida, celery, chamomile, fenugreek, horse chestnut, licorice root, lovage root, parsley, passionflower herb, quassia, red clover, and rue.
    - Salicylate containing
        - Meadowsweet, poplar, and willow bark
    - Anti-Platelet
        - Ginkgo, bromelain, clove, onion, and turmeric
    - Borage seed oil, bogbean, capsicum

http://www.medscape.com/viewarticle/406896

Warfarin Monitoring

- Continuous weekly/biweekly INR and PTT

- Consistency with diet and supplementation

Biomedical Treatment of AFib

- Cardioversion
- RFA
- Surgery

Cardioversion

- **Electrical** – electrical shock is delivered to the heart in hopes of resetting the heart's rhythm.

- **Chemical** – antiarrhythmic agents (oral or IV)

Anti-arrythmic Agents

- **Class I** (a,b,c) – Na+ channel blockers, some with K+ blocking activity (procainamide, lidocaine, propafenone)
- **Class II** – Beta Blockers (metoprolol, propranolol – also partial Na+ channel blocker)
- **Class III** – K+ channel blockers (amiodarone – multiple class actions)
- **Class IV** – Ca++ channel blockers (verapamil)
- **Class V** – work by unknown mechanism (adenosine, digoxin)

- *Beta Blockers and Calcium channel blockers are most commonly prescribed for AFib

Beta Blockers

- Block catecholamine action on adrenergic beta receptors
- Inhibits fight or flight response
- Beta 1 receptors are located primarily in the heart and kidneys
- **Cardioselective** – metoprolol, atenolol, bisoprolol, nebivolol
- **Beta Blockers and Cancer**
  - *BCa*
    Therapeutic Advances in Medical Oncology 2012; 4(3):113-125
  - *Oca*
    Cancer 2015;121:3435-43.

Calcium Channel Blockers

- **Amlodipine** (Dihydropyridines) - Primarily for HTN

- **Verapamil** (Phenylalkylamines) - selective for myocardium

- **Diltiazem** (Benzothiazepines) – cardiac depressant, vasodilation

- **Gabapentin, Pregabalin** (Gabapentenoids)

- Ethanol

K+ channel blockers

Amiodarone

- Progenitor Molecule = Khellin
- AV node blocking effects – mixed action
- Mostly used in post-surgical setting
- High incidence of side effects
- Resembles thyroxine

Adenosine

- AV node-dependent SVT's
- Atrial tachycardia
- Antagonized by methylated xanthines
- Side effects – chest pain, lightheadedness, SOB, worsening of symptoms, low BP

- Traditional acupuncture triggers a local increase in adenosine in human subjects J.Pain. 2012 Dec;13(12):1215-23.

Caffeine   Adenosine

Digoxin and Digitalis

- Digoxin
- Increases myocardial contractility
- Narrow Therapeutic Index
- Antidigoxin

- Digitalis Lanata
  - Cardiac Glycosides
  - "The direct heart stimulant" Ellingwood 216
  - Suppresses HIF-1 by >88% (reducing hypoxia)
    (Proc Natl Acad Sci U S A. 2009 Mar 3;106(9):E26)

Invasive Therapies

- **Maze procedure** – open-heart surgery. Incisions with scalpel create scar tissue which does not conduct electrical impulse.
- **A/V node ablation** – destroys tissue between atria and ventricles. Followed by pacemaker.
- **Radiofrequency Ablation (RFA)** to pulmonary veins

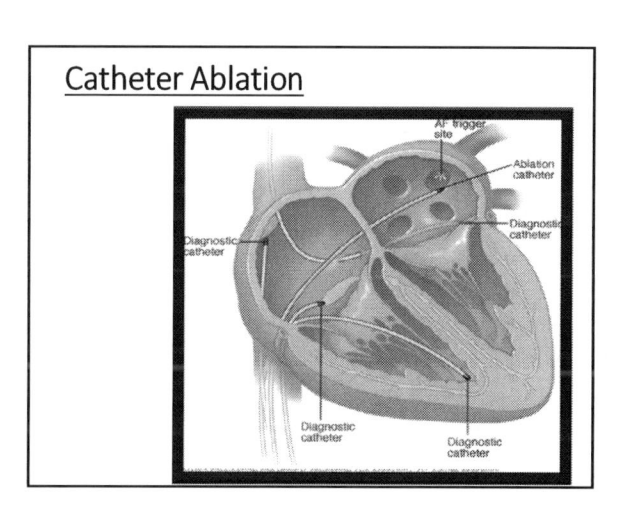

Catheter Ablation

Pulmonary vein isolation

Four main pulmonary vein junctions are found in the left atrium. All four are 'electrically isolated' as they might be involved in 'triggering' atrial fibrillation.

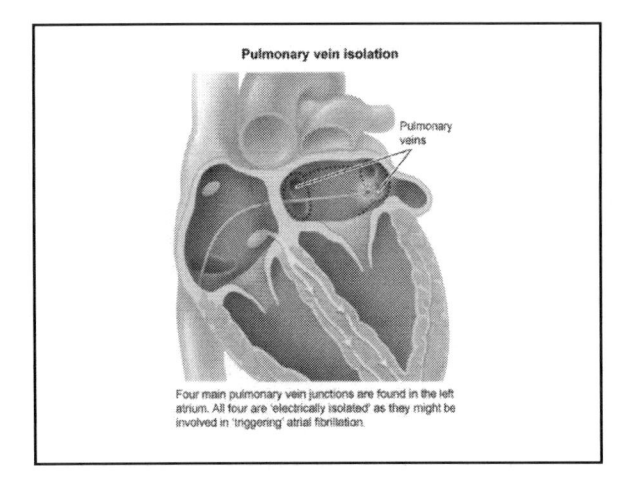

Ablation Procedure

and

Pacemakers

Pacemakers

- Pacemaker leads
- Pacemaker
- Right atrium
- Right ventricle

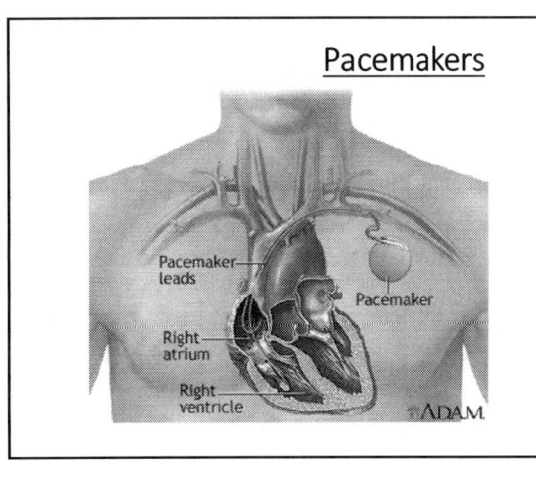

Is AFib a Disease?

- Modern cardiology has viewed atrial fibrillation as a *disease* rather than seeing it as a *result of other diseases*.
- Explains why our treatments (drugs and ablation) have performed so poorly
- "A wrong-target problem"
- A barometer for something wrong in the body
- "The atria fibrillate for a reason. And that reason is the main therapeutic target."
- Focal (easy) solutions for systemic diseases due to lifestyle are destined to fail.

Basic Health Promotion for Afib

- "Lifestyle diseases, via pressure and volume-induced atrial stretch, inflammation, or neural imbalances, induce disease in and around the cells of the heart."

- Proper diet and lifestyle changes significantly affect Afib outcomes

- Fibrosis can regress

theheart.org on Medscape > Trials and Fibrillations With John Mandrola

---

Aggressive Risk Factor Regression

- 281 patients undergoing AF ablation
  - 149 with a body mass index ≥27 kg/m^2

- AF frequency, duration, symptoms, and symptom severity decreased more in the RFM group compared with the control group (all p < 0.001)

- Arrhythmia-free survival was greater in RFM patients compared with control subjects (p < 0.001).

J Am Coll Cardiol Volume 64, Issue 21, 2 Dec 2014, Pages 2222-2231

Weight Loss and AFib

- In 355 patients with BMI >/= 27
- "Long-term sustained weight loss is associated with significant reduction of AF burden and maintenance of sinus rhythm. (Long-Term Effect of Goal directed weight management on Atrial Fibrillation Cohort: A 5 Year follow-up study [LEGACY Study]

J Am Coll Cardiol Volume 65, Issue 20, 26 May 2015, Pages 2159–2169

An integrative Approach

- Antiarrhythmic therapy as short-term
- Address other lifestyle issues:
  - Sleep disorders
  - Alcohol intake
  - Over-exercise and overwork
  - Stress
- Positive impacts on Afib:
  - Improves glucose handling
  - Lower blood pressure
  - Relieve inflammation

TCM Assessment of AFib

- Constitutional Picture
- Pulse diagnosis
- Tongue picture
- Comprehensive system review
- BP, HR
- Pattern differentiation and accurate TCM Dx
- Treatment Principles
- Multi-modal therapy

---

8 Principles

- Yin or Yang
- Hot or Cold
- Excess or Deficiency
- Internal or External

TCM Pattern Differentiation

- Heat in the Heart
- Phlegm obstructing the Heart
- Blood Stagnation
- Kidney and Heart Disharmony
- Kidney Yin Deficiency
- Kidney Yang Deficiency
- Liver Qi Stagnation
- Liver Fire
- Liver Yang Rising
- Spleen Qi Deficiency
- Phlegm Damp Syndrome

Botanical Medicine

- Treat the whole person

Excess or Deficiency?

- Too much
- Not enough

Excess Tongue Picture

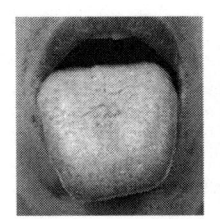

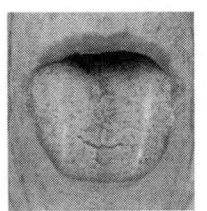

Deficiency Tongue Picture

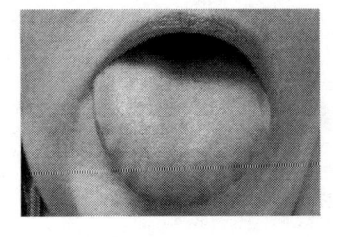

Heart Tonic Herbs

- Hawthorn (*Crataegus oxyacantha*) leaf, flower and berry
- Lily of the Valley (Convolaria)
- Cactus (Selenicereus)
- Arjuna (*Terminalia Arjuna*)
- Dual Action:
  - Chinese salvia (*Salvia miltiorrhiza*)
  - San Qi (*Panax Notoginseng*)
- Coleus (*Coleus forskohlii*)
- Rhodiola rosea

More on Heart Tonics

- Vascular-heart stimulants
  - Lily of the valley (*Convallaria majalis*)
  - Foxglove (*Digitalis*)
  - Scotch broom (*Cytisus scoparius*)
  - Squill (*Urginea scilla*)
- Peripheral stimulating tonics
  - Night blooming cereus (*Cereus grandiflorus*)
  - *Ginkgo biloba*
  - Gotu kola (*Centella a.*)
  - Prickly Ash (Zanthoxylum)

Hawthorne – Crataegus Oxyacantha

Crataegus in History

- **"Shan Zha" uses in TCM:**
  - Removes food stagnation
  - Promotes digestion
  - Invigorates the blood
  - Removes blood stasis
  - Eliminates accumulations
- Used as cardiac tonic in Greece since first century A.D.
- The Eclectics considered it to be the most valuable tonic-herb for conditions of the heart in the late 19th century.

Chemical Constituents

- **Flavonoids** – "most important"
  - Vitexin
  - Hyperoside
  - Rutin
- **OPC's**
  - Catechin/epicatechin
- **Triterpenic acids**
  - ursolic, oleanolic, and crataegolic acid
- **Phenol carboxylic acids**
  - chlorogenic and caffeic acids

Evid Based Complement Alternat Med. 2013; 2013: 149363.

Hawthorne Effects Researched

- Antioxidant activity
- Positive inotropic
- Anti-inflammatory
- Anticardiac remodeling
- Antiplatelet aggregation
- Vasodilating
- Endothelial protective

Evid Based Complement Alternat Med. 2013; 2013

More Hawthorne Effects

- Reduction of smooth muscle cell migration and proliferation
- Protective against ischemia/reperfusion injury
- Antiarrhythmic
- Lipid-lowering
- Decrease of arterial blood pressure

Evid Based Complement Alternat Med. 2013; 2013

Hawthorne in Practice

- Dosage: As a single agent in tincture can be used in tsp doses

- Often used as highest dosed herb in herbal formulas

- Synergy with other agents

Lily of the Valley Convolaria Majalis

- "It strengthens the heart's action, slows a rapid and feeble pulse, corrects the rhyme and rhythm, improves the tone and increases the power of the heart..."
- "adds power and regularity to the action of the heart"

Ellingwood p 223

Convolaria Indications

- Simple cardiac arrhythmia – with or without lesions of the orifices or valves of the heart, and with or without hypertrophy of the heart
- "pale, flabby mucous membranes of the mouth, broad, thick tongue, with a heavy, dirty white coating.
- "Not for cases in which the tongue is red and thin with elongated papillae, redness of the tips and edges" (Heat in the Heart in TCM)
- AF prevalence increases sharply with age, with 80% of cases occurring in people >65 years

Br J Gen Pract. 2016 Feb;66(643):62-3

Cactus
Cereus Grandiflorus

- "Increases the musculo-motor energy of the heart, elevates the arterial tension, increasing the height and force of the pulse wave."
- "It acts directly on the cardiac plexus, regulating the functional activity of the heart."
- For "feebleness" of the heart muscle
- Specific for valvular insufficiency.
- Soothes gastric irritability.
- Ellingwood 212

Cactus Indications

- Cactus is a great therapy for people who are experiencing heart issues due to deficiency.
- Poor circulation, fragile nervous system.

Contraindications

- It is contraindicated in excess conditions.
- Hypertension, redness in the face, anger, strong nervous system.

Avena Sativa

- Nutritive for the nervous system
- Calming action through empowering the nerve force. According to Ellingwood:

"It is a remedy of great utility in loss of nerve power and in muscular feebleness from lack of nerve force". It is good to *combine with cactus in cases where there is a weak heart.

AFib tincture for Deficient Heart

- Hawthorne 50ml
- Cactus 15ml
- Lily of the Valley 15ml
- Scotch Broom 10ml
- Salvia M. 10ml
- Leonurus 10ml
- Rhodiola 10ml

Dosage: 4 droppers 3 x day. Best at least 30 minutes before or 1 hour after meals.

Start with this formula and take for 7 days, then report with results and we'll see if we need to make any modifications

Vascular Astringent Tonics

- *Collinsonia*
- Horse chestnut (*Aesculus hippocastanum*)
- Butchers broom (*Ruscus aculeatus*)
- Witch hazel (*Hamamelis*)
  - Escins - group of saponin compounds found in horse chestnut
  - Ruscogenins, a group of saponin compounds found in Butchers broom
  - Aesculin - coumarin derivative
  - Traditionally used for diseases of the venous system, including varicose veins, thrombophlebitis, bruises, painful leg cramps that occur at night, brain trauma, edema of the ankles, postoperative edema

Heart Clearing and Calming Herbs

- Lycopus Virginica
- Zizyphus Spinosa – clears Heat from the Heart, and Nourishes Heart Blood
  - sedative, hypnotic and antiarrhythmic effects
- Salvia Miltiorrhizoma
- Zizyphus Spinosa
- Rauwolfia Sepentina

Motherwort
Lycopus Virginica

- "In diseases of the heart, either functional or organic, marked by irritability and irregularity of the organ, dyspnea, feeling oppression in the cardiac region, it's administration is followed by gratifying results."
  (Ellingwood) p224
- Calming, with blood moving properties

- "Man Jing Zi"

"Dan Shen" - *Salvia Miltiorrhiza*

- Bitter and Slightly Cold
- Invigorates Blood
- Removes Blood Stagnation
- Clears Heat
- Soothes irritability

- Chief herb in classical formula: "Xue Fu Zhu Yu Tang" - "Remove Stasis In The Mansion of Blood Decoction"

Salvia Miltiorrhiza Biomedical

- Reduces inflammation and lowers CRP in a controlled pilot study
- Antiinflammatory effects
- Lowers Homocysteine
- Liver and Heart protective
  Phytother Res. 2009 Dec;23(12):1721-5.
- Used to treat: Angina, palpitations, menstrual problems, insomnia, liver diseases, and cancer in China for centuries.

AFib Tincture for Excess Condition

- Hawthorne 40 ml
- Salvia Miltiorrhiza 30 ml
- White Peony 20 ml
- Zizyphus 15 ml
- Bupleurum 10 ml
- Rauwolfia Serpentina 5 ml (often drop dosed in separate tincture)
- Dosage: 4 droppers 3 x day. Best at least 30 minutes before or 1 hour after meals.

AFib Specific Nutrients

- Magnesium taurate
- Potassium taurate
- CoQ10
- Carnitine
- Taurine
- EFA's
- B Vitamins
- Amino Acids

Magnesium

- Fourth most abundant cation in the human body
- Modulates vascular smooth muscle tone, endothelial cell function, and myocardial excitability. Cardiol Rev. 2014 Jul-Aug;22(4):182-92
- Increases efficacy of antiarrhythmic agents
  The America Journal of Cardiology Volume, 99, 12, 15 June 2007, Pages 1726–1732
- Circulating and dietary magnesium are inversely associated with CVD risk Am J Clin Nutr. 2013 ul;98(1):160-73.
- Safe and effective for cardiac arrhythmias Dtsch Med Wochenschr. 2013   May;138(22):1165-71.
- Regulates potassium Kardiologiia. 2013;53(10):38-48.

Magnesium deficiency

- Modern farming
- PPI's (proton pump inhibitors)
  Ren Fail. 2015 Aug;37(7):1237-41. J Clin Pharmacol. 2015 Nov 18. World J Nephrol. 2012 Dec 6;1(6):151-4. Clin Exp Rheumatol. 2014 Nov-Dec;32. Int J Gen Med. 2013 Jun 28;6:515-8. Expert Opin Drug Saf. 2013 Sep;12(5):709-16.
- Diuretics
- Digoxin – dysrhythmias due to Mg depletion
  J Emerg Med. 2013 Aug;45(2):e31-4
- Dialysis
- Muscle cramps, cardiac arrhythmias and epilepsy
- Dose 5-1500mg/day

The Framingham Heart Study

- Hypomagnesemia has been linked to the pathogenesis of arrhythmias in experimental studies
- Individuals in the lowest quartile of serum magnesium were ~50% more likely to develop AF compared with those in the upper quartiles.

Circulation. 2013 Jan 1;127(1):33-8.

Potassium K+

- Low serum levels of potassium were associated with a higher risk of atrial fibrillation.
- The Rotterdam Study Int J Cardiol. 2013 Oct 15;168(6):5411-5
- Potassium/Magnesium Taurate
- 2-600mg/day

Coenzyme (Co) Q10

- Ubiquinol and ubiquinone – distinct functions
- Ubiquinol is more bioavailable and remains active in the body longer
- Positively influences cellular metabolism and combats signs of aging at the cellular level
- Is involved in redox control of cell signaling and gene expression and acts as a direct antioxidant
- Dose 1-400 mg/day in oil

Coenzyme Q_{10} and Vit K2

- Structurally related to menaquinone (vitamin K2)
- Vit K2 puts calcium on the bones
- Vitamin K-like effects of Coenzyme Q_{10} have been demonstrated in vitro and in four case reports describing possible warfarin and Coenzyme Q_{10} interactions

Res Commun Chem Pathol Pharmacol. 1976; 13:109-14.
Ugeskr Laeger. 1998; 160:3226-7 (English abstract).
Lancet. 1994; 344:1372-3.

L-Carnitine

- Antiarrythmic
  Arch Int Pharmacodyn Ther. 1975 Oct;217(2):246-50.
- Improves fatty acid utilization and energy production.
- Increases cellular respiration, membrane potential and cardiolipin levels.
- Low levels of L-carnitine in heart muscles resulted in significant heart damage
- Less discomfort and experienced fewer heart emergencies
- Dose 1-2 grams per day
  Japanese Circulation Journal; 56(1): 86–94.(1992) *Drugs Under Experimental and Clinical Research;* 18(8): 355–65. (1992)
  Postgraduate Medical Journal; 72(843): 45–50. (1996)

Taurine

- Affects Ca^{2+} metabolism in heart
  - prevents arrhythmogenesis by limiting cardiac hypertrophy and calcium overload of the myocardium
    Res. Commun. Chem. Patho. Pharma., 43(2):343-346, 1984.
- Preserves K^+ in the heart
  Life Sci., 33:1649-1655, 1983.
- Reduces sympathetic tone
  Surgery, 99(4):491-500 1986 Apr.
- Prevents arrhythmia in ischemic conditions
  - Membrane stabilizer
  - O2 free radical scavenger
    Eur. J. Pharmacol, 98:269-273, 1984.
  Dose 1-6 grams per day

EPA and DHA

- Eicosapentanoic and Docosahexanoic Acids
- Antiarrhythmogenic
- Attenuate structural atrial remodeling
- Suppress ectopic firing from pulmonary veins
- "Studies using adequate four-week pretreatment with n-3 PUFA before cardioversion of AF showed a reduction of the AF incidence".
  Int J Mol Sci. 2015 Sep 22;16(9):22870-87.

Dosage: EPA – 750-1500mg/day
DHA – 500-1000mg/day

Nutrition for Valvular Heart Disease

- Valve regurgitation – mitral, aortic, tricuspid

- Stenosis
  - Vitamin K2

- Myopathies
  - B12
  - Mg
  - Carnitine
  - Branched Chain Amino Acids

AFib Treatment Principles

- Address clotting risk
- Stabilize the heart
- Identify underlying causes
- Treat the whole person

Chronic Prostate Conditions BPH, and Prostate Cancer

Local to Systemic

Botanical to Biomedical

Therapeutic Avenues and Considerations.

Presented by Jason Miller LAc. MAcOM

Turbidity

"Approximately one third of the U.S. population has metabolic syndrome, which is defined as the co-occurrence of at least three of the following five conditions: raised blood pressure, elevated waist circumference, low HDL or "good" cholesterol, raised triglyceride levels and raised fasting plasma glucose levels."

[American Association for Cancer Research (2011, April 3)]

Prostate Cancer Risk Factors

- Obesity
- Diabetes
- Family Hx
- Lack of sunlight and Vit D (deficiency linked to aggressive disease)
- Smoking
- Pesticides
- Shift Work
- Lipid imbalances
- Viral infections (new research)

STRESS

- B Adrenergic up-regulation
- Immune dysregulation
- Endocrine disharmony
- Catabolic
- Loss of apoptosis
- Studies indicate that shift workers have a higher incidence of PCa Cancer

Epidemiol Biomarkers Prev. 2006 Jan;15(1):3-5.

Lack of Sleep

- 3rd most important key to life after air and water
- Adrenal Rhythm
- Decreased Oxygen
- Hypoxia
- HIF1a

Low Testosterone and the Prostate

- Hypogonadism
- Testosterone – contraindicated with prostate cancer or BPH
- Perceived risks are high
- These risks may be exaggerated

Testosterone and PCa

- "There is no evidence that exogenous testosterone stimulates the development of severe symptomatic prostate hyperplasia, nor does exogenous testosterone seem to increase the risks of clinically significant prostate cancer."
  Amer Acad Derm 2001 Sep; 45(3): 116-24.

- After following 154 men with low-risk prostate cancer for 38 months, the investigators found that
  - Low levels of free testosterone were significantly linked with an increased risk of developing more aggressive disease.
  - "These results suggest low levels of testosterone are associated with more aggressive prostate cancer,"

  May 5, 2014, BJU International

More Testosterone and PCa

- "Patients with lower levels of serum testosterone had a higher risk of prostate cancer than did patients with high serum testosterone."
  Korean J Urol. 2010 Dec;51(12):819-23.

- Low testosterone levels are associated with an increased percentage of prostate cancer-positive biopsies.
  J Steroid Biochem Mol Biol. 2006 Dec;102(1-5):261-6.
  J Urol. 2000 Mar;163(3):824-7.

And More...

- Low serum testosterone is a risk factor for development of prostate cancer.

  1. Morgentaler, A., Bruning, C. O. 3rd & DeWolf, W. C. Occult prostate cancer in men with low serum testosterone levels. JAMA **276**, 1904–1906 (1996).
  2. Labrie, F. et al. Serum prostate specific antigen as pre-screening test for prostate cancer. J. Urol. **147**, 846–851 (1992).
  3. Cooner, W. H. et al. Prostate cancer detection in a clinical urological practice by ultrasonography, digital rectal examination, and prostate-specific antigen. J. Urol. **143**,1146–1150 (1990).
  4. Seaman, E. et al. PSA density (PSAD). Urol. Clin. North Am. **20**, 653–663 (1993).
  5. Hoffman, M. A., DeWolf, W. C. & Morgentaler, A. Is low serum free testosterone a marker for high grade prostate cancer? J. Urol. **163**, 824–827 (2000).

Low Testosterone and PCa Aggression

- Correlated with higher Gleason score.
  Prostate **47**, 52–58 (2001).
- Occult prostate cancer in men with low serum testosterone levels. JAMA **276**, 1904–1906 (1996).
- "Patients with prostate cancer and low free testosterone had more extensive disease."
- "All men with a biopsy Gleason score of 8 or greater had low serum free testosterone."
  J. Urol. **163**, 824–827 (2000).
- High-grade prostate cancer is associated with low serum testosterone levels.
  Prostate. 2001 Apr;47(1):52-8.

Testosterone & Cardiovascular Health

Sufficient to high testosterone:
- < Blood pressure
- < Total cholesterol (TC), LDL-cholesterol (LDL) & triglycerides (TG)
- < Visceral body fat
- < Waist-hip ratio (WHR)
- < Serum insulin
- < Fasting and post-prandial glucose,
- > HDL-cholesterol (HDL)
- > Insulin sensitivity

Exogenous Testosterone Therapy

Anabolic Hormone Enhancing Plants

- Rhaponticum Carthamoides (Leuzea)
- Panax Ginseng
- Tribulis Terrestris
- Eurycoma Longifolia Jax
- Pfaffia Paniculata (Suma)
- Epimedium
- Pantocrine (Deer antler)
- Mumie
- Royal Jelly

Two Primary Reproductive Changes

- 5 alpha reductase enzyme elevation leading increased levels of DHT

- Up-regulation of aromatase enzyme leading to more conversion of Testosterone to estrogen

DHT – Dihydrotestosterone

- Active intracellular androgen
- Formed from testosterone by 5 alpha-reductase.
- DHT concentrations appear a little higher in BPH tissue than in normal tissue
- DHT-receptor complex modulates gene expression.

    Eur Urol. 1991;20 Suppl 1:68-77.

Estrogen in PCa and BPH

- Elevated Estrogen to Testosterone ratio
- Testosterone is metabolized into estrogens, stimulating the growth of the fibromuscular tissue of the prostate.

    Vitam Horm. 1975;33:39-60.

- Both types of estrogen receptor subtypes (ERα and ERβ) are present in the prostate

    J Clin Endocrinol Metab 1999: Feb; 84(2):573-7.

Plastics

- Estrogen mimics
- Endocrine disruptors
- From water bottles to laundry detergents

    Endocrinology 1998 Oct; 139(10): 4252-63.

- Bisphenol A (BPA) exposure during adulthood alters expression of aromatase and 5α-reductase isozymes

    PLoS One. 2013;8(2) (animal)
    FEBS J. 2013 Jan;280(1):93-101 (animal)

Endocrine disruptors

- Endocrine disruptors are synthetic chemicals found in pesticides and some plastics.
- Interfere with hormone balance
  - disturb proper endocrine health
    - reduction in male hormones
    - higher levels of fat and estrogens
  - increase body mass index
  - increase the risk of several cancers
  - fibroid tumors
  - endocrine-related diseases
  - infertility
  - Etc. ad nauseum…

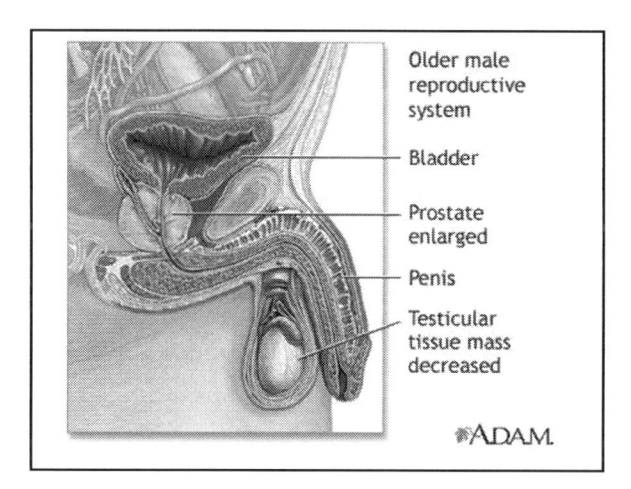

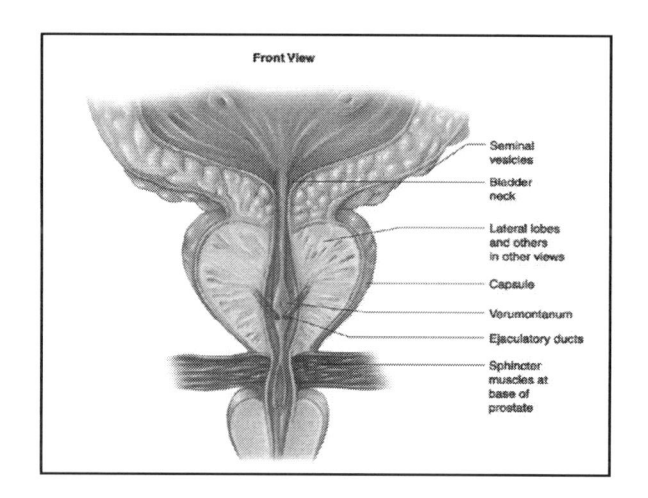

Prostate Functions

- Secretes a milky substance that constitutes about 15 to 30 percent of semen
- Nourishes and protects sperm
- Muscles associated with the prostate aid in the expulsion of both urine and semen through the urethra

Prostate Dysfunctions

- **Prostatitis** – acute or chronic, often acute. 8% of all urology visits. J. Urol. 159 (4): 1224–8
- **BPH** – chronic endocrine condition
- **Prostate Cancer** – chronic disease

BPH

- Benign prostatic hyperplasia (BPH) is a "histological diagnosis that refers to the proliferation of smooth muscle and epithelial cells within the prostatic transition zone, leading to an increase in the size of the prostate". Urol Clin North Am. 1995 May; 22(2):237-46.
- Clarification – hyperplasia versus hypertrophy

The Enlarged Prostate

1. Static component
2. Dynamic component

Textbook of Benign Prostatic Hyperplasia. Isis Medical Media. London. 2002

- LUTS
- Urinary Obstruction
  - Bladder
  - Kidneys

Biomedical Therapies for BPH

- Alpha blockers – Tamsulosin
- 5 Alpha Reductase inhibitors – finasteride, dutasteride.
- Catheters - self and Foley
- TURP
- HOLEP
- Laser Vaporization
- Thermotherapy
- Prostatectomy

Ther Adv Urol. 2011 Dec; 3(6): 263–272

Hormone Inhibition for BPH

- **Pharmaceutical 5 Alpha Reductase Inhibitors**
- Proscar (Finasteride) also Rx'd as Propecia
- Avodart (Dutasteride)

- **Pharmaceutical Aromatase inhibitors**
- Aromasin – steroidal inhibition
- Arimidex
- Femara

TURP - Transurethral Resection of the Prostate

- **Indications:** acute urinary retention, bladder stones, obstructive kidney failure, and hematuria.
- **Side Effects:** perioperative bleeding, blood transfusions, transurethral resection (TUR) syndrome, prolonged catheterization, long hospital stay, urinary incontinence, and retrograde ejaculation.

Textbook of Benign Prostatic Hyperplasia. Isis Medical Media. London. 2002

Recent Developments

- Prostatic Artery Embollization
- UroLift
- Gat/Goren Method

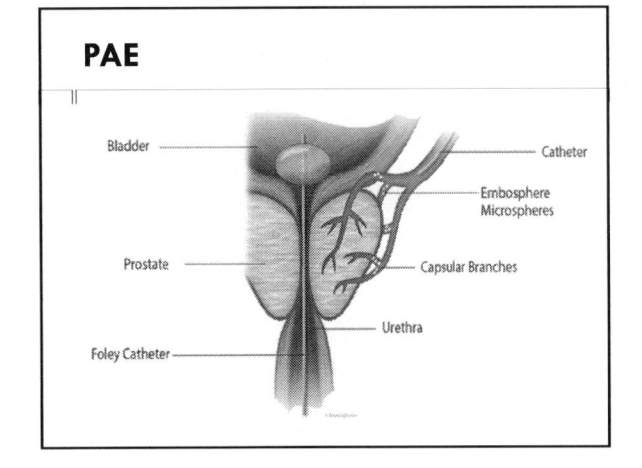

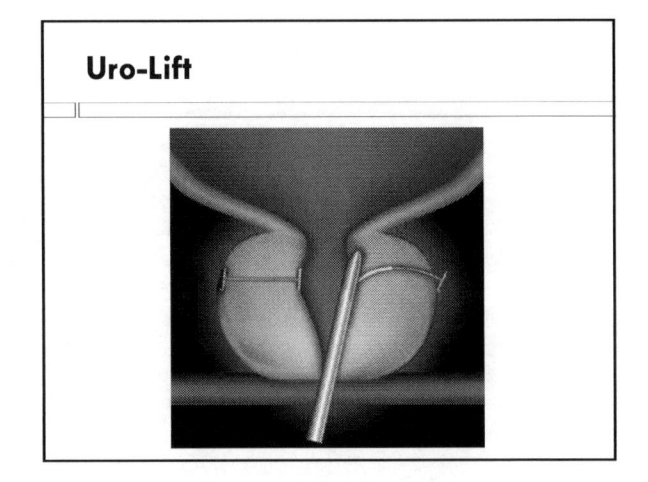

PAE

Uro-Lift

Gat/Goren Method

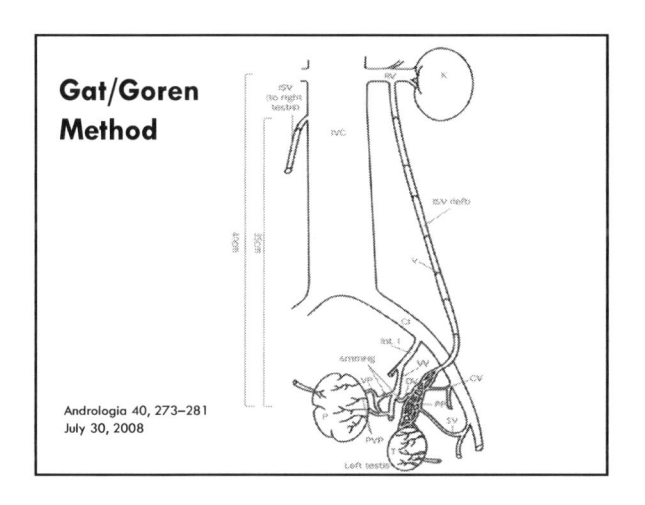

Andrologia 40, 273–281
July 30, 2008

Chronic Venous Insufficiency

- Approximately one third of men and women aged 18-64 years had trunk varices
- "Changes in lifestyle or other factors might be contributing to an alteration in the epidemiology of venous disease."
  J Epidmiol Community Health. 1999 Mar;53(3):149-53.
- Hippocrates

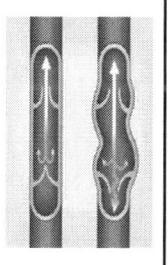

Vascular astringent tonics

- *Collinsonia*
- Horse chestnut (*Aesculus hippocastanum*)
- Butchers broom (*Ruscus aculeatus*)
- Witch hazel (*Hamamelis*)

Sitting and Sedentary Lifestyle

"Prolonged sitting was associated with higher mortality from all causes, as well as increased incidence of cancer, cardiovascular disease, and type 2 diabetes, even among people who exercise regularly, according to a meta-analysis published in the January 20 issue of the Annals of Internal Medicine."

Ann Intern Med. 2015;162:123-132, 146-147.

Exercise and Prostate Cancer

- "In both younger and older patients, there was a statistically significant increase in testosterone levels after exercise"
  J App Physiol 2001; 90(4): 1497-1507
- Regular high-intensity exercise increases testosterone
  J App Physiol 1999 Sep; 87(3): 982-92

Holistic Approach to BPH

- Treat the patient as an individual
- Address pathological factors
- Correct endocrine imbalances
- Improve cellular detoxification
- Improve lean body mass
- Improve sleep and reduce stress
- Balance adrenal function
- Support androgens – normalize testosterone

TCM Pattern Differentiation

- Spleen Qi Deficiency
- Phlegm/Damp Syndrome
- Liver Qi Stagnation
- Qi Stagnation
- Blood Stagnation
- Kidney Essence Deficiency
- Kidney Yang Deficiency
- Kidney Yin Deficiency

Some Relevant Biomarkers in Prostate Health

- **Prostate Screening**
  - PSA free and total
- **Blood Sugar Related**
  - Fasting glucose, insulin
  - HgA1c
  - C-peptide
  - Free and total
- **Hormonal**
  - Free and Total testosterone
  - DHT
  - SHBG
  - Estradiol
  - Estrone Sulfate
  - Thyroid panel
  - DHEAs
- **CVD related**
  - MTHFR SNP
  - Homocysteine
  - Hs CRP
  - Cholesterol Panel
  - Fibrinogen
- **Nutrient Specific**
  - Serum Zinc
  - Ceruloplasmin
  - 25-OH Vit D
  - 1,25 diOH Vit D

PCa - Prostate Cancer

- Nearly all men in the course of their lifetimes will experience a health issue relating to the prostate, and although prostate cancer (PC) is the second leading cause of cancer-related deaths in US men, most men die *with* PC, rather than *of* the disease.

- One in 6 American men will be diagnosed as having prostate cancer during their lifetime.

Prostate Biopsy

- Definitive diagnostic test for PCa
- Risk factors associated with biopsy:
  - Infections
  - Bleeding
  - Inflammation
  - Coagulation
  - "Puncturing the capsule"
- Liquid Biopsy

Gleason Score

- Tissue pathology report from needle biopsy
- Scored from 1-10
- </= 6 is low grade
- 7 is intermediate grade
- >7 is high grade
- Is Gleason 6 cancer?

"...men with low-risk disease (Gleason score 6, PSA < 10 ng/mL, and clinical stage T1c to T2a) who are untreated have a similar cancer-specific survival when compared with those treated over 10 to 15 years after diagnosis."

JCO **December 10, 2012** vol. 30 no. 35 **4294-4296**

Gleason </= 6 and Overtreatment

- PSA > Biopsy > Treatment

- approximately half of newly diagnosed men have Gleason score ≤ 6 at diagnosis, and 80% to 90% depending on age undergo some form of treatment even when age at diagnosis is > 75 years.

- The Fear Factor

JCO **December 10, 2012** vol. 30 no. 35 **4294-4296**

Biomedical Therapy for PCa

- Local Therapy
  - Radical Prostatectomy
  - Radiation

- Systemic Therapy
  - ADT

Data from the Prostate Cancer Outcomes Study (PCOS)

- 1655 men who were diagnosed with localized prostate cancer in 1994 or 1995, when they were between the ages of 55 and 74 years underwent surgery or radiation therapy.
- Followed for 15 years
- Dysfunction:
  - Urinary incontinence – 18.5% PE, and 9.4% RT
  - Bowel urgency – 21.9% PE and 35.8% RT
  - Erectile

Prostatectomy/Radiation and ED

- "At 15 years, erectile dysfunction was "nearly universal," affecting 87.0% of those in the prostatectomy group and 93.9% of those in the radiotherapy group."
  N Engl J Med. 2013;368:436-445

- "A significant proportion of these men are not going to die from their disease and I think if a man has low grade prostate cancer, these data should really make him think carefully before he signs on to have any surgery or radiation because a lot of these quality of life side effects could be avoided by choosing active surveillance."
  Prostate Cancer Tx Side-Effects Study: New 15-Year Data. Medscape. Jan 30, 2013.

Prostatectomy

- "Men with localized prostate cancer who elect to have prostatectomy or radiotherapy will experience problems with urinary, bowel, and sexual function in the long term"
- Following radical prostatectomy, *death from cardiovascular diseases, other cancers, and other causes* is far more common than death from prostate cancer".

  Prostate Cancer and Prostatic Diseases (2012) 15, 106–11

TGFbeta 1

- Preoperative plasma levels of transforming growth factor β1 (TGF-β1) "strongly predicts" cancer progression in patients who undergo radical prostatectomy
  Urology. 2004 Jun;63(6):1191-7.
  Clin Cancer Res. 2004 Mar 15;10(6):1992-9
  J Clin Oncol. 2003 Oct 1;21(19):3573-9.

Radiation Aftermath

- 32,000 men treated between 2002 and 2009 in Ontario, Canada
- 22% of the men had some form of hospitalization for 1 of these outcomes: urologic, anal, and rectal procedures; the incidence of secondary cancers; and the incidence of open surgical treatments.
  Lancet Oncol. 2014;15:223-231.

ADT - Androgen Deprivation Therapy

Triple Hormone Blockage:
Lupron, Casodex, Avodart

- In conventional medicine, after PCa has returned following surgery or radiation therapy, or even as a first treatment in older men, hormone (androgen) blockage therapy is then the next route of treatment.
- More than 500,000 men are treated with a GnRH agonist annually in the US

    Nat Clin Pract Urol. 2005;2(12):608-615.

Clinical Genitourinary Cancer, Vol.12, No. 6, 399-"©-407" 2014 Elsevier

---

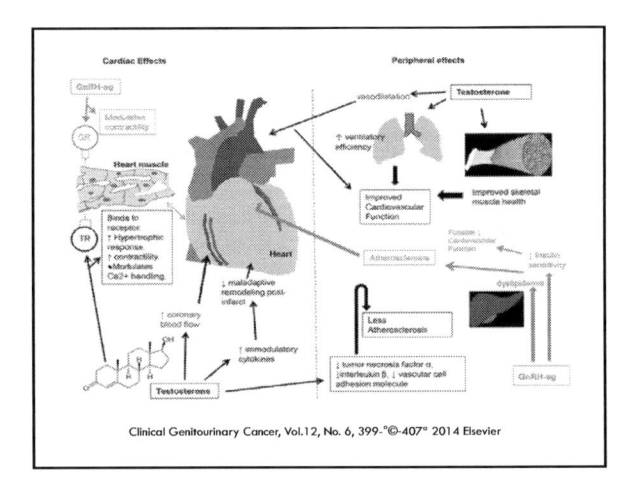

Degaralix

- **Degarelix** as improvement to Lupron – no testosterone surge up front - cross over study showed improvement in several areas.
    Nat Clin Pract Urol. 2005;2(12):608-615.

- Still need to implement Intermittent therapy

ADT?

- Primary ADT is not associated with improved long-term overall or disease-specific survival for men with localized prostate cancer. Primary ADT should be used only to palliate symptoms of disease or prevent imminent symptoms associated with disease progression. JAMA Intern. Med. doi:10.1001/jamainternmed.2014.3028

- Many studies elucidate the role of ADT in worsening CVD

ADT Side Effects

- Hot Flashes 80%
- Sexual Dysfunction
- Skeletal Morbidity - 6 x fracture risk
- Anemia <10% Hgb
- Cognitive
    - Depression
    - Anxiety
    - Insomnia
    - < QOL
- CVD Morbidity
    - Metabolic Syndrome
    - > risk fatal MI's

    ISRN Urology, vol. 2013, Article ID 240108, 8 pages, 2013.

Additional Problems with ADT

- Strong Environmental pressures lead to mutational changes
    Cancer Epidemiol Biomarkers Prev Mar 1994 3;177

- It appears that IADT is as effective long-term as ADT as a palliative treatment for many patients, and has reduced side effects.
    Oncologist 5, 45-52, 2000.

PCa Specific Biomarkers

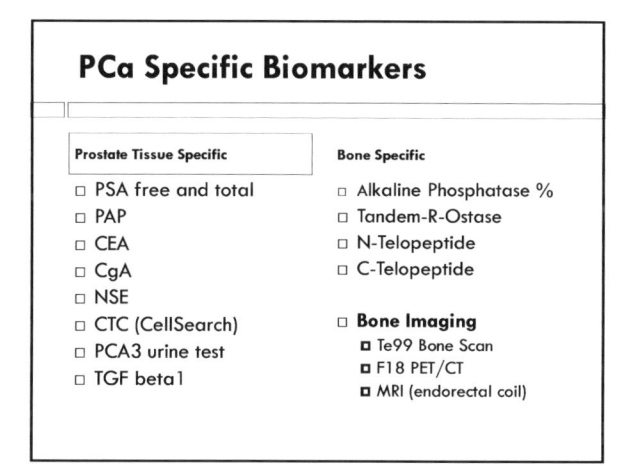

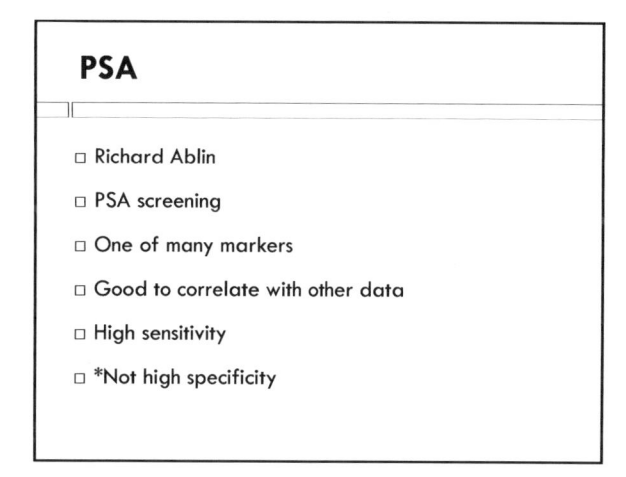

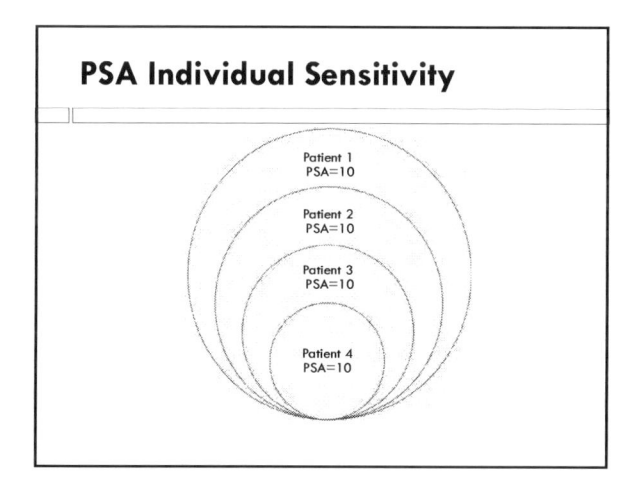

Prostate Tissue Specific
- PSA free and total
- PAP
- CEA
- CgA
- NSE
- CTC (CellSearch)
- PCA3 urine test
- TGF beta1

Bone Specific
- Alkaline Phosphatase %
- Tandem-R-Ostase
- N-Telopeptide
- C-Telopeptide
- **Bone Imaging**
  - Te99 Bone Scan
  - F18 PET/CT
  - MRI (endorectal coil)

PSA

- Richard Ablin
- PSA screening
- One of many markers
- Good to correlate with other data
- High sensitivity
- *Not high specificity

PSA Individual Sensitivity

Patient 1 PSA=10
Patient 2 PSA=10
Patient 3 PSA=10
Patient 4 PSA=10

Key Botanicals in BPH/PCa

- Panax Ginseng
- Saw Palmetto (Serenoa Repens)
- Pygeum Africanum
- Urtica Dioica
- Curcubita Pepo
- Tomato extract (Lycopene)

Panax Ginseng in TCM

- "Pan – axos"
- Used as a "male tonic herb" for millenia
- Tonifies the "source Qi"
- TCM Actions from The Herbal Classic of the The Divine Plowman:
  - Supports the five visceral organs
  - calms the nerves
  - Tranquilizes the mind
  - Stops convulsions
  - Expunges evil spirits
  - Clears the eyes, and
  - Improves the memory

Panax Ginseng in BPH/PCa

- More than 500 scientific papers published on it throughout the world.
- Enhances HPA Axis
- Stress Response Modifier
- Anabolic
- Counteracts fatigue
- Immune enhancement
- Reduces CVD risk
- Anti-cancer effects documented in several cancers
- Ginseng shows anti-proliferative activity against a human prostate cancer cell line

Serenoa Repens – Saw Palmetto

- Anabolic, nutritive tonic
- Phytosterol/fatty acid make-up = anti-catabolic, anabolic
- Given by eclectics as a reproductive system tonic. *Often prescribed for impotence
- Modern extracts should be 85-95% fatty acids
- "Liquid supplements contained the highest fatty acid and phytosterol quantities"

Nutrients. 2013 Sep; 5(9): 3617–3633.

Serenoa Repens Extract

- Long-term treatment reduces urinary obstruction
- Improves symptomatology and QoL in BPH
- Positive effect on sexual function, demonstrated by the statistically significant increase in the IIEF.

Urol Int. 2011;86(3):284-9. Epub 2011 Feb 8

- Marked reduction of LUTS in 85% of evaluable cases, especially with regard to pain and irritative symptoms.

Urologia 2010; 77(1): 43 - 51

Saw Palm Research in BPH

- Eur Urol. 2003 Nov;44(5):549-55.
- Ann Pharmacother. 2002 Sep;36(9):1443-52.

Nettles - Urtica Dioica

- Urtica dioica has beneficial effects in the treatment of symptomatic BPH.
- Decrease in prostate volume
- Increases QOL
- Normalizes SHBG

2010 Jul-Sep;77(3):180-6.
J Herb Pharmacother. 2005;5(4):1-11.

Nettles - Urtica Dioica

- The root of nettles is the primary part used for prostate health and prostate cancer inhibition
- Phytosterols: B-sitosterol and sitosterol B-glucoside are found in the root
- Nettles for both PCa and BPH
- Root extract 6:1, or fluid-extract
- 1-3 grams/day as single agent
- *In formulas less is needed

Nettles - Urtica Dioica

- **Studies on nettles in BPH:**

- Planta Med. 1999 Oct;65(7):666-8. (mice)
- Urologe A. 2004 Mar;43(3):302-6. (human)
- World J Urol. 2005 Jun;23(2):139-46. (human)
- Fortschr Med. 2005 Oct 6;147 Suppl 3:103-8.

Pygeum Africanum

- Improved all the urinary parameters investigated
- Prostatic echography revealed reduction of peri-urethral edema
- 300 mg BID to TID (standardized to 25% total sterols)
  Arch Ital Urol Nefrol Androl. 1991 Sep;63(3):341-5
- Many studies have shown the effectiveness of Pygeum extract in treating BPH
  Arch.It.Urol. LX (1988) 313-322.
  Ann. Urol 18 (1984) 193-195.
  J Urol. 1997, Jun;157(6):2381-7. (rats)

Curcubita Pepo

- Improved urinary function in human trial with 2000 men with enlarged prostates.
- Documented by German Commission E
- Delta 7 sterine
- Sterol compound
- Competes with DHT
  J. MedFood. 2006 Summer;9(2):284-6

Key Botanicals in PCa

- Milk Thistle
- Turmeric
- Green tea
- Scutellaria Baicalensis
- Medicinal Mushrooms
- Polygonum Cuspidatum

Milk thistle (*Silymarin marianum*)

- Organic Milk thistle Extract – 80% Silymarin
- Dose 1-3 g/day
- Represents a mixture of four isomeric flavonoids: silibinin, isosilibinin, silydianin and silychristin.
- Silibinin
  ToxicolAppl Pharmacol. 2006 Nov 15
- Many animal and in vitro studies demonstrate anti-PC activity through many mechanisms.

Milk thistle (*Silymarin marianum*)

- NF-kappaB (nuclear factor-kappa B) pathways,
- 2) VEGF modulation,
- 3) EGFR modulation,
- 4) Insulin-like growth factor-1 receptor (IGF-1R) signaling,
- 5) Modulates cell-cycle regulators, including cyclin-dependent kinases (CDKs), Kip1/p27 and Cip1/p21, and cyclins for its anticancer efficacy against PCA,
- 6) Telomerase inhibition,
- 7) Reduces lipids
- 8) Inhibitis RANKL-induced osteoclastogenesis
- Human Study - 2.6 fold increase in the PSA doubling time from 445 to 1150 days for the supplement and placebo periods
  Eur Urol. 2005 Dec;48(6):922-30; discussion 930-1.

Turmeric (*Curcuma Longa*)

Active compounds: curcuminoids (I-IV), and sesquiterpenes: turmerone

Curcumin

Turmeric

- **TCM Category** - Promote Blood Circulation to Dispel Stasis
- **TCM Actions:** Promotes Blood circulation, Removes Blood Stagnation, Promotes Qi circulation, Expels Wind and relieves Wind-Damp pain
- **Biomedical Actions:** anti-inflammatory, antioxidant, antineoplastic, antiviral, immune-modulation
- Better anti-PC in mice with PEITC (cabbage sprouts)
  - journal Cancer Research, 1/15/06 cancerres.aacrjournals.org
  - Pharm Res. 2008 Apr 25

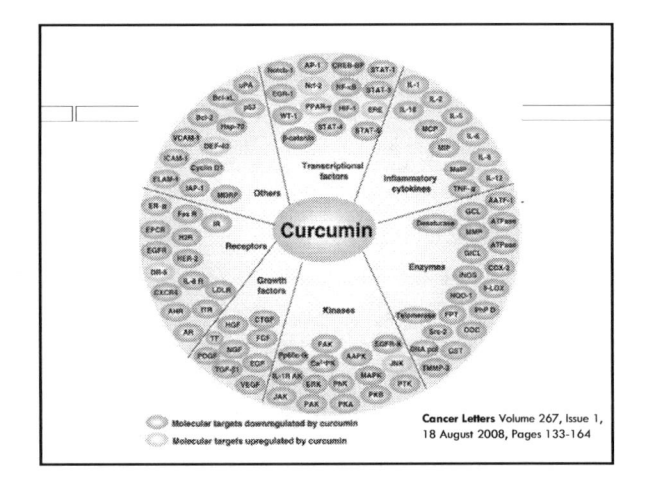

Cancer Letters Volume 267, Issue 1, 18 August 2008, Pages 133-164

Green Tea - Camillia Sinensis

- EGCG
- Anti-PC *Curr Opin Urol.* 2004 May;14(3):143-149.
- Anti-inflammatory
- Reduces oxidative damage
- Modulates IGF's
- Inhibits aromatase
- human study preventive effect in PCa (600mg TID)
  - Eur Urol. 2008 Apr 4
- Combine with curcumin, selenium, lycopene, and Grape skin and seed.
  - Cancer Lett. 2006 Jul 18;238(2):202-9.
- Dosing should be in the range of 1-2 grams per day of powdered extract containing between 40% and 65% EGCG

Some Well Researched Synergists

- Green Tea with Quercetin
  - PLoS ONE 7(4): e35368.
- Turmeric with Resveratrol
  - Oncogene (2000) 19, 4159-4169
- Green tea with Zinc
  - Mol Nutr Food Res. 2008 Apr;52(4):465-71.
- Green Tea with Lycopene
  - Asia Pac J Clin Nutr. 2007;16 Suppl:453-7.

Huang Qin - (Scutellaria Baicalensis)

- Also known as Baikal Skullcap or Golden Root
- **TCM Category** - Herbs that Clear Damp-Heat
- **Actions** - Clears Heat, Dries Dampness, Disperses Fire, Expels toxins, Stops bleeding, Prevents miscarriage.
- Grows in China and Russia

Huang Qin – "Scute"

- **Biomedical Actions:** anti-microbial, anti-pyretic, cholagogic, hepato-protective, anti-hypertensive, and anti-inflammatory (McGuffin, Hobbs, Upton. American Herbal Products Association (AHPA) Safety & Labeling Guidelines SubCommittee)
- Anti-inflammatory and anti-cancer effects appear to be mediated via repression of 5 and 12-lipoxygenase (LOX) and inhibition of interleukin-1B, and prostaglandin E_2
- Inhibits carcinogen-induced iNOS, COX-2, NF-kB activation
  - (Chen Y, Biochem Pharmacol. 2000 Jun 1;59(11):1445-57.)
- Anti-inflammatory/anticancer properties are attributed to its main active constituents: Wogonin, Baicalein and Baicalin

Medicinal Mushroom Extracts

Bioremediators
- Multiple in vitro and in vivo studies in support.
  - Biochem Biophys Res Commun. 2002 Nov 8;298(4):603-12.
- Traditional usage data very strong
- Reishi (ganoderma lucidum) – reduced DHT in rats
  - J Ethnopharmacol. 2005 Oct 31;102(1):107-12.
- 3-6 grams per day 4:1-15:1 Good to get full spectrum products as well as beta glucan rich fraction
- Turkey Tail (Trametes) – extensive anti-cancer data PSP
- Cordyceps
- Chaga – extensive anti-cancer data (betulinic acid)

Hu Zhang - (*Polygonum cuspidatum*)

- Richest known source of **resveratrol**
- Traditionally used to treat cancer
- Addresses three underlying factors
  - Phlegm
  - Blood stasis
  - Heat toxins
- Several compounds have shown anti-cancer actions, including resveratrol, emodin and chrysophanol

TCM Actions:

Expels toxins	Moves Blood
Transforms Phlegm	clears Heat
Calms cough	Drains Dampness.

Biomedical Actions of Resveratrol

- Direct antioxidant
- Estrogenic and anti-estrogenic activities
- Cancer prevention: effects on biotransformation enzymes, preservation of normal cell cycle regulation, inhibition of proliferation and induction of apoptosis, inhibition of tumor invasion and angiogenesis, anti-inflammatory, organ system protective
- Anti-HIV Effects (anti-viral)
- Reverses drug resistance of taxol in prostate cancer by down-regulating tyrosine kinases and STAT1
  - Mol Cancer Ther. 2007 Nov;6(11):2938-47

Resveratrol Actions Continued

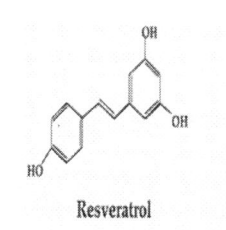

Resveratrol
(Trans-3,4',5-Trihydroxystilbene; MW 228.2)

- Inhibits Vascular Cell Adhesion Molecule Expression
- Stimulation of Endothelial Nitric Oxide Synthase (eNOS) Activity
- Inhibits Platelet Aggregation
- Inhibits ischemia
- **Normalizes Gene Expression**
- Protected mice against diet-induced-obesity and insulin resistance, and significantly extended lifespan

Key Nutrients/Extracts for BPH/PCa

- Zinc
- Vitamin D
- Vitamin K
- Magnesium
- Selenium
- Vit E (tocotrienols)
- Resveratrol
- Lycopene
- Chrysin
- I3C and DIM
- Beta-sitosterol
- Ursolic Acid

Zinc

- #1 Prostate Nutrient
- Needed for some 300 enzyme-systems used by the body.
- Essential co-factor in the production of seminal fluid;
- Is involved with the metabolism of testes, pituitary, thyroid, and adrenals;
- Down regulates transcriptional growth factors including NF-kB. Carcinogenesis. 2006 Oct;27(10):1980-90.
- Blocks dietary copper

Vitamin D

- Higher serum levels of Vit D correlate with higher levels of Testosterone.
- Men with sufficient 25(OH)D level (> or =30 mi /l) had significantly higher levels of testosterone and significantly lower levels of SHBG than those who were deficient.
- Seasonal concordance

Clin Endocrinol (Oxf). 2010 Aug;73(2):243-8.

Vitamin K

- Vit K takes calcium out of the arteries and puts it on the bones.
- Calcium supp's should be taken with caution due to their effects on the CV system
- Increased calcium intake leads to increased risk of MI.
- "poor prostate health is essentially a vitamin K insufficiency disorder"

Heart. 2012 Jun;98(12):920-5.
Med Hypotheses. 2015 Mar;84(3):219-22.

Vitamin K2 Research (MK4 and 7)

Vit K2 prevents and reverses Arterial calcification

- Arterioscler Thromb Vasc Biol. 2004 Jul;24(7):1161-70.
- Atherosclerosis. 2009 Apr;203(2):489-93.
- Acta Physiol Hung. 2010 Sep;97(3):256-66.
- Atherosclerosis. 2008 Jul 19.
- Blood. 2007 Apr 1;109(7):2823-31.

Beta-sitosterol

- Significant improvement in symptoms and urinary flow parameters in BPH
  Lancet. 1995 Jun 17;345(8964):1529-32.
- Effective option in the treatment of BPH.
  J Urol. 1997 Sep;80(3):427-32.
- The beneficial effects of beta-sitosterol treatment recorded in the 6-month double-blind trial were maintained for 18 months.
  BJU Int. 2000 May;85(7):842-6.

Chrysin

- Chrysin (w/Bioperine) 500 to 1000 mg 1-2 x day
- Potent Natural Aromatase Inhibitor
- Combine with:
  - Green Tea Extract (98% polyphenols, 80% catechins, 50% EGCG) 500 -1000mg BID
  - Quercetin 500-1000mg BID

Vegetables to the Rescue

- **Lycopene** from tomatoes reduces oxidative damage and regulates redox coupling in the prostate, reduces PSA.
  Cancer Res 1999;59:1225-1230.
  J Natl Cancer Inst 2001;93:1872-1879.
  Neill MG, Fleshner NE. An update on chemoprevention strategies
- Whole food source better (tomato products)
  Exp Biol Med (Maywood). 2002; 227:869-80.

Dose 20-30mg/day in formula

Vegetables to the Rescue

- Cruciferous vegetables contain **sulforaphane**, and **diindole methane (DIM)** which are protective against PCa

    Cancer Epidemiol. Biomarkers Prev. 5: 733–748.

- **Sulforophane** and cancer prevention (Animal studies)

    Proc Natl Acad Sci USA 1994;91:3147-3150.
    Proc Natl Acad Sci USA 1992;89:2399-2403.
    Proc Natl Acad Sci USA 2001;98:15221-15226.

I3C/DIM and ITC's

- Increases the ratio of 2- hydroxyesterone to 16-alpha-hydroxyesterone
- "Based on our results, a model for cancer protective effects of DIM and I3C was proposed"

    Carcinog. 2011 Apr 22.
    Cancer Causes Control 2002 Dec; 13(10): 947-55.

- DIM over I3C as isolate
- ITC's - Isothiocyanates

Additional Therapeutic Strategies

Countering Environmental Disruption

- Isothiocyanates (ITCs)
    - sulforaphane (SFN), phenethyl isothiocyanate (PEITC), allyl isothiocyanate (AITC), and 6-(methylsulfinyl)hexyl isothiocyanate (6-MITC)
- Diindolemethane (DIM)
- Calcium D Glucarate
- Selenium, cysteine, B-6 and 12, folate
- Phenolic compounds (catechins, flavones, isoflavonoids etc.)
- Lignans (flax seed, burdock seed)
- Adaptogens —protective, anti-toxic agents
    - (schisandra seed - schisandrins)

Additions for CVI

- Collinsonia
- Aesculus
- Butcher's Broom
- Hamemelis
- Polyphenols
- Anthocyanins

Combating Estrogen Mimics and Endocrine Disruptors

- Support liver function
- Alteratives
- Adaptogens
- Phenolic-rich plant extracts
    - Resveratrol
- Isothiocynate-rich compounds
    - Sulforaphane
- Milk Thistle
- Sulfur rich amino acids
- Plants that induce NRF-2

Urine pH

- Give patient pH strips
- Have them take their reading 3-4 x daily
- Adjust intake of acid or base buffers
- Normal pH is about 6.5
- In some cases, it is good to maintain a higher pH for awhile ~ 7 is good.

Carbonates for pH control

Trisalts
- Magnesium
- Potassium
- Calcium

Baking soda
- Sodium Bicarbonate

Prevention of Radiation Induced Fibrosis

- Trental 400mg BID

- Vit E 1,000iu QD

- Significant regression of radiation-induced fibrosis has been achieved after treatment combining pentoxifylline and alpha-tocopherol (vitE).

  J Clin Oncol. 2005 Dec 1;23(34):8570-9.

Prostate Cancer Controversies

Avodart/Proscar Issues

- Prostate Cancer Prevention
- Studies revealed increased risk for high grade tumors N Engl J Med 2003; 349:215-224
- Reduced the risk of prostate cancer by 25%, but with an apparent increased risk of high-grade disease.
- Several studies have since disputed this finding
  Clin Cancer Res. 2009;15:4694-4699.
  Cancer Prev Res August 208 1;174
- Prostate Cancer Prevention Controversy- LFE (2013)

Avodart over Proscar

- Longer half-life = 3 weeks versus short half-life of several hours
- Blocks Type 1 and 2 isoenzymes – Blocks only Type 2
- Both isoenzymes appear increased in high-grade compared with low-grade localised cancer
- Dual inhibition of both isoenzymes with dutasteride may, therefore, be effective in preventing or delaying the growth of prostate cancer.
  Eur Urol. 2008 Feb;53(2):244-52
- Off/on label issues

Red Meat and PCa?

- Correlation does not imply causation.

- Data shows that people who eat red meat also: smoke more, eat fewer fruits and veggies, while eating more processed flour and sugar, as well as bad oils.

    Mayo Clin Proc 76, 576-581, 2001. JAMA 281 (17), 1591-1597, 1999.
    Int J Cancer 2000;85:60-67.
    Cancer Metastasis Rev 2003;22:83-86.
    J Natl Cancer Inst 1995;87:652-661.

Selenium and Vit E

- Controversial studies implicating these nutrients with PCa – problems with studies – overwhelming data shows benefit.
    Biometals. 2010 Aug;23(4):695-705.

Vitamin E

- Alpha and gamma-tocopheryl succinate (mixed tocopherols)
    - Reduces the abundance of androgen receptor (AR) in prostate cancer cells
- Combine with Selenium

- Dose 2-400 iu/day (non synthetic)

Therapy with DHEA

- When giving DHEA – use DIM for estrogen conversion from 16 alpha hydroxy to 2 hydroxy;
-
- Chrysin, EGCG, and quercetin as aromatase inhibitors

- Can be combined with Pharm ARI's

The Doctrine of Signatures: Flower Essences to Support Reproductive Health by Rhonda PallasDowney

The Doctrine of Signatures refers to the personality and characteristics of a plant as a statement about its medicinal qualities and properties. The plant's signature is an encompassing evaluation of the plants parts- leaves, root, stem, flowers, buds, seeds, pods, and fruits – as well as its constitution, shape, color, texture, appearance, and the environment in which it grows.

Reproductive health is defined as a state of physical, mental, and social well-being in all matters relating to the reproductive system, at all stages of life (www.reproductive-health-journal.com/about/faq/whatis).

Although reproductive health is most associated with women, especially at puberty and the childbearing years, reproductive health includes the spectrum of human development, beginning with childhood, adolescence, adulthood, and then sets the stage for our health beyond the age of reproductive health for both men and women.

The regeneration of our cells is an important factor in our body's support of the aging process. For example, 95% of the body's cells die and are replaced within a year. How you treat your body can affect the ability to healthy functioning of the reproduction of cells.

The reproduction of cells help stimulate the regeneration of our body's functions throughout the aging process. The liver, for example, has the best rate of regeneration than any other organ in our bodies, as it rebuilds itself in about 6 weeks.

The skin is also an area of the body that regenerates quickly, as the surface layer of the skin is recycled nearly every 2-4 weeks. Our blood, DNA, bones, lungs, stomach lining, and brain, are capable of rebuilding/reproducing cells.

At each stage of our lives, no matter who we are, we are faced with the choices we make and the lifestyles we live, to regenerate and rebuild our bodies, and to shift our thoughts and well being to a creative and energetic conscious awareness.

Our mind, body and spirit are intimately connected. The energetics of flower essences and plant energy can be very powerful, yet simple, when we take time to understand what we are truly experiencing. When the energy system is out of alignment within our bodies, whether it be an emotional, spiritual, or physical feeling, flower essences can help us to learn not just the symptoms occurring but more importantly to identify, understand, and connect to the main cause of the discomfort. Where did it come from?

Flower essences support inspiration, insights, and positive awareness to patterns of imbalance that contribute to these symptoms and help us take action towards healing.

In this lecture we will step into a deeper connection and intimacy associating the relationship between the Doctrine of Signatures promoting the support and awareness of the energetics (both visible and invisible) of healthy regeneration of the mind- body-spirit with the following 6 plants:

Mullein (Verbascum thapsus)
Pomegranate (Punica granatum)
Strawberry Hedgehog (Echinocereus engelmannii)
Vervain (Verbena macdougali)
Yellow Monkeyflower (Mimulus guttatus)
Wild Rose (Rosa arizonaca)

Mullein (Verbascum thapsus)
Primary Quality: Security

Family: Snapdragon or Figwort (Scrophulariaceae)
Other Names: Velvet Dock, Velvet Plant, Flannel Leaf, Flannel Mullein, Blanketweed, Woolly Mullein, Candlewick, Candelaria, Torchweed, Torches, Donkey's Ears, Hag's Taper, Common Mullein, Our Lady's Candle, Gordolobo, Candle Flower.
Verbascum is a Latin word, used in Pliny's writing, which comes from the word **barbātus** and means "bearded." **Thapsus** was a town in Sicily, or the word may come from the isle of Thapsos, which is now Magnise. The Latin word **mollis** means "soft," and refers to its velvety leaves, on which the English name is based.

Where Found: Waste areas, river bottoms, along roadsides, railroad tracks,
hedgerows, dry meadows and open grassy places, pastures, gravelly and chalky banks around settlements, and disturbed earth throughout North America. Can be found between juniper-pinyon and ponderosa belts in the West. Native to Europe and naturalized in the U.S.

Elevation: averages 4,500' to 7,000'

Energy Impact (Chakra Correspondence): second and third chakras

Key Rubrics for Positive Healing Patterns: intimacy, listening, purpose, positive masculine energy, protection, security, sensitivity

Key Rubrics for Symptoms and Patterns of Imbalance: lack of intimacy, lack of direction and purpose in life, insensitivity

Other Rubrics: acceptance, abandonment, aggressive, anger, anxiety, appreciation, assimilation, awareness, calm, centered, change, clarity, cleansing, communication, confidence, conscience, courage, creativity, depression, discernment, fear, focus, gentleness,
goals, groundedness, guidance, highest good, impatience, indecisive, inner self, inner truths, joy, light, nonacceptance, nurturing, optimism, overbearing, patience, personal space, phallic, quieting, sadness, self-acceptance, sexual expression, softness, solar plexus chakra, soothing, spleen chakra, strength, truth, unconscious, values

Traditional Use
Mullein is a powerful, multifacetated plant that goes back into ancient history. In Homer's Odyssey, Ulysses used mullein as a protection against the enchantress Circe. In Europe and India, mullein was used to get rid of evil spirits.
   In medieval Europe, the tall dried stems were dipped in tallow to make tapers or torches and were used in funeral and religious processions. The Spaniards called it "candelaria," and the English named it

"torchweed." The dried down on mullein's leaves and stem was used to make wicks for candles, hence the name "candlewick." "Hag's taper" is a country name referring to "hag" as witch and "taper" as hedge taper (candle); witches were said to have used hedges (where mullein plants grew) as their shelter and they, too, made use of the light provided by the mullein candlestick.

Pliny and Dioscorides suggested preserving food by wrapping it in mullein's leaves. Dioscorides used mullein to treat scorpion stings, eye complaints, toothaches, tonsillitis, and coughs. Galen wrote about mullein's use to aid digestion and cleansing, and Culpeper recommended it as a treatment for gout, obstructions of the bladder and veins, and inflammations of the throat. The Appalachian Indians made an infusion of the leaves to treat dysentery, and the early settlers tied mullein leaves to their feet and arms to cure malaria. The Hopi Indians dried the leaves and used them as a smoking tobacco and as a cure for people who were mentally unbalanced or "to revive the unconscious."

Mullein has also been recommended as a remedy for edema, based on its properties as an absorbent. Mullein flower oil has long been known as a German folk remedy to treat earache and to remove warts, and the use of oil prepared from mullein flowers dates back to the Renaissance. Dr. Constantine Hering, the "Father of American Homeopathy," took it with him to America as one of his few herbal remedies. According to Moore, the roots can be used as a diuretic, to treat incontinence, and to tone the bladder following childbirth. The use of mullein leaves was included in the National Formulary in 1916–36. Rich in mucilage, mullein leaves were traditionally smoked to relieve chest complaints, lung congestion, and asthma.

Leaves and flowers are used as an antispasmodic, astringent, mild diuretic, mild sedative, demulcent, emollient, expectorant, and tonic, as teas, extracts, tinctures, infusions, gargles, or as a syrup. Mullein is known as the "natural wonder herb"; it
has narcotic properties that aren't habit-forming or poisonous. Herbalists use mullein to treat a wide variety of ailments, including coughs, colds and pectoral complaints, bronchitis, asthma and catarrh, coughing or bronchial spasms, nervous disorders, hemorrhages from the lungs, shortness of breath, diaper rashes, tonsillitis, migraines, earaches, colic, emphysema, glandular swelling, swollen joints, problems of the mucous membranes, pulmonary diseases, venereal disease, and whooping cough. Mullein is also a painkiller and can be used as a sedative to induce sleep.

The leaves, as an external woundwort, can be placed on burns, injuries, sprains, and broken bones to encourage healing and to relieve nerve pain. The leaves can also be placed in shoes when the soles are thin, or around a blister to prevent rubbing while walking, or as an emergency Band-Aid[tm]. They are also a handy replacement for toilet paper when out in nature. The flowers can also be used in a facial cream to soothe the skin or as an infusion to brighten hair. Seed oil soothes chilblains and chapped skin, and the plant is also used as a dye.

Homeopathic Use

Tincture of the fresh plant is made from its leaves when it begins to flower. Dr. Samuel Hahnemann proved Verbascum as a "cough remedy" and generated a broad list of symptoms. Verbascum is primarily used to treat facial pains on the left side and trigeminal neuralgia (nerve pain in the face). It is also used to treat itching of the anus, incontinence, colic, earache, respiratory tract and bladder problems, catarrhs and colds, hoarseness, bronchitis, constipation, cough, deafness, hemorrhoids, and nerve pains.

Positive Healing Patterns
- Promotes strength with softness, enhancing intimacy, humbleness, and gentleness.
- Is especially helpful to men who are seeking true intimacy and security in their relationships, or for women who want to strengthen yet soften their masculine nature.
- Guides us toward our inner light, encouraging focus and sense of purpose.

- Reminds us to listen to our inner selves and to others as they communicate their inner depths and feelings with us.
- Awakens our unconscious mind and heightens our conscience. Teaches us to live and act according to our inner truths and values.
- Activates creativity, sexual expression, joy, and optimism.
- Assists us in assimilating emotional and mental states that no longer serve us. Through the process of assimilation, we are able to incorporate our highest good and absorb it at the highest level possible.
- Soothes, calms, and nurtures our emotional and mental states.

Symptoms and Patterns of Imbalance
Mullein may be an appropriate flower essence for those who
- Lack acceptance and awareness of their own inner worth and values
- Have feelings and thoughts of depression, fear, abandonment, sadness, irritability, anxiety, and/or impatience and who are unwilling or tired of listening to other people's problems, so they deal with others in a grumpy and impatient way
- Are overbearing and aggressive and who force issues with others
- Lack intimacy in relationships and want to soften their masculine nature yet stay strong in their positive masculine traits
- Lack incentive, focus, purpose, and direction and have lost touch with their own inner light and truths.

Features of the Original Flower-Essence Water
Odor: slight honey-scented aroma is more profound in the water
Taste: slightly sweet
Sensations: Soothing, cool, and gentle in the throat and in swallowing. Gives a relaxing, soothing feeling in the abdomen and solar plexus.
Water Color: clear

Physical Makeup
Root, Stem, Leaves/Leaflets, Height: Mullein forms a light-colored taproot and a basal rosette of large, soft, downy, woolly leaves that grow near the ground the first year of the plant's life. The second year, a tall, stout, thick, staff-like fibrous stalk emerges from the center of the basal rosette and can grow from 2 to 6 feet tall. The unbranched, woolly, phallus-shaped stalk produces large, thick, foxglove-like leaves that are soft and densely hairy, covering both sides with a flannel-like gray coat. The lower leaves are large and oval/lanceolate and have leafstalks. The upper leaves are stalkless and gradually become smaller and more ovate. The leaves alternate and have noticeable indented wavy veins. A unique feature of this medicinal mullein plant, compared to other mullein species, is that the leaves narrow at the base into two wings that pass down the stem. The leaves are highly absorbent and they pass rainwater down the stem and into the roots, allowing the plant to grow in dry places. The woolly down on the leaves also prevents the leaves from drying out. By placing the fresh
leaves in your mouth and breathing in, a cool, moist, soothing sensation is felt. The fresh leaves have a slightly bitter taste. The soft fine hairs on the leaves and stalk also protect the plant from insects and grazing animals due to the irritation caused to the mucous membranes from the down. Mullein's average lifespan is two years, although some plants can survive up to three or four years. Propagation is by seed and the plant self-sows abundantly. New plants can usually be found near the old ones.

Flower Color: Lemon-yellow

Flowers: The slightly honey-scented, bright lemon-yellow flowers open randomly and are densely packed around the woolly cylindrical terminal spike for a foot or more. The tight flower buds, small lemon-yellow flowers, and round tiny-seeded pods all intermingle toward the top of the dense spike. The cup-shaped lemon-yellow flowers are stalkless, have five rounded slightly uneven petals, and are about 1 inch wide. They have five slightly orange stamens with deeper orange anthers.

Blooming Period: July and August

Doctrine of Signatures

- Mullein's stalk is stout, thick, and tall, and its base is especially strong. The entire plant is soft, fuzzy, hairy, and velvety. The plant's character of strength along with its softness represents its ability to cut through coughing and bronchial spasms that damage the soft hairs lining the mucous membranes. The velvety soft, hairy, downy leaves resemble the soft hairs of the mucous membranes. The mullein's phallus-shaped terminal spike filled with flowers also represents strength with softness, promoting intimacy and gentleness.
- The densely packed lemon-yellow cuplike flowers, flower buds, and seeds are securely protected in the soft, woolly, phallic spike, demonstrating emotional openness yet a tightness offering security, protection, and personal space. This signature relates especially to men who are seeking true intimacy and security in expressing a soft, gentle, humble nature, or for women who want to strengthen yet soften their masculine nature. This signature also may refer to males with both strength with softness, or to helping males relate with others in strength and softness, learning to give lots of "warm fuzzies."
- Mullein's use as a torch or candlestick — in addition to the way the densely packed lemon-yellow flowers and buds circle around and upward toward the top of the spike giving off a yellowish light — is a signature of its ability to promote focus, purpose, and Light, thus guiding us toward our own inner selves and light and encouraging us to share our light with others in an effortless and steadfast way.
- The softly colored lemon-yellow flowers correspond with our third chakra and our emotional relationship with ourselves and others. These emotions may include depression, fear, abandonment, irritation, and sadness, yet with the ability to relax and let go. They also help us awaken and stir our unconscious minds which, in turn, heightens our consciousness and teaches us to live and act according to our inner truths and values. The orange stamens and anthers refer to our second chakra, or creative and sexual selves, activating feelings of optimism and joy.
- The woolly, earlike signature reminds us to listen to our inner selves and to others as they communicate with us.
- The incredible absorbency of mullein leaves is a powerful signature of the plant. They act as a relaxant, and they promote absorption in cases of cellular dropsy, chronic disease, pleuritic effusions, and similar accumulations of fluid. Perhaps, on another level, this signature can be related to a person's process of assimilating emotional and mental states that no longer serve the individual. Through the process of assimilation, the individual is able to take in and incorporate what he or she is able to absorb at the highest level possible.
- The taste of the leaves is slightly bitter and their temperature is slightly cool. The leaves have a mucilaginous quality, and the roots and flowers give off a soothing, aromatic scent. These qualities give a signature of the plant's physical ability to soothe irritated membranes, reduce fever, increase secretion, and clear the lungs. The flower-essence water is more aromatic than the flower itself, and the taste of the water is gentle, quieting, soft, and somewhat sweet. The sensation of drinking the water is soothing on the throat, and its gentleness and smoothness is felt all the way down to the abdomen and solar plexus.

Pomegranate (Punica granatum)
Primary Quality: Abundance

Family: Pomegranate (Punicaceae)
Other Names: Apple of Carthage, Grenadier. Latin name derived from **poma granata,** meaning "many-seeded apple." Botanical name also refers to the source of the plant, which was a Roman colony in North Africa named Punicus or Carthage.

Where Found: Pomegranate is native to Asia, especially Iran, Afghanistan, and the Himalayan slopes. It grows wild on the shores of the Mediterranean and in Arabia, Persia, and Japan, and it is cultivated in the East and West Indies. Pomegranate is cultivated in the western U.S., from the Northwest Coast to Arizona and New Mexico, wherever the climate is sufficiently warm to allow the fruit to ripen. In higher latitudes, it is raised in gardens or hothouses for its beautiful flowers even though it doesn't bear fruit.

Elevation: most climates across the North American continent

Energy Impact (Chakra Correspondence): first, second, and third chakras

Key Rubrics for Positive Healing Patterns: abundance, creativity, loving, nurturing, passion, resourcefulness, self-empowerment, sexuality

Key Rubrics for Symptoms and Patterns of Imbalance: hidden talents, lack of creativity, lack of passion and joy in life, inability to locate resources
Other Rubrics: abundance, adolescence, appreciation, balance, beauty, calm, career, change, clairvoyance, dreams, emotional, female, freedom, fruitful, grounded, heart, home, joyful, kundalini, life force, menopausal, menstrual, mother, optimistic, positive, power, pregnancy, premenstrual, protection, psychic energies, purpose, reproductive, respect, root chakra, solar plexus chakra, spleen chakra, transformation, transition, understanding, underworld, values, wisdom, womb

Traditional Use
The pomegranate has long been known as an ancient symbol of fertility due to its striking red color and seed arrangement.
It is also an ancient design motif. Pomegranate was included in the Egyptian Ebers Papyrus, written in 2000 b.c., and also in the Old Testament (Numbers 13:23). Pomegranate was suspected to be the "forbidden fruit" eaten by Eve in the Garden of Eden, and it was included in the design on the pillars of King Solomon's temple.

In Greek mythology, Persephone was said to have eaten six seeds of a pomegranate after she fell into Hades, the underworld. As a symbol of union,
the pomegranate bound her to Pluto, the god of the underworld, in his hidden kingdom for six months from fall to spring (each seed representing one month). Despite this, the symbol of Persephone eating the seeds is also about a birthing period and her return to self. The underworld helped her discover her hidden wisdom, beauty, and power, and allowed her to confront her fears in the darkest moments of her life. In spring, Persephone was free and emerged with the newly found gifts she had given herself.

The medicinal history of pomegranate dates back to Pliny in the first century. The root bark has been used since ancient times to expel worms from the intestinal tract; it has been found most beneficial in cases of tapeworm. In 1804, an East Indian practitioner cured an Englishman of a tapeworm with an infusion of the root bark and used it as a purgative. The bark's active ingredient — liquid alkaloid pelletierine — was discovered in 1878; it was once used in human medicine and is now used in veterinary medicine.

If you bite into the rind of a pomegranate, you will experience its highly astringent nature. About 30 percent of the rind is composed of tannin, a powerful astringent substance. Powdered fruit rind is also used as an astringent, and has been used to treat dysentery, diarrhea, excessive perspiration, and for intermittent fevers, and as a gargle for sore throats. Pomegranate is used in Ayurvedic medicine as a blood purifier to enhance the memory.

Pomegranate fruit is eaten whole, and it is juiced to make delicious drinks and desserts, especially in the Middle East where it has been cultivated for over 5,000 years. Middle Eastern cooks boil the sour pulp to make a pomegranate syrup, which has a distinguished scent and adds flavors to stews and meat dishes. Its sweet juice is also used to make grenadine, a flavoring for cocktails, sherbet, and pickles. The sour East Indian condiment anardana is made from the dried seeds of pomegranate and used for stuffings in flavorful breads and pastries. Fabric dyes are also made from the fruits, rind, and bark.

Caution: Large doses of the rind or root bark infusion can cause nausea, cramps, and vomiting.

Homeopathic Use
The homeopathic remedy Granatum is used to get rid of tapeworm with itching of the anus and constant hunger. It is also used to treat persistent vertigo with salivation and nausea, pain in the shoulder so heavy that clothing is intolerable, aching in all the finger joints, and convulsive movements of the extremities.

Positive Healing Patterns
- Activates the awakening and experience of the kundalini life-force.
- Stirs passion, sexuality, and creative awareness and expression of feminine energy, which nurtures and connects us to the Great Earth Mother; this is helpful for both men and women.
- Teaches us to protect, respect, and honor our vulnerability; to discover our inner wisdom, beauty, and power in the seemingly darkest moments of our lives; and to make use of these gifts externally by setting healthy boundaries, learning to express our emotions and creativity in safe ways, and feeling free in who we are.
- Attracts an abundance of positive, fruitful inner and outer resources; guides us in personal balance within ourselves, at home, with our family, in our job, and our role within the larger community.
- For women, Pomegranate especially helps us understand how our emotional and mental states affect who we are and how we feel in our physical, sexual, and feminine bodies. It is helpful to women of all ages and in all life cycles — adolescence or premenstrual, menstrual, or menopausal.
- Helps us express a positive nature of joy, optimism, and freedom.

Symptoms and Patterns of Imbalance
Pomegranate may be an appropriate flower essence for those who
- Do not feel connected with their creative, sexual, passionate, and feminine nature (men or women)
- Are overly emotional, moody, or mental, especially around premenses, menses, or menopause, or for young teenage girls who generally seem to be "out of whack" emotionally
- Have difficulty finding and nurturing their inner and outer resources, and who feel out of touch or out of balance with their own values and needs; this may relate especially to the struggle between being out in the world with a career or at home with children and family.

Features of the Original Flower-Essence Water
Odor: subtle yet sweet
Taste: slightly sweet, fruity, and delicate; taste lingers at the back of the tongue

Sensations: Tingling and numbing sensation that moves downward. Feels grounded, soothing, and relaxing. Feel warmth in the ovaries that moves upward to abdomen area and continues to move upward to the shoulders.
Water Color: slightly yellow

Physical Makeup
Root, Stem, Leaves/Leaflets, Height: Pomegranate is a small, deciduous, shrubby tree growing up to 20 feet in height. The trunk's bark is pale brown and is often uneven, and its many slender branches bear spines or thorns at the tips. Leaf buds and young shoots are red, and the bright green leaves are opposite, entire, oblong or lance-shaped, and pointed at the end. They are smooth, thick, and shiny and have short leafstalks. Pomegranate bears fruit about the size of an apple or orange, and its fruit is a globular berry. The fruit is crowned at the calyx, and it has a thick, reddish yellow, leatherlike peel or rind; it resembles a swollen womb. When the fruit is broken in half, you can see that the brightly colored red, angular seeds are grouped in many compartments or cells. The seeds are fruity, juicy, and very flavorful. The inside rind contains an acidulous pulp that tastes bitter. Pomegranate trees like full sun and lots of water in order to yield plenty of fruit.
Flower Color: Orange-red to scarlet-red
Flowers: The fragrant, showy orange-
red to scarlet-red single flowers are somewhat large and emerge at the ends of the young branches. The flowers have five to seven rounded, waxy, wrinkly paperlike petals that grow from the upper part of the tube of the calyx, which is bright red, thick, and fleshy. A somewhat prolific group of yellow stamens with yellow anthers grows from the center of the flower.
Blooming Period: April to June

Doctrine of Signatures
- The colorful orange-red to scarlet-red flowers, leaf buds, and young shoots, and the red, juicy, flavorful seeds relate primarily to the first or root chakra and second or spleen chakra, which is the seat of the kundalini within the body. This is where our life-promoting energy lies, which influences our circulatory system, our reproductive system, and how our lower extremities operate. The color orange relates to the spleen chakra and is linked to sensation and emotion, which influences creativity. The rounded, feminine appearance of the flower highlights qualities associated with being a woman. The juicy, fruity taste of the fruit, as well as its appearance, stirs passion, sexuality, and creative feminine energy, which nurtures and connects us to the Great Earth Mother. Even the calyx is bright red and fleshy. The astringent nature of the fruit — "the red-juice-dripping, seed-filled pomegranate" distinctly implies the womb and the power, wisdom, and beauty to be discovered by women in their own hidden underworld kingdom. This also relates to the changes within the female body, such as when the blood stops, the process of fertilization, and then when the blood begins a new cycle again.
- The previous signatures may also refer to the intuitive, psychological, and feminine qualities within males. By awakening the "inner feminine," a male can nurture his ability to discover and embody these feminine qualities. The Pomegranate flower essence can also be beneficial for men in the arousal of their passionate and sensual natures.
- The way in which the juicy, red seeds are grouped in compartments yet individual is a signature of their magnetic nature, in which they both attract and give out energy. This magnetic signature represents an abundant gathering of positive and fruitful inner and outer resources, teaching balance in this way.
- The thorns at the tips of the branches and the thick, leatherlike, orangish-reddish rind on the fruit are a signature of protection. They demonstrate a safeguard from being manipulated, taken

advantage of, bullied, or eating fruit prematurely or before it is ready and willing. This signature teaches respect and honors vulnerability, healthy boundaries, and safe expression of emotions.
- The smooth, shiny leaves are a signature of the plant's positive nature. The leaves appear luminous, especially on bright sunny days. They express themselves with joy, optimism, and freedom.
- The golden yellow stamens that emerge from the flower's center and the slightly yellow flower-essence water correspond to the third or solar plexus chakra, which is linked to our emotional and mental states and to psychic energies and clairvoyance. The significance of the yellow stamens and the yellow water relates to our ability, especially as women, to understand through experience how certain emotional/mental states can cause who and how we are in our physical, sexual, and feminine bodies. The yellowish rind on the inside of the pomegranate fruit is bitter and represents an emotional bitterness to watch out for. This signature is another link to being an especially influential remedy for women of all ages and in all life cycles.

Strawberry Hedgehog (Echinocereus engelmannii)
Primary Quality: Passion

Family: Cactus (Cactaceae)
Other Names: Strawberry Cactus, Hedgehog Cactus, Engelmann Hedgehog, Engelmann's Cactus, Torch Cactus, Strawberry Echinocereus. The botanical name
Echinocereus engelmannii was given in honor of George Engelmann, a botanist and doctor from Germany who came to the United States in 1832 at the age of twenty-three. He gradually succeeded in an obstetric practice in St. Louis while maintaining an interest in plant life and botany. Many botanical explorers sent specimens for him to identify, and he has long been remembered for his botanical work with the cactus family.
The "strawberry" part of the plant's common name comes from the dark red mahogany-colored fruits that are juicy and rich in sugar and may be eaten like strawberries. "Hedgehog" refers to the plant's stems, which are rounded like a hedgehog.

Where Found: low-moisture and well-drained soils, rocky flats, sandy desert areas, and hillsides in Arizona and California deserts

Elevation: sea level to 5,000'

Energy Impact (Chakra Correspondence): first, third, and fourth chakras

Key Rubrics for Positive Healing Patterns: compassion, love, intimacy, sexuality, self-worth

Key Rubrics for Symptoms and Patterns of Imbalance: aggression, insecurity, insensitivity, inhibition, shut-down sexuality

Other Rubrics: balance, creativity, expression, fear, female, femininity, freedom, giving, heart chakra, kundalini, male, mother, nurturing, passion, procreation, protection, receiving, relationship, reproduction, respect, root chakra, security, sensitivity, sensuality, solar plexus chakra, spleen chakra, trust

Traditional Use
The Strawberry Hedgehog cactus is a survival plant of the desert. Although it reduces in size in the summer heat, it recovers in size and moisture with the downfall of rain. Thorns can be removed by cutting off the outer skin from the cactus while the stem is still rooted. Placing the thorns back into the

ground allows them to propagate. The inner cactus flesh can then be used for sunburns, bites, stings, open wounds, cuts, abrasions, and even to treat earaches. The flesh, as a food, can be eaten raw in hot weather and either cooked or roasted in cold weather. Although the texture is slimy, it is a good emergency food in the desert. The Pima Indians regarded the fruit as a delicacy, and the fruits are important in the diets of birds and rodents.

Homeopathic Use: Unknown to author.

Positive Healing Patterns
- Promotes relationship and sexual openness based on trust, security, protection, intimacy, and expressing love with a partner freely and passionately.
- Increases our sensitivity, creativity, appreciation, and awareness of ourselves and our partner.
- Gives a strong balance of male and female roles in positive ways.
- Assists those who want to experience the kundalini life-force during sexual interactions.
- Promotes heart-centered energy that opens us up to love, compassion, and passion.

Symptoms and Patterns of Imbalance
Strawberry Hedgehog may be an appropriate flower essence for those who
- Feel closed down, insecure, inhibited, or blocked sexually and emotionally and lack self-worth and appreciation of self, especially women
- Fear yielding, giving, or receiving
- Are insensitive of their partner's needs
- Want more sexual excitement and satisfaction
- Are obsessively sexual and aggressive, and desire immediate sexual gratification without a whole-body experience
- Are in need of healing and loving their mothers, especially for women.

Features of the Original   Flower-Essence Water
Odor: roselike, subtle, and soft
Taste: very pleasant and roselike with
a full yet light taste that stays in the mouth
Sensations: Obvious light tingling in the vagina; feel the lips of the vagina open as if to receive and give energy; also feel a warm tingling in the heart chakra.
Water Color: clear

Physical Makeup
Root, Stem, Leaves/Leaflets, Height: Grows in open clumps that form a loose or thick cluster up to 3 inches wide and 20 inches long, looking like spine-covered cucumbers standing on end. They are green and cylindrical, and grow up to 3 inches in diameter. The straight spines are usually yellow, although they can vary in color from white or gold to pinkish to black, and they tend to point downward. There are ten to fourteen protruding ribs on each stem with areoles (small open spaces) set about $1/2$ inch apart. Each areole consists of eight to twelve $1/2$-inch-long radial spines, and up to six central spines that can be up to 3 inches long. The plant's ribs appear tough, yet they are very delicate and are protected by the spines.
Flower Color: Magenta
Flowers: The deep magenta flower
makes an opening in the skin of the cactus right above the areoles (the small open spaces), where two to six central spines come together along the plant's ribs. The flowers carry a very sweet fragrance. They are delicate, transparent, and elastic. The cup-shaped flowers are up to 3 inches wide. The inner petals

are more intense in their magenta color, and the outer petals are a softer pink. There are dozens of soft, airy, lemon-yellow stamens that grow close in the center and around the pistil, then spread out in a circle inside the base of the flower. Inside the very center is a profound green pistil that is firm yet soft and looks like a miniature tree with nine to eleven small fingerlike segments. The sepal is thorny with alternating whitish long and short spines. The flowers bloom for several consecutive days, attracting bees and beetles to their abundant pollen and sweet nectar. The blooms are followed by green spiny fruit, which becomes red when ripe and grows up to $1/4$ inch long and 1 inch in diameter. The ripe, succulent fruit is juicy and rich in sugar, and may be eaten like strawberries.

Blooming Period: March to April

Doctrine of Signatures
- It is amazing that a beautiful, sensual, soft flower can emerge from a cucumber-like organ that is covered with needles. The cylindrical stem of the cactus is actually very delicate, and the needles provide protection. This signature in and of itself is certainly symbolic of both the male and female, and gives a strong balance of male and female roles in positive ways. The needed protection of the spines or needles indicates sensitivity toward each other. Even the flower is able to find its place to emerge from the skin of the stem at a cluster of spines, protected yet free to express itself. The stem (resembling the male organ) is able to receive the flower's sweet nectar from within the skin, even with the spines all around. And the stem is able to give to the flower so that the flower can emerge from the stem's sustenance. What a fascinating signature!
- As if the above signature weren't enough, we're going to take this a few steps farther. The deep magenta petals are more intense on the inside of the flower, like the deeper, brighter reddish colors inside the vagina, especially when a woman is sexually excited and passionate. The womb is protected, and the vagina opens up like a flower in its peak blossom! The strawberry hedgehog's flowers are elastic, giving a feeling of stretching. Yes, this is true. The petals are strong, yet yielding and gentle. The outer petals are a softer pink like the vulva and its surrounding area. This signature certainly points to female sensuality and passion. Another added attraction to this signature is the male-looking pistil in the center of the flower. The pistil is firm yet soft, and emerges right from the very center of the flower as yet another gift from Mother Nature. Also, it's another indication of the balance of giving and receiving sexual energy.
- The magenta flower and the red, juicy fruit correspond with the first or root chakra, the seat of the kundalini life-force and sexual energy within our bodies. It's linked to the reproductive system, and influences the functions of the testicles and ovaries. It stems from who we are and is related to our self-worth and our appreciation of self so that we can open up and experience our sexuality at its fullest. This signature relates to the experience of kundalini, sexuality, and creativity in a highly evolved and positive way. A more challenging aspect would be for those who are obsessively sexual, aggressive, insensitive, and only desire immediate gratification without a whole-body experience. The softer pink outer petals represent the fourth or heart chakra, which gives the ability to transmute and open the sexual energy into a hot-pink, passionate love. My friend Eileen refers to this as "being in love with the act of living in the moment." These signatures relate to more than just sexual passion and expression. They also relate to the heart-centered energy that opens us to love and to the nurturing we may need so that we can love. The femininity of the flower relates to the female as the mother and also represents the healing of our love toward our mothers and ourselves.
- The red, juicy, succulent fruits also represent sensuality and sweet passion.
- The soft lemon-yellow stamens that emerge profusely from the center of the flower's cup correspond to our third or solar plexus chakra and the emotions we feel in relation to ourselves, our sexuality, and our passion.

Vervain (Verbena macdougali)
Primary Quality: Inspiration

Family: Verbena or Vervain (Verbenaceae)
Other Names: New Mexico Vervain, Spike Verbena, Tall Verbena, Blue Vervain, Macdougal Verbena. Derived from the Latin word **verbenae** and named for Dr. David Trembly Macdougal (1865‹1958), a plant physiologist with the Carnegie Institute and an authority on desert vegetation.

Where Found: most common in Arizona and the southern Rockies, in valleys, roadsides, mountain meadows, and open flats

Elevation: 6,000' to 8,000'
Energy Impact (Chakra Correspondence): sixth and seventh chakras

Bach Flower Remedy: Verbena officinalis is used to treat those who are strongly opinionated with tendencies to preach or teach and philosophize. They are easily provoked by injustices, and when taken to the edge have tendencies to be overly enthusiastic, argumentative, and overbearing.

Key Rubrics for Positive Healing Patterns: accomplishment, direction, insight, inspiration, leadership, motivation, purpose, uplift

Key Rubrics for Symptoms and Patterns of Imbalance: complicated thoughts, being judgmental, lack of motivation, nervous exhaustion, being opinionated, rigidity, tending to be overstressed

Other Rubrics: achievement, balance, brow chakra, crown chakra, elegance, extreme, goals, grace, groundedness, heart, idealism, integration, integrity, moderation, nervousness, relaxation, relief, simplicity, spiritual, stress, strive, tension, uplifting, vision

Traditional Use
The genus Verbena is referred to as "holy bough," and vervain is known as "the enchanter's plant." It has been associated with mysticism and magic for centuries. The Romans placed vervain plants on their altars, and the ancient Egyptians devoted the plant to the goddess Isis. The Druids of Celtic Britain used vervain to purify the water used in sacred rituals; the word vervain is believed to be of Celtic origin, meaning "a stone-expeller." It was used to treat urinary stones and gravel. Vervain is also associated with Christ's crucifixion; according to myth, it stopped the bleeding from Christ's wounds. In medieval days, necklaces of vervain were worn as lucky charms for protection
from headaches and snakebites. Known as the "herb of Venus," vervain was also used in love potions and lucky charms. In
seventeenth-century England, Culpeper used vervain to treat "pain in the secret parts."

Today vervain has multiple medicinal uses: sedative, mild tranquilizer, diaphoretic, emetic, diuretic, bitter tonic, and antispasmodic. It is used to treat the onset of a cold, especially if accompanied by upper respiratory inflammation. Vervain induces sweating, and it relaxes and settles the stomach. It eases nervous tension, depression, insomnia, headaches, jaundice, and stomach, bowel, and menstrual cramps. A salve made of vervain leaves is used to treat sprains, deep bruises, and muscle tension. Drinking a tea will assist in reabsorption of blood from ruptured tissues. A decoction of leaves and flowers can also be added to bathwater as an enchanting way to relieve tension.

The Navajo and other Native American tribes used vervain petals as a source of blue pollen to replace larkspur when unavailable, and they used the crushed petals ceremonially like corn pollen. The Navajo also used vervain as a medicine in their Water Way, Life Way, and Plume Way ceremonies.

Homeopathic Use
Mother tincture is prepared from the entire fresh plant. It is used to treat disorders of the nervous system, such as nervous depression, nervous exhaustion, insomnia, and epilepsy and other spasms. It raises the absorption of blood and relieves pain in bruises. It is also used as a remedy to treat various skin irritations, such as from poison oak.

Positive Healing Patterns
- Encourages direction, leadership with open-mindedness, encouragement, and a sense of crowning achievement. Promotes an inner excitement to "reach for the stars," and to be and feel inspired.
- Gives the insight and perspective to see ahead and to strive for accomplishments not yet present.
- Helps bring an organizational framework to goal-setting and lifestyle that promotes simplicity, moderation, elegance, grace, integrity, and integration.
- Helps us remain relaxed, peaceful, and grounded while striving for goals and ideals or in relating to others.
- Allows us stay open and tolerant with others, letting others make their own choices.

Symptoms and Patterns
of Imbalance
Vervain may be an appropriate flower essence for those who
- Tend to be overcomplicated, overjudgmental, overopinionated, argumentative, and rigid, and take extreme measures to make their point from a place of personal (ego) will
- Lack direction and motivation, along with a lack of desire or an inability to see the whole picture
- Tend to be over-idealistic and are not down-to-earth
- Act overenthusiastically and lack physical, emotional, and mental strength, especially due to stress and nervous exhaustion.

Features of the Original Flower Essence Water
Odor: subtle and slightly bitter
Taste: full, pleasant, soft, and slightly sweet; doesn't taste like it smells
Sensations: Slightly warming and calming; tingling from toes to head; gives a feeling of balance, integration, and focus.
Water Color: clear

Physical Makeup
Root, Stem, Leaves/Leaflets, Height: The strong, thick, square stem is sticky and composed of many layers. The stem is hairy all around. The branching stems arise from spreading roots. Dark green lance-shaped, mintlike leaves are widely spaced and grow in opposites. The leaves are up to 4 inches long, with larger
leaves at the base and smaller leaves toward the top. The prominently veined leaves are prickly yet fuzzy, and are irregularly toothed. The entire plant has a slight bitter smell. Its average height is 2 to 3 feet.
Flower Color: Lavender to purple
Flowers: The flowers grow on a long, erect spike. Forming a ring around the spike, the flowers first open at the bottom of the spike and then appear to progress up the spike as the season progresses. Seed pods appear below and flower buds appear above. The singular, tiny flower is composed of five petals or

lobes, with three petals bending downward and two petals bending upward. The center of each tiny flower (about ¼ inch wide) is whitish yellow and star-shaped. The flowers have a slightly bitter smell.
Blooming Period: June through September

Doctrine of Signatures
- The formation of the spike and the ring of flowers progressing upward signifies integrity, direction, leadership, inspiration, and a sense of crowning achievement (seventh chakra). This also represents the plant's ability to see ahead and to strive for accomplishments not yet present. It also demonstrates the plant's openness and its capacity for calmness and a higher perspective for the good of all.
- The lavender/purple color relates to the sixth chakra and signifies spiritual vision, peacefulness, inspiration, and purpose.
- The tiny star shape in the center of the flower also symbolizes an upward direction, as if encouraging us to "reach for the stars" and to stay open and receptive to the good of all.
- The organizational structure of this plant as a whole — especially the neat appearance of the spiraling spikes along with each circle of flowers and each layer that makes up the stem — represents simplicity, moderation, elegance, and integration without overcomplication or extreme measures.
- The leaves growing in opposites represent balance, and the soft hairiness of the leaves and stem represent nerve endings and the plant's ability to relieve stress and tension. Along the wiry stems are knots that resemble a ladder, hinting of the tension that increases or escalates when a feeling of peacefulness is absent.
- The spreading roots and the sturdy branching stems symbolize the plant's ability to remain grounded while striving for ideals and goals, as represented by the spiraling spike.

Wild Rose (Rosa arizonaca)
Primary Quality: Love

Family: Rose (Rosaceae)
Other Names: Arizona Rose. The name "rose" comes from an ancient root **wrod,** the modern translation of which is **vard,** an Old English word meaning "thornbush."

Where Found: ponderosa forests and shady streamsides
Elevation: 4,000' to 9,000'

Energy Impact (Chakra Correspondence): third and fourth chakras

Bach Flower Remedy: **Rosa canina** is one of Dr. Edward Bach's thirty-eight flower remedies. Wild rose is for the "apathetic" — "those who without apparently sufficient reason become resigned to all that happens, and just glide through life, take it as it is, without any effort to improve things and find some joy."

Key Rubrics for Positive Healing Patterns: beauty, compassion, devotion, freedom, protection, vitality

Key Rubrics for Symptoms and Patterns of Imbalance: apathy, avoidance, depression, dissociation, disinterest, grief, weariness

Other Rubrics: aliveness, anxiety, appreciation, brokenheartedness, celebration, cheerfulness, creativity, displaced, dreams, gratefulness, healing, heart chakra, joy, love, misery, motivation, pain, passion, release, resignation, solar plexus chakra, sorrow, suffering, surrender, vibrancy

Traditional Use
The rose began its long European history in Greece, where its legend goes back to the Greek historian Herodotus. Its cultivation then spread to southern Italy, and from there to Persia and China. For over 3,000 years the rose has been the "queen of flowers." People of all lands have honored and cherished the rose. Cleopatra enticed Mark Anthony knee-deep in rose petals on her palace floor to gain his affections. The Romans crowned bridal couples with roses, and Roman banquets were decorated with rose centerpieces. Roses were a sacred flower to Aphrodite, the Greek goddess of love and beauty. Even as early as the tenth century, rose water (made by placing rose petals in water) was prepared as a purification.

The Muslim conqueror Saladin had the Omar mosque purified in rose water upon entering Jerusalem in 1187. In the sixteenth century, an essential oil called an "attar" or "otto" was prepared from rose petals; its production has been a prominent industry in France ever since. The rose became known as the "gift of the angels" due to its safe, soothing healing qualities. Rose water became popular for cooking, and is an ingredient in a candy called "Turkish delight." Wine prepared from rose petals was made in ancient Persia, and rose petals have historically been used in jams, vinegar, and pies, and as a garnish.

American Indians gathered the wild rose for ornaments and for medicinal uses. Young braves picked wild roses for their brides. Wooden needles from the rose bush were used for leatherwork. They used rose petals with bear grease to treat mouth sores, and they made a rose powder to treat fever sores and blisters. Sore eyes were treated with rose rainwater (rose petals in rainwater), and the inner bark of the rose root was used to treat boils. Indians also cooked the seeds and ate them to relieve muscular pains. The leaves were made into a poultice and used to soothe insect stings.

Most parts of the Rose plant can be made into a wash to cleanse cuts, wounds, and infections and the petals can be used as a bandage. Medicinally, rosehips are recommended in a tea as a source of vitamin B-complex and vitamins A, E, C and rutin, and as a mild laxative and diuretic. Rose hips tea is also said to expel kidney stones. The petals offer a flavor to medicines in the form of a syrup and have been used in tonics and gargles to treat catarrhs, sore throats, mouth sores, and stomach problems. Flowers steeped in hot water are a good treatment for diarrhea and gallstones. The flowers also relieve nervousness. Rose petals have been used to ease uterine cramps and labor pains, and to soothe the mother after childbirth. Roses are considered cooling and are used for soothing the mind in Ayurvedic medicine.

The petals are also common in potpourris. One of the most popular, best-loved fragrances is that of the rose. Its soothing aroma is associated with love and femininity and is found in perfumes, bath oils, soaps, hair tonics, skin lotions, ointments, creams, and air fresheners. One of the most costly oils is made from damask roses, which are cultivated in Bulgaria. Chewing on the fresh petals offers a pleasant taste, and placing rose petals in a tub of butter or margarine for a few days makes a delightful spread.

Homeopathic Use
Unknown to author.

Positive Healing Patterns
- Promotes a vibrancy, a feeling of wanting to do something.
- Helps us go beyond our miseries to face the deepest pains, especially those associated with "heartaches," in order to release them and move forward in life.
- Offers devotion and love toward life and living.
- Helps us find our passion for being alive.

Symptoms and Patterns of Imbalance
Wild Rose may be an appropriate flower essence for those who
- Show disinterest or indifference in themselves and their life circumstances
- Feel they live in misery, whose heart is closed down, and who may have limiting conditions such as a terminal illness, a permanent disability, or the loss of a loved one
- Have chosen to live among the thorns and do nothing about it
- Are weary, lack vitality, and lack love and joy in living.

Features of the Original Flower Essence Water
Odor: especially sweet
Taste: especially sweet
Sensations: Soothes the throat and very pleasant to drink. Is quieting and soft.
Water Color: clear

Physical Makeup
Root, Stem, Leaves/Leaflets, Height: This rosebush grows from 1 to 3 feet high. The stems are brownish in color and many-branched. Its thorns are up to $1/4$ inch long and they are hooked. The bright green leaves are made up of three to nine toothed leaflets that are somewhat oval and range from $3/4$ inch to $2\ 1/2$ inches long.
Flower Color: Pink
Flowers: The flower carries a sweet rose fragrance and has five wavy petals. The petals grow up to $2\ 1/4$ inches wide. A clump of many yellow stamens with yellow anthers give a "loose" appearance as they emerge from the inside. The fleshy, rounded, orangish red hip is small, dry, and hard, and a one-seeded berry-like fruit follows.
Blooming Period: June through August

Doctrine of Signatures
- The wild rose bush has many branching stems that are covered with prickly thorns. I have walked in the wilderness and studied many wild rose bushes. The rose always seems to be protected amidst the thorns. When reaching for the rose, one must take great care to not get pricked by a thorn. This has always reminded me to have a clear intention and to pay attention when I pick a rose flower or when I'm near a rosebush. There have been times when I have gently pulled aside branches so that the flowers have more room to breathe. And although the flower seems to say "Leave me alone," at first, it also seems relieved to have received some attention and to have more space to grow in. The thorns are the plant's expression of protection; they represent our need to protect ourselves from life's blows, our pains, our challenges, and our suffering. The flower's destiny is to live among the thorns. As people, we will always have our challenges, pains, and suffering. The question is whether to accept that there can be anything else in the midst of these pains. Some people like living in their own misery and indifference as a form of protection: "Nothing can get better, so there's no need to hope for anything that might not happen." Yet the flower itself holds a vibrancy, an energy that says, "It's time to get up and go."
- The pink color of the flower corresponds to the heart or fourth chakra, the center that awakens our compassion, our love, our joy for life, and the way we love ourselves. It relates to loving emotions such as grieving the loss of a loved one, feeling a lack of love in life and for one's self, and perhaps feeling self-pity and despair with no interest in change one's circumstances.
- The clump of yellow stamens relates to the third or solar plexus chakra, which is associated with psychosomatic diseases caused by feelings that can break down and lead to apathy, dissociation from others, disinterest, indifference, lack of motivation, and lack of positive change.

- The wild rose bush represents a signature of abundance and growth, freedom and beauty. It demonstrates the power of our emotions and thoughts, once stuck among the thorns, to find a new freedom toward personal growth and change, and a true desire to make the best of living.

Yellow Monkeyflower (Mimulus guttatus)
Primary Quality: Trust

Family: Snapdragon or Figwort (Scrophulariaceae)
Other Names: Common Monkey Flower, Seep-Spring Monkey Flower, Spotted Monkey Flower, Yellow Monkey Flower, Mimulus
Where Found: Along mountain brooks, streams, wet meadows, marshy places, springs, and seeps with preference to the shade and flowing waters, from Montana to Alaska and throughout the West. Native to North America.

Elevation: 500' to 9,500'

Energy Impact (Chakra Correspondence): first, second, third, and fifth chakras

Bach Flower Remedy: One of the first three flower essences discovered by Dr. Bach, Mimulus is used to treat those who have known conditions of fears and anxieties, such as fear of darkness, life, other people, heights, death, being alone, illness and pain, animals, insects, accidents, and lack of physical security. Mimulus types tend to be physically sensitive,
timid, and shy, or they may appear cheerful or extroverted and hide their fears.

Key Rubrics for Positive Healing Patterns: cleansing, confidence, courage to
communicate, self-expression, self-assertiveness, self-respect, and trusting in one's self

Key Rubrics for Symptoms and Patterns of Imbalance: abandonment, doubt,
fear, restlessness, timidity, unworthiness, lack of confidence to communicate needs

Other Rubrics: anger, anxieties, avoidance, burden, calm, challenge, change, community, conscious, courage, criticism, darkness, defensiveness, emotions, expression, family, flow, focus, frustrated, mental, moodiness, overcome emotions, release, root chakra, self-confident, shy, solar plexus chakra, sorrow, spleen chakra, strength, support, throat chakra, uncertainties, water, worthiness, voice

Traditional Use
The roots were used as an astringent. The leaves taste somewhat buttery and were included in the diet of Native Americans, who also crushed the raw leaves and stems to use as a poultice to treat rope burns and wounds. The fresh plants can be eaten raw for salad and greens; the leaves can also be cooked as potherbs.
Homeopathic Use
Unknown to author.

Positive Healing Patterns
- Offers a gentle kindred spirit, giving courage and trust to believe in oneself.
- Helps us identify, understand, and face our fears and emotions.
- Gives the strength to focus mental faculties and to feel and act creatively in thoughts, feelings, and communication.

- Nurtures our communication skills and teaches us courage and honesty in everyday expression of ourselves, without fear of others. Gives us the confidence to speak our truths and to trust in who we are.

Symptoms and Patterns of Imbalance
Yellow monkeyflower may be an appropriate flower essence for those who
- Need to overcome known fears or emotions
- Have difficulty expressing their fears to others
- Tend to be timid, shy, and fearful of expressing themselves, or who hide behind false masks to cover their fears and their true expression of self
- Need courage and strength to know and understand themselves in order to fully embrace their fears and express their fears to others.

Features of the Original Flower Essence Water
Odor: subtle mellow smell, difficult to identify
Taste: subtle, smooth, mellow taste, more noticeable at the palate than the roof or opening of the mouth
Sensations: tingling on palate and back of tongue that moves downward
Water Color: clear
Physical Makeup
Root, Stem, Leaves/Leaflets, Height: The root is easily pulled and develops from fallen stems where they contact the soil. The smooth, hollow, bending stems root at the nodes and develop clumps on cliffs and along rocks in wet places. The stems grow from 2 inches to 3 feet tall.
The dark-green, oval, veiny leaves have toothed margins and grow in opposites. The smooth rubbery leaves grow up to 4 inches long, and the upper leaves are sessile.
Flower Color: Yellow with reddish orange spots
Flowers: The yellow flower with its red spots resembles a monkey's face, which is how the name of the flower was derived. The two-lipped slightly fuzzy flower is about $1^1/_2$ inches long and $1^1/_4$ inches wide, with five petals or lobes. The upper lip has two broad lobes that join to form a tunnel and point upward, and the lower lip has three broad lobes that point downward. Both the calyx and the corolla have reddish orange spots, with larger spots toward the outside and smaller spots toward the inside of the flower. Two pairs of threadlike stamens with yellow anthers emerge from the center.
Blooming Period: March to September

Doctrine of Signatures
- One signature of the plant is that it grows in or near flowing waters. Water represents emotions, moods, and gentle nurturing. Since the plant prefers waters that flow, this is an indication of the capability to move out of or flow with moods, thoughts, and feelings without staying stuck in them.
- The plant's ability to root at the stem's nodes and to develop clumps where it contacts the soil is a signature that demonstrates the connection made with earth, air, fire, and water. It also shows a strong desire to live near each other, in need of family and community support.
- The yellow color of the flower refers to the third or solar plexus chakra and mental faculties; it deals with thought patterns associated with feelings, such as uncertainties, fears, emotional upsets, and mood changes. The reddish orange spots indicate a connection with the earth as well as with fire and water, and demonstrate strength and courage. The spots get smaller as they go deeper inside the tunnel and eventually become hidden, resembling how we have to seek deep within ourselves to gather our courage and strength.
- The name of the plant has a legendary meaning of fear as related to the monkey. If you look at the monkeyflower from a side view, you will see that the flower petals express a mouthlike opening that appears shy and fearful, as if it is a monkey gaping with fear. The

funnel-like part of the petals
resembles a throat that opens into a mouth. I see these signatures as offering the ability to speak freely and to speak one's truths, without fear of shyness or dread.
- The flower petals are mildly flavored, yet they taste noticeably stronger at the palate. This signature refers to the throat and communication from deep within.

The plants/flower essences references in this article are written in the book *The Healing Power of Flowers* by Rhonda PallasDowney, of Woodland Publishing, and includes the following bibliography.

Complete bibliography available in the downloadable version of this book, for purchase at www.botanicalmedicine.org

Adolescent Angst: The Teenage Brain on Hormones

By Dr. Kenneth Proefrock

"Scientists used to think that the human brain development was pretty complete by age 10, that a teenage brain was just an adult brain with fewer miles on it."
Francis Jensen, neurologist, Boston Children's Hospital

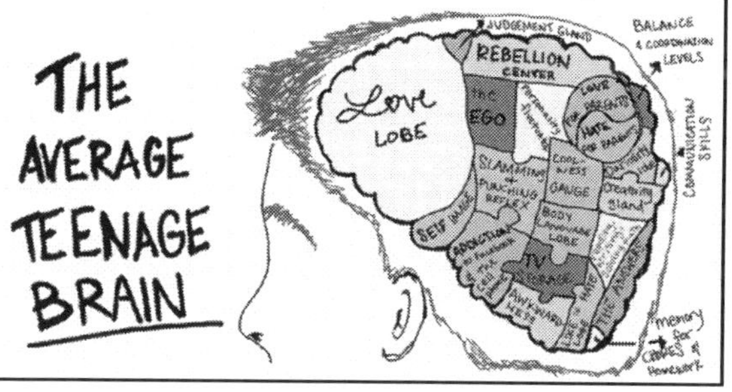

"*Neuroscience, the scientific study of the biology of the brain, has made great strides over the past decade in revealing that remarkable changes occur in the brain during the second decade of life. Contrary to long-held ideas that the brain was mostly grown up – "fully cooked" – by the end of childhood, it is now clear that adolescence is a time of profound brain growth and change.*"

Weinberger, Elevag, & Giedd, 2005

The cerebral cortex

Parietal lobe — Perception, spatial awareness, manipulating objects, spelling

Wernicke's area — Understanding language

Broca's area — Expressing language

Frontal lobe — Planning, organising, emotional and behavioural control, personality, problem solving, attention, social skills, flexible thinking and conscious movement

Occipital lobe — Vision

Temporal lobe — Memory, recognising faces, generating emotions, language

---

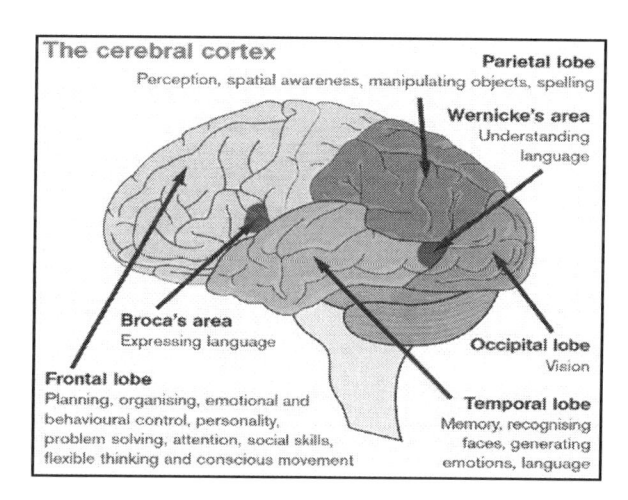

Brain architecture is shaped by rapid periods of over production followed by periods of pruning

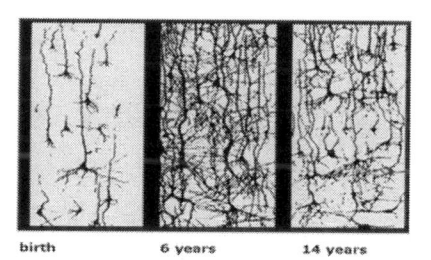

birth — 6 years — 14 years

During a neural growth spurt, axons and dendrites explode with new connections. Electrical activity triggered by *sensory* experiences, fine tunes the brain's circuitry, determining which connections will be retained and which will be pruned

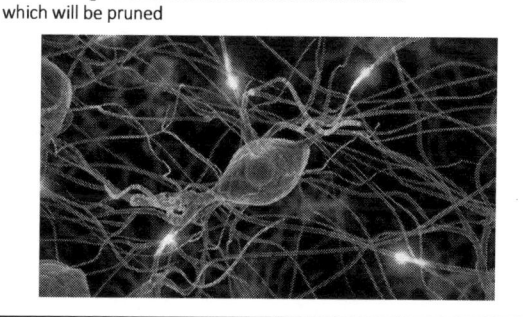

A reciprocal dynamic develops as millions of sensory nerves deep inside and covering the surface of the body contact the environment and abstract meaning from the sensory information gathered moment by moment. The structure of each major system of the brain is designed from a genetic blueprint. How each area unfolds is shaped by adapting to sensory, emotional and, later, abstract symbolic 'experiences'.

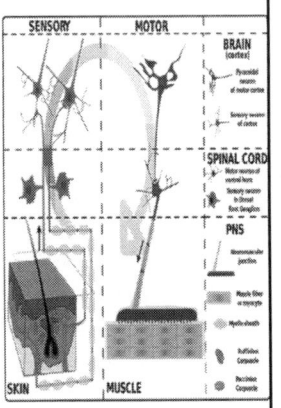

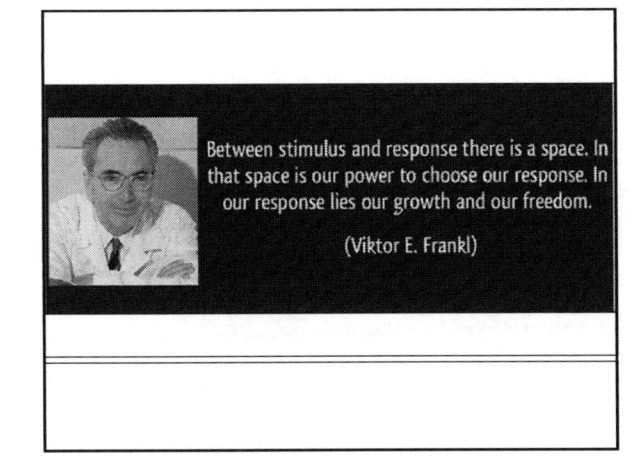

Between stimulus and response there is a space. In that space is our power to choose our response. In our response lies our growth and our freedom.

(Viktor E. Frankl)

Experience-Dependent Processes

- Experience-dependent plasticity is the process through which neural connections are created and reorganized throughout life as a function of an individual's experience.

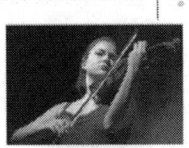

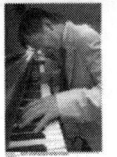

Intimate body contact, breastfeeding, being held, movement and affectionate play provide naturally a constant source of multi-sensory experiences that feed development. From this point of view not breastfeeding, no skin to skin contact, not being held, not moving and playing affectionately are forms of sensory deprivation, which affects neural remodeling.

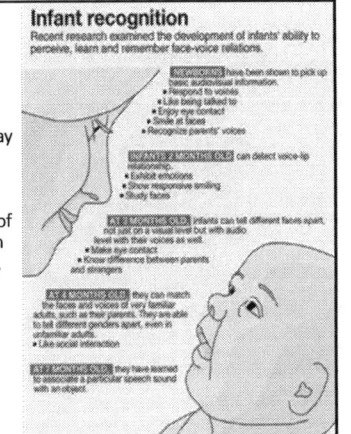

Conceptions of embodiment

Embodiment of Self
As long as you have the same body, you will be the same self

What happens when your body is changing daily?

We look to our social network for clues to our sense of self
—often at odds with familial network—
"I am not that anymore"

So many variables affect brain development, it is a miracle that we are as alike as we are...

How do You Know Who you are?

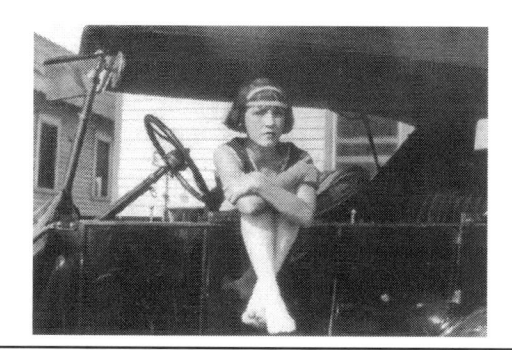

The leading edge of the peripheral cytoplasmic domain of a neuronal growth cone.

Microtubule behavior integrated over 10 minutes in the peripheral growth cone lamellipodium (top).

Axonal and Dendritic microtubules dynamically remodel, assembling and disassembling at an incredible rate (bottom).

The Subtleties of Consciousness and Sense of Self may well manifest right here…

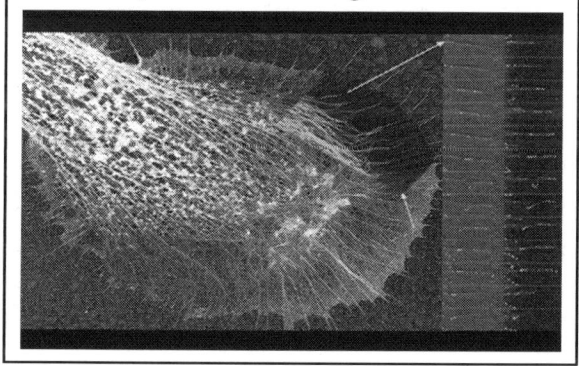

The quality of the neural architecture is dependent on the quality of the raw materials used to build it and the experiential feedback that affects remodeling

Chemical exposure, stress, lack of sleep, nutritional imbalances and temperature extremes reduce neurological richness

---

Memory

- Implicit Memory
  - A type of memory in which previous experiences aid the performance of a task without conscious awareness of these previous experiences
  - Didn't require focal attention to be encoded or retrieved
  - Fear - amygdala
- Explicit Memory
  - Conscious, intentional recollection of previous experiences and information
  - Requires focal attention to be encoded
  - Impaired when there is excessive catecholamines and cortisol
  - Hippocampus

Explicit and Implicit Memory

CORTEX: higher level thought processes, planning, problem solving

HIPPOCAMPUS: Explicit memory - governs recollection of facts, events or associations

AMYGDALA: Implicit memory – No conscious awareness (procedural memory – e.g., riding a bike and emotional memory - e.g., fear)

Chronic stress = overstimulation of the Amygdala, resulting in the release of cortisol, possible shrinkage or atrophy of the Hippocampus and Cortex, affecting memory and cognition, and leading to anxiety or depression.

Northern Illinois University Center for Child Welfare & Education - 2013 (Adapted from: Brunson, Lorang, & Baram, 2002)

Limbic System

The limbic system has been referred to as the emotional center of the brain. The amygdala is part of the limbic system. It is responsible for signaling to other brain areas in response to emotionally significant visual stimuli (Phan et al., 2002). The amygdala works more efficiently under stress

Hippocampus

The hippocampus is also part of the limbic system. The hippocampus is involved in learning and memory (McEwen, 2001; 2004). The hippocampus plays a critical role in explicit memory, which is concerned with facts and events (Sapolsky, 2003).

Basal Ganglia

Compulsive Difficulty linking natural consequences with choices
Increased violence and aggression
Seek immediate gratification
Loss of natural empathy and sympathy for others
Loss of willpower
Self-centered
Much more likely to engage in addictive behaviors

Amygdala Hijack

STRESS The amygdala and basal ganglia are affected oppositely of the prefrontal cortex in response to stress.

"Chronic stress appears to expand the intricate web of connections among neurons in our lower emotional centers, whereas the areas engaged in flexible, sustained reasoning begin to shrivel" (Arnsten, 2012, pg. 51).

Amygdala hijack is an immediate and overwhelming emotional response Out of proportion to the stimulus because it has triggered a more Significant emotional response

In low to moderate stress, the PFC inhibits the amygdala

In extreme stress, the amygdala shuts down the cortex

Evolutionary response—no time for thinking

The wave of neurotransmitters affects the basal ganglia differently than the prefrontal cortex. It works more efficiently. With the basal ganglia in charge, the individual becomes more compulsive and driven by immediate gratification. They essentially become more like animals driven by reward stimulation.

Brain Architecture is developed from back to front during adolescence

In order of developmental priority:
1) Physical coordination-Cerebellum
2) Emotion—Amygdala-midbrain
    passionate, committed but overreactive
3) Motivation-Nucleus acumbens-midbrain
    not always goal directed or prioritized
4) Judgment/Reasoning—Prefrontal Cortex
    Decisions, impulse control, forethought, planning

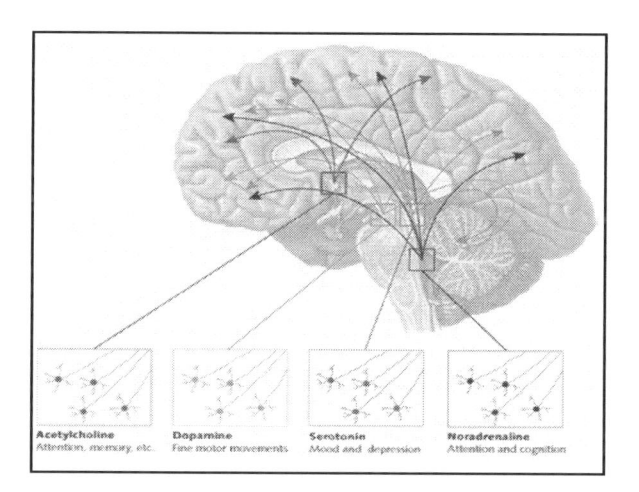

Acetylcholine

The most abundant neurotransmitter in the body
Present at neuromuscular junctions
Involved in the processing of information throughout the nervous system

Serotonin (5-HT) - summary

- 5-HT has a primarily **inhibitory** function & often acts in opposition to acetylcholine, noradrenaline & dopamine
- important role in sleep, mood, pain & temperature regulation
- also modulates cognitive function – especially memory, response inhibition & perception of emotional stimuli (e.g. faces)
- 5-HT levels can be manipulated by dietary interventions – **tryptophan supplements** increase 5-HT, **tryptophan depletion** reduces 5-HT
- **acute tryptophan depletion** (ATD) is associated with **negative mood** (irritability, aggression, depression)
- increased serotonergic neurotransmission is associated with **positive mood** & **pro-social behaviour**, and is the basis for action of **SSRI anti-depressants** (e.g. Prozac) & subjective effects of **psychedelic** drugs (LSD, Ecstasy)
- long-term, heavy use of Ecstasy is associated with increased incidence of **mood & sleep disorders**, and with **impaired cognitive function** (especially in **frontal executive & memory** tasks)

Cortisol—The Stress Hormone

- The wave of neurotransmitters activates the hypothalamus. The hypothalamus activates the adrenal cortex, which secretes cortisol.
- Cortisol can directly reduce the functioning of the prefrontal cortex by blocking transporters that clear norepinephrine and dopamine, therefore increasing the levels of neurotransmitters (Grundaman et al., 1998).
- Brief exposure to cortisol during 10 days was found to result in marked reduction of the neuronal complexity in the prefrontal cortex, causing less efficient information transmission

---

The amygdala and basal ganglia are affected oppositely of the prefrontal cortex in response to stress.

"Chronic stress appears to expand the intricate web of connections among neurons in our lower emotional centers, whereas the areas engaged in flexible, sustained reasoning begin to shrivel" (Arnsten, 2012, pg. 51).

The hippocampus has abundant glucocorticoid receptors and is very sensitive to the stress hormone cortisol (McEwen, 2001; 2004).

*Remember that the hippocampus has to do with remembering facts and events.

- Cortisol and stress suppress neurogenesis and cause neurons to retract (McEwen, 2001; Radley, 2005).
- Chronic stress can cause permanent damage to the hippocampus (McEwen, 2001).
- Animal models have shown that periodic stress responses over a period of three weeks were sufficient to cause neural retraction (Brown et al.,

Methylation Balance

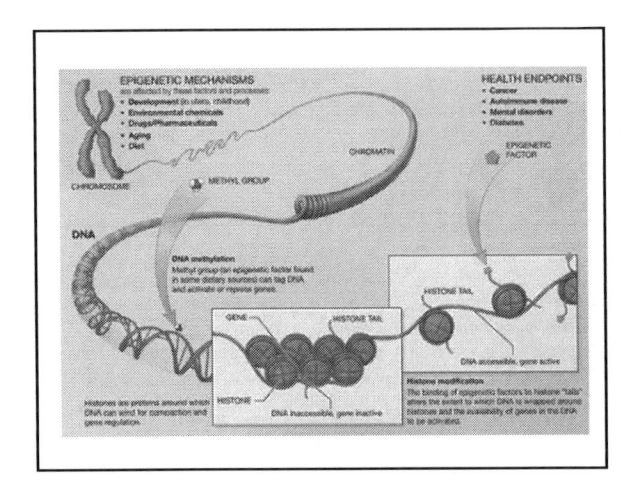

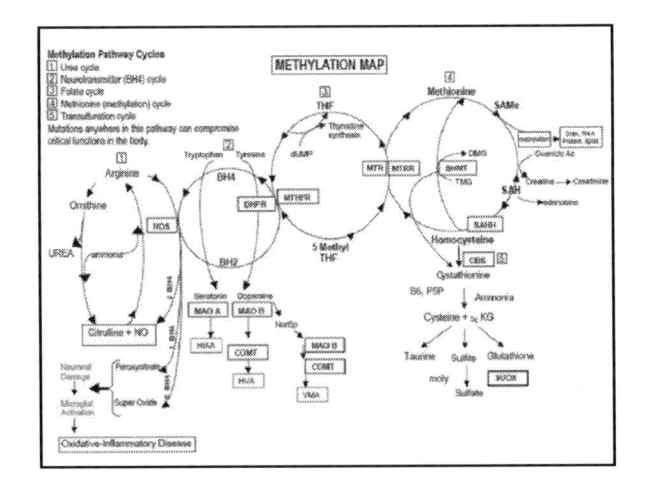

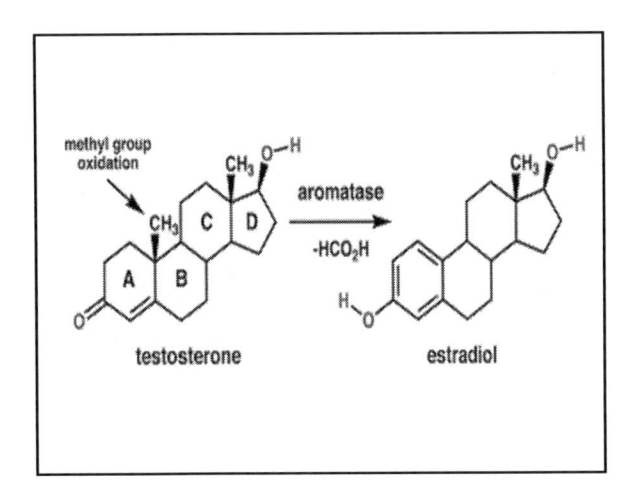

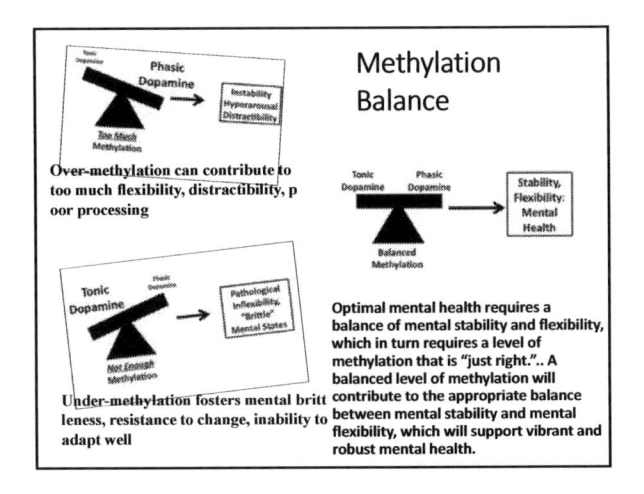

Over-methylation can contribute to too much flexibility, distractibility, poor processing

Under-methylation fosters mental brittleness, resistance to change, inability to adapt well

Optimal mental health requires a balance of mental stability and flexibility, which in turn requires a level of methylation that is "just right."... A balanced level of methylation will contribute to the appropriate balance between mental stability and mental flexibility, which will support vibrant and robust mental health.

Gastrointestinal Distress

Overarching Strategy:
Fortifying the Microbiome
  Fermented foods
probiotics
Stabilizing Mast cells
  Scutellaria biacalensis
  Albizia lebbeck
  Cromolyn sodium/Ammi visnaga
  Quercetin
Rebuilding compromised membranes
  Ulmus/Althea/Calendula
  Glycyrrhiza/glycyrrhizic acid
  L-Glutamine/N-Acetyl-L-Glutamine
Hyaluronic Acid

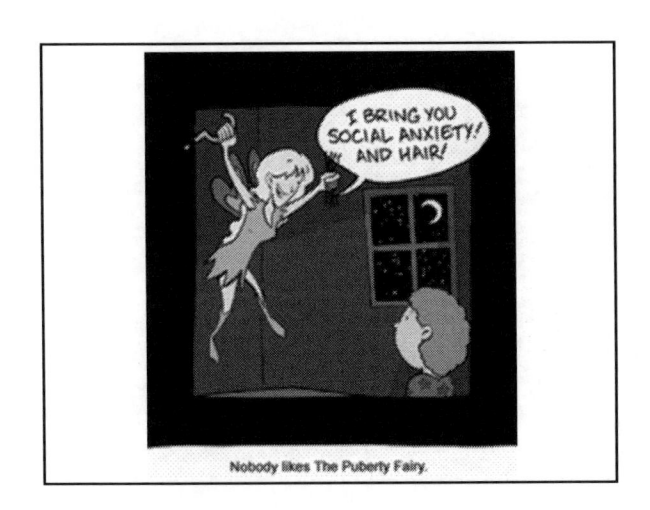

Nobody likes The Puberty Fairy.

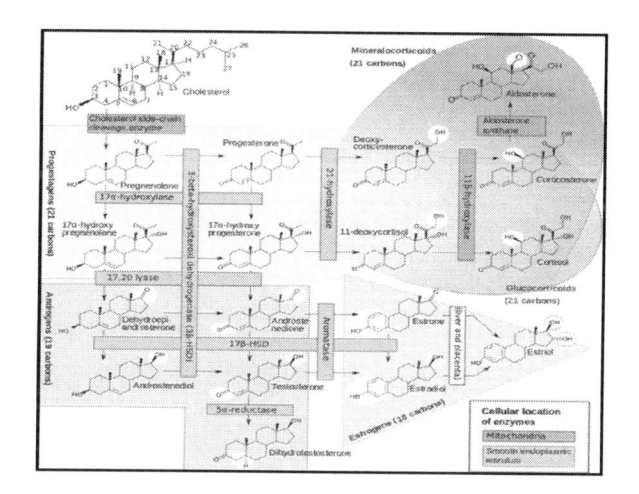

Cortisol—stress hormone
The wave of neurotransmitters activates the hypothalamus. The hypothalamus activates the adrenal cortex, which secretes cortisol.

Cortisol can directly reduce the functioning of the prefrontal cortex by blocking transporters that clear norepinephrine and dopamine, therefore increasing the levels of neurotransmitters (Grundaman et al., 1998).

Brief exposure to cortisol During 10 days was found to result in marked reduction of the neuronal complexity in the prefrontal cortex, causing less efficient information transmission (Brown et al., 2005).

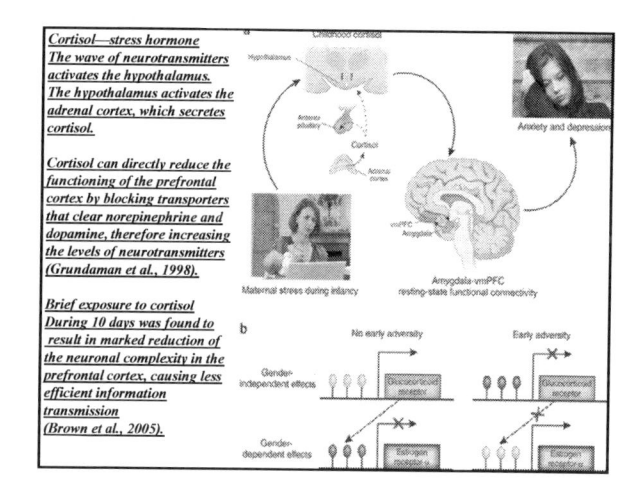

The prefrontal cortex is exquisitely sensitive to the detrimental effects of stress. In some cases, even mild uncontrollable stressors may lead to Compromised cognitive abilities, including deficits in working memory, cognitive flexibility, and emotional control.
(Arnsten, 2009)

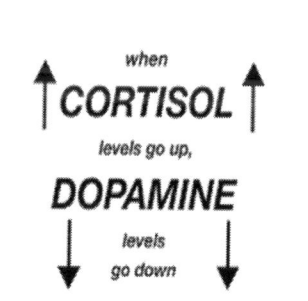

when ↑ **CORTISOL** ↑ levels go up,

DOPAMINE ↓ levels ↓ go down

Phosphatidyl-Serine
100 mg 3 times a day

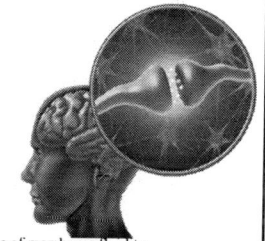

Phosphatidylserine prevents the decline in learning capacity that occurs with age
Prevents the decline in the
number of brain dendrites that occur as a result of inflammatory processes
Improvement and stabilization of mood

Involved in Myelin Sheath repair, maintenance of membrane fluidity
Improves the durability of neurotransmitter receptor sites   Facilitates dopamine release and acetylcholine production
Augments the function of Nerve Growth Factor (NGF) reduces seizure frequenc

---

Inositol

Direct architectural precursor to the phospholipids which comprise neural cell membranes.

Helps to maintain proper electrical energy and nutrient transfer across the neuronal cell membrane.

Establishes healthy, stable, neuronal cell membranes, which facilitate predictable and self-reflective nervous impulses.
1500-2000 mg/day

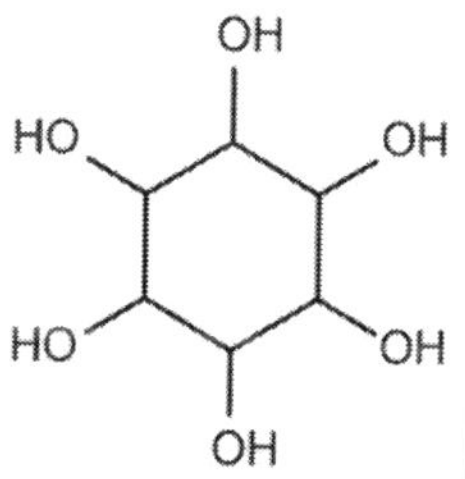

Choline

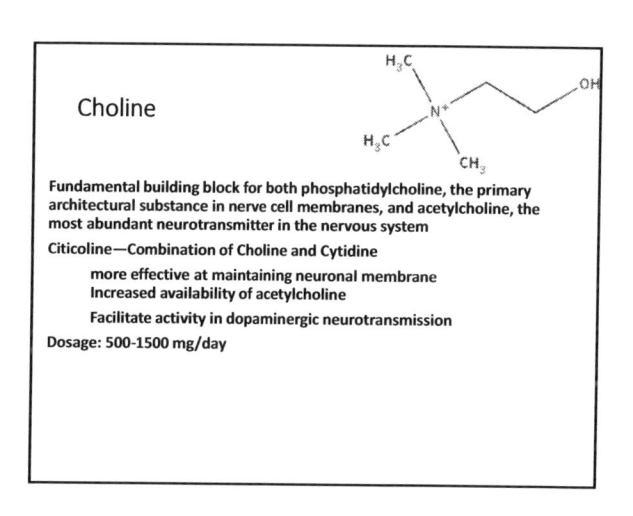

Fundamental building block for both phosphatidylcholine, the primary architectural substance in nerve cell membranes, and acetylcholine, the most abundant neurotransmitter in the nervous system
Citicoline—Combination of Choline and Cytidine
    more effective at maintaining neuronal membrane
    Increased availability of acetylcholine
    Facilitate activity in dopaminergic neurotransmission
Dosage: 500-1500 mg/day

Saw Palmetto-Serenoa repens

King's American Dispensatory (1898) says of the extract:
It is also an expectorant, and controls irritation of mucous tissues. It has proved useful in irritative cough, chronic bronchial coughs, whooping-cough, laryngitis, acute and chronic, acute catarrh, asthma, tubercular laryngitis, and in the cough of phthisis Pulmonalis. Upon the digestive organs it acts kindly, improving the appetite, digestion and assimilation. However, its most pronounced effects appear to be those exerted upon the urogenital tracts of both male and female, and upon all the organs concerned in reproduction. It is said to enlarge wasted organs, as the breasts, ovaries, and testicle, while the paradoxical claim is also made that it reduces the hypertrophy of the prostate

---

Serenoa repens-Saw Palmetto

Saw palmetto is used in several forms of traditional herbal medicine. Native American people used the fruit for food and as a treatment for urinary and reproductive issues. The Mayans drank it as a tonic and the Seminoles used the berries as an expectorant and antiseptic.

Inhibits conversion of Testosterone to DHT, decreasing severity of acne and hair loss.

Increases conversion of Testosterone to Estrogen

Dosage is typically 320 mg/day

Vincamine

Peripheral Vasodilator that improves blood flow into the brain
Derived from Vinca Minor—up to 50% of the indole alkaloids in the plant are vincamine.
Vinpocetine fraction of vincamine even more specific at improving memory
Dosage 5-50 mg/day
Consider an acetract of Vinca for tincture extracts.

Acetyl-L-Carnitine

- Acetyl-L-Carnitine (ALCAR) is an amino acid that has the capacity to cross the blood brain barrier, traverse the mitochondrial inner membrane of neuronal cells and provide a transport mechanism for fatty acids into the neuron, while it regenerates acetyl CoA in the cytosol
- Structurally similar to the neurotransmitter acetylcholine (Ach), and acts as an agonist when binding Ach receptors. It provides a supportive effect on choline acetyltransferase, the enzyme responsible for Ach synthesis and release.
- ALC is nutritionally protective to neurons, partly due its antioxidant nature as well as its ability to reduce glutathione and Co Q10, it also improves cerebral blood flow.
- ALC participates in cellular energy production, maintenance and repair of neurons and receptors.
- Clinically shown to improve axonal redundancy, increasing the numbers of connections between neurons
- Dosage 1500 mg/day

Selegiline

MAO, type B inhibitor

Dextro-amphetamine (Phenethylamine derived)

Developed in 1964-65 by Dr. Joseph Knoll as a "psychic energizer," designed to integrate some amphetamine-like brain effects with antidepressant activity

Profoundly neuro-protective from a wide range of chemical and physical assaults

Useful in Parkinson's Disease and drug resistant depression

Available as a transdermal patch--Emsam

Leonotis leonurus-Wild Dagga

Phenibut

Phenyl derivative of GABA-
B-Phenyl-Gamma Amino Butyric Acid (GABA)
Non-sedating Anxiolytic
The pharmacological effects of phenibut are similar to but less potent than baclofen
Phenibut exerts its effects by being an agonist at the metabotropic $GABA_B$ receptor and at higher doses also the ionotropic $GABA_A$ receptor.
Some studies suggest that phenibut can antagonize the effects of Phenethylamine (PEA) and has been shown to increase dopamine activity.

Glycine

Inhibitory neurotransmitter for the locus ceruleus release of norepinephrine

Smallest amino acid...life would never have occurred if not for glycine

Deeply calming

Stabilizes seizure conditions lessens intensity and frequency of seizures

Looks like sugar, tastes like sugar

Dosage: ½ tsp. 3 times a day 1 tsp before bed

Theanine

Water soluble amino acid derived from black and green teas

Non-sedating reducer of anxiety

Dosage 50 -200 mg 1-3 times per day

Improves the restorative quality of sleep

Acorus calamus-Vacha

The common Sweet Flag grows wild on the edges of swamps throughout North America, Europe, and Asia and has a long history of use as a medicine.

In Ayruveda, it is primarily applied to open the mind, improve concentration, clarity and speech. It is useful in treating mental depression and sluggishness. It is said that it actually scrapes away the stagnation from the subtle channels of the mind.

It has a long history of use in children with developmental delays, Vacha specifically nourishes the Sadhaka pitta, strengthening the ability of the mind to receive information and recall from memory. Small amounts of root powder are easily added to other teas or herbs, dosage is 1-3 grams per day. The Essential oil diffused into the environment is also helpful.

Sceletium Tortuosum--Kanna

Sceletium has been used in South Africa since prehistoric times as a social lubricant, mood elevator, and as a means to reduce anxiety, stress and tension, and times, as an appetite suppressant. In intoxicating doses it can cause euphoria, initially with stimulation and later with sedation. Long-term use in the local context followed by abstinence has not been reported to result in a withdrawal state. The plant is not hallucinogenic, and no severe adverse effects have been documented.

Historically *Sceletium* was chewed, smoked or used as snuff producing euphoria and alertness which gently fade into relaxation. If chewed in sufficient quantity *Sceletium* has a mild anaesthetic effect in the mouth, and is used by the San tribes for dental concerns and teething babies. Sceletium tea has a tradition of use for weaning alcoholics from alcohol. Fermenting Kanna makes it more potent.

Sceletium is rich in "mesembrine-type alkaloids" (mesembrine, mesembrenone, mesembrenol and tortuosamine) which are considered to be responsible for the psychoactive properties of the plant. The ability of these alkaloids to remedy CNS-related disorders is assumed to be, at least, related to their role in serotonin re-uptake inhibition and phosphodiesterase 4 (PDE4) inhibition. Mesembrine has been demonstrated to be a potent serotonin-reuptake inhibitor.

Sceletium Alkaloids
1–1.5% total alkaloids
Around 0.3% mesembrine in the leaves and 0.86% in the leaves, stems, and flowers of the plant.

Tortuosamine
Mesembrenone
Mesembrenol
Mesembrine

Sulbutiamine/Benfotiamine

Fat soluble forms of Thiamine (B1)

Lipophilicity allows for better neurological uptake and utilization

- Sulbutiamine has CNS effect reduces mental fatigue
- Benfotiamine has effect in peripheral nervous system
  - neuropathy
  - neuralgias

Centrophenoxine

Dimethylaminoethanol (DMAE) and parachlorophenoxyacetate (pCPA)

DMAE acts as a vasodilator at the synapse and is a precursor to choline in nerve tissue

pCPA is a dendritic growth factor and metabolic effector of nerve metabolism

Extremely effective at reducing lipofuscin accumulation in nervous tissue related to tissue level inflammation

Choline can ultimately become acetylcholine or phosphatidylcholine which bridges a magical gap between architectural compound and communication compound.

Allows for an increase in repair of the synapses that connect nerve cells to each other, under conditions that cause untreated synapses to deteriorate in number, structure and function.

Dosage 250-1000 mg/day

The racetams

- Piracetam
  - Facilitates activity in cholinergic, noradrenergic, and dopaminergic systems
  - Maintain neuronal receptor sensitivity (N-methyl-D-aspartate and cholinergic)
  - Protect neurons from toxins, removal of glutamate from freshly damaged tissue
  - Improves the fluidity of neuronal cell membranes
  - Reduces frequency and severity of seizures
  - Reduces long-term neuronal damage from hypoxia
    - Dosage: 850-2400 mg/day
  - Limits Neuronal damage—fosters early restoration of neural activity

---

The Other racetams

While all of the racetams are neuroprotective and all behave as cognitive enhancers, each one has unique effects

Pramiracetam-Fat-soluble, very well absorbed and very potent
- Dramatically increases choline uptake in the brain
- Typical dosages of 75-1500 mg/day

Oxiracetam-Water-soluble, like piracetam
- Far more protective against chemical and hypoxic insults
- Specifically helpful in social recognition conditions
- Typical daosage 1500-2500 mg/day

Aniracetam-The Swiss pharmaceutical company Hoffman-La Roche developed Aniracetam (1-p-anisoyl-2-pyrrolidinone) in the 1970s as a fat soluble alternative to Piracetam. It is faster acting, allows for better impulse control and has a notable anti-anxiety and anti-depressant effect.
- Typical dosages 1500-2500 mg/day.

Levitaracetam—Keppra—Conventional anti-epileptic drug...toxic and the only racetam to enjoy FDA approval

Sunifiram-perhaps the most potent, has a slight stimulating effect—dosage is 5 mg twice daily

---

Bacopa monniere--Brahmi

Brahman is the Hindu name given to Universal Consciousness, the name, Brahmi, is derived from the fact that this botanical can lead us to its understanding

Traditionally used to improve memory, learning ability and concentration. It has been used in Ayurveda for the treatment of mental illness, epilepsy, mania and hysteria. It is also a tonic and aid to recovery from exhaustion, stress and debility.

Often combined with milk or ghee to enhance its tonifying, nerve nourishing and cooling effects.

Combines well with Mucuna, Shankapushpi, and Ashwagandha for nerve regeneration.

Dosage is 2-6 gms per day

Mucuna pruriens- Kappi Kacchu

Traditionally used to treat tremors and spasms

Contains L-Dopa—in some cases up to 60%

Classically combined with *Tribulus terrestris*, intestinal MAO breaks L-Dopa down before it can be properly absorbed, Tribulus contains a number of harmala alkaloids that act as MAO inhibitors, improving L-Dopa effectiveness

Dosage: 60 mg-300 mg L-Dopa

The pharmaceutical carbidopa at 75 mg/day augments central nervous system L-Dopa effectiveness by inhibiting peripheral decarboxylation

Modulating Neuroendocrine Responses to Stress with Botanical Agents

Kenneth Proefrock NMD

Endocrine response is a redundantly controlled process

Pituitary Regulation of hormonal output is an interdependent and hierarchical process

Increased cortisol release serves to inhibit conversion of T4-T3 and suppresses LH/FSH levels...
One rationale for this effect is to preserve resources during stressful circumstances

Prolactin similarly suppresses FSH/LH and TSH...preserve resources while breast feeding

We are hard-wired for survival...

Stress begins with perception...Safe vs unsafe

Functions of the Prefrontal Cortex

- Responsible for executive functions (goal-directed behavior) which are:
  - Decision making
  - Initiation and control over the execution of deliberate actions
  - Targeting attention
  - Problem solving
  - Planning initiation of activities
  - Processes in Working memory
  - Social Behavior/Reasoning
- When an action is executed, the prefrontal cortex is informed, & allows appropriate monitoring
- Feedback-feedforward loop helps judge activity & reveals possible deficiencies

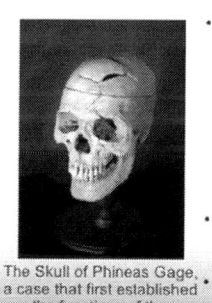

The Skull of Phineas Gage, a case that first established the functions of the Prefrontal Cortex

---

Reticular Activating System

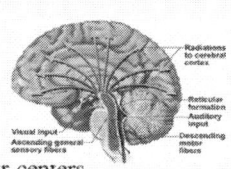

- Regulate balance & posture
  - relaying information from eyes & ears to cerebellum
  - gaze centers allow you to track moving object
- Includes cardiac & vasomotor centers
- Origin of descending analgesic pathways
- Regulates sleep & arousal
  - injury leads to irreversible coma
  - general anesthetics blocks this system
- Habituation – acts as a sensory filter

Reticular Activating System

Maintains the conscious, alert state that makes perception possible

Activated by sensory information being relayed through the cerebral cortex

Is your world a safe place or an unsafe place?

Consists of Brainstem reticular formation

Ascending projection system

Non-specific thalamic nuclei

Diffuse, Non-specific, Thalamocortical projections

NEURAL BASIS OF CONSCIOUSNESS

- Maintenance of consciousness depends on interaction between ascending reticular activating system (ARAS) and the cerebral hemispheres.
- ARAS extends from the lower border of pons to the ventromedial thalamus and then project to whole of the cerebral cortex.
- It receives collaterals from the spinothalamic and trigeminal thalamic pathways.
- Disorders that distort normal anatomical relationships of the midbrain, thalamus, and cortex appear to impair arousal.

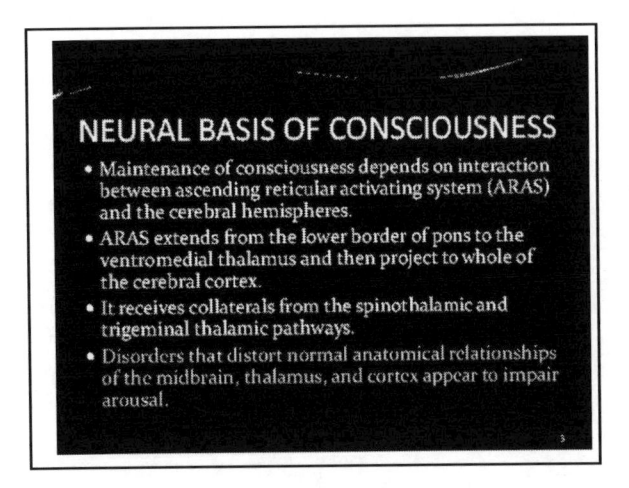

Locus Coeruleus

The primary hub of norepinephrine production

Very primitive and reflexive neural tissue—responds to environmental unsafeness

Locus Coeruleus

Heavily involved in learning and memory, especially avoidance learning

Implicit memory of unsafeness or discomfort supersedes explicit memories

Norepinephrine comes from dopamine—and at the expense of dopamine

---

As RAS provides evidence of perceived unsafeness,

Locus Coeruleus responds with a surge of norepinephrine

Hypothalamus then responds with a surge of CRF, causing ACTH output from Anterior Pituitary and a surge of cortisol from adrenal glands.

Cortisol is a glucocorticoid, it raises blood sugar, and induces a catabolic state of metabolism.

Insulin typically over responds to blood sugar changes and induces a

hypoglycemic state that is, in its turn, contributory to anxiety with another

norepinephrine surge.

This roller coaster goes on throughout the day, day after day.

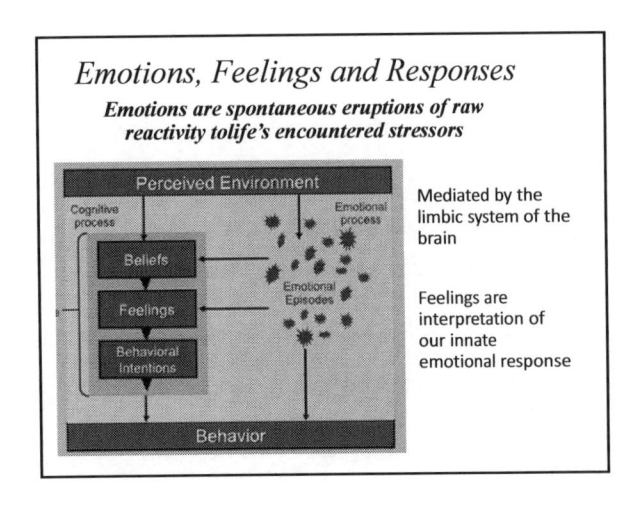

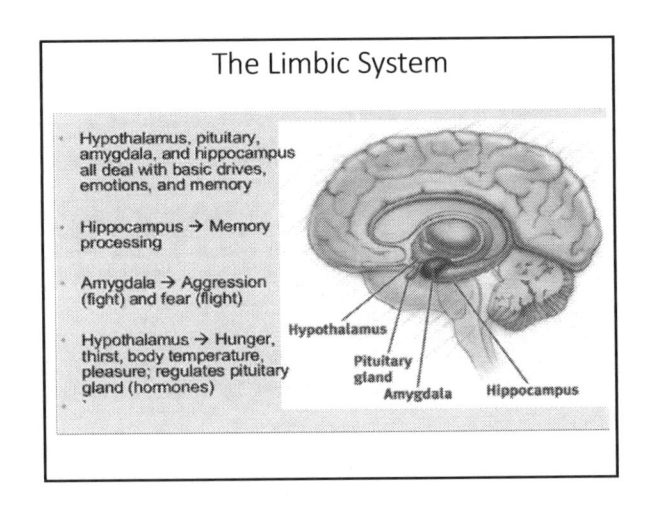

Emotions, Feelings and Responses

Emotions are spontaneous eruptions of raw reactivity to life's encountered stressors

Mediated by the limbic system of the brain

Feelings are interpretation of our innate emotional response

The Limbic System

- Hypothalamus, pituitary, amygdala, and hippocampus all deal with basic drives, emotions, and memory
- Hippocampus → Memory processing
- Amygdala → Aggression (fight) and fear (flight)
- Hypothalamus → Hunger, thirst, body temperature, pleasure; regulates pituitary gland (hormones)

The Limbic System

Hippocampus—Medial temporal lobe, involved in the formation of memories—Explicit vs implicit memory

Amygdala- Adjacent to the hippocampus and involved in emotional responsiveness—Reactive vs Responsive emotionality

Centers of emotion and learning—gratification/reward and aversion

Hippocampus

The hippocampus has abundant glucocorticoid receptors and is very sensitive to the stress hormone cortisol (McEwen, 2001; 2004).

*Remember that the hippocampus has to do with remembering facts and events.

- Cortisol and stress suppress neurogenesis and cause neurons to retract (McEwen, 2001; Radley, 2005).
- Chronic stress can cause permanent damage to the hippocampus (McEwen, 2001).
- Animal models have shown that periodic stress responses over a period of three weeks were sufficient to cause neural retraction (Brown et al.,

The Basal Ganglia

Cerebellum
- Major role in timing of motor activities and in rapid, smooth progression of movements
  - Monitors and makes corrective adjustments to motor plan

Basal ganglia
- Helps plan and control complex patterns of movement
  - Relative movement intensities, directions, and sequence
- No direct projections to lower motor neurons of skeletal muscle
- Movement influenced by regulation of activity of upper motor neurons

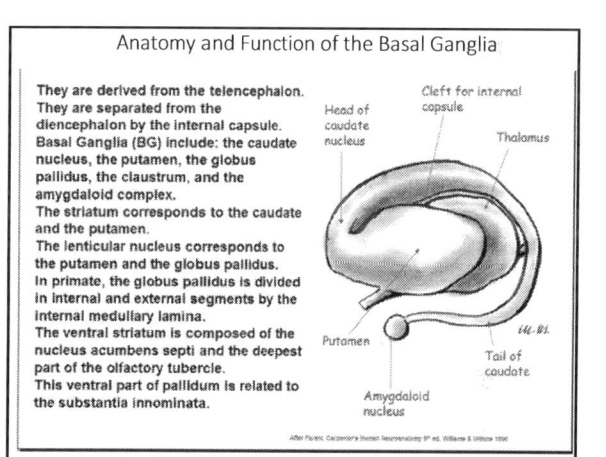

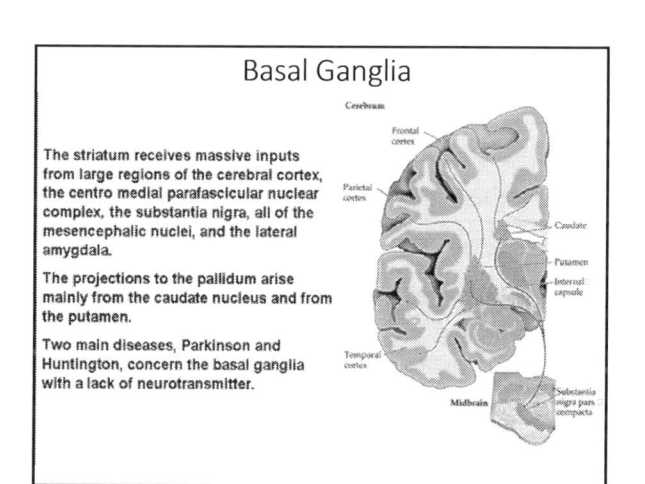

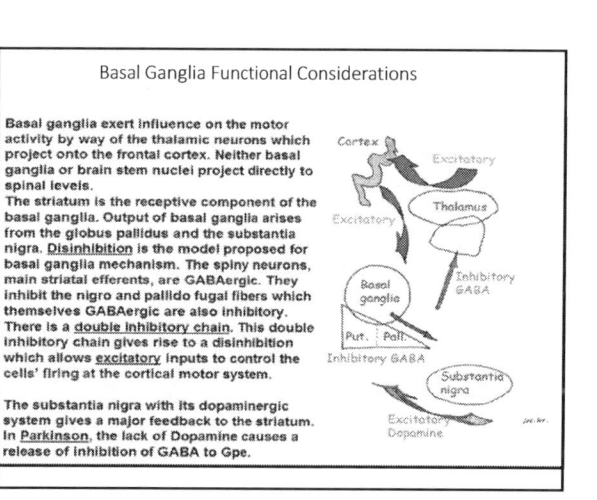

Anatomy and Function of the Basal Ganglia

They are derived from the telencephalon. They are separated from the diencephalon by the internal capsule. Basal Ganglia (BG) include: the caudate nucleus, the putamen, the globus pallidus, the claustrum, and the amygdaloid complex.
The striatum corresponds to the caudate and the putamen.
The lenticular nucleus corresponds to the putamen and the globus pallidus.
In primate, the globus pallidus is divided in internal and external segments by the internal medullary lamina.
The ventral striatum is composed of the nucleus acumbens septi and the deepest part of the olfactory tubercle.
This ventral part of pallidum is related to the substantia innominata.

Basal Ganglia

The striatum receives massive inputs from large regions of the cerebral cortex, the centro medial parafascicular nuclear complex, the substantia nigra, all of the mesencephalic nuclei, and the lateral amygdala.

The projections to the pallidum arise mainly from the caudate nucleus and from the putamen.

Two main diseases, Parkinson and Huntington, concern the basal ganglia with a lack of neurotransmitter.

Basal Ganglia Functional Considerations

Basal ganglia exert influence on the motor activity by way of the thalamic neurons which project onto the frontal cortex. Neither basal ganglia or brain stem nuclei project directly to spinal levels.
The striatum is the receptive component of the basal ganglia. Output of basal ganglia arises from the globus pallidus and the substantia nigra. Disinhibition is the model proposed for basal ganglia mechanism. The spiny neurons, main striatal efferents, are GABAergic. They inhibit the nigro and pallido fugal fibers which themselves GABAergic are also inhibitory. There is a double inhibitory chain. This double inhibitory chain gives rise to a disinhibition which allows excitatory inputs to control the cells' firing at the cortical motor system.

The substantia nigra with its dopaminergic system gives a major feedback to the striatum. In Parkinson, the lack of Dopamine causes a release of inhibition of GABA to Gpe.

183

The wave of neurotransmitters affects the basal ganglia differently than the prefrontal cortex. It works more efficiently. With the basal ganglia in charge, the individual becomes more compulsive and driven by immediate gratification. They essentially become more like animals driven by reward stimulation.

Stress

The amygdala and basal ganglia are affected oppositely of the prefrontal cortex in response to stress.

"Chronic stress appears to expand the intricate web of connections among neurons in our lower emotional centers, whereas the areas engaged in flexible, sustained reasoning begin to shrivel" (Arnsten, 2012, pg. 51).

Relevant Neurochemistry

The Mono-amines-
- Dopamine
- Serotonin
- Norepinephrine

GABA
Acetylcholine
- nicotinic
- muscarinic

Glutamate
Adrenalin/Epinephrine
Endorphins
Histamine

Mono-Amines

Neurotransmitters and neuromodulators that contain one amino group connected to an aromatic ring by a two-carbon chain.

All monoamines are derived from aromatic amino acids like phenylalanine, tyrosine, tryptophan, and the thyroid hormones by the action of aromatic amino acid decarboxylase enzymes.

Monoaminergic systems, i.e., the networks of neurons that utilize monoamine neurotransmitters, are involved in the regulation of cognitive processes such as emotion, arousal, and certain types of memory.

It has been found that monoamine neurotransmitters play an important role in the secretion and production of neurotrophin-3 by astrocytes, a chemical which maintains neuron integrity and provides neurons with trophic support.

Drugs used to increase the effect of monoamine may be used to treat patients with psychiatric disorders, including depression, anxiety, and schizophrenia

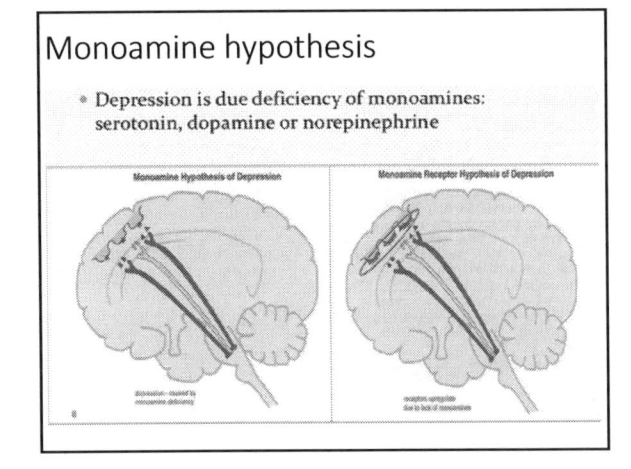

Monoamine hypothesis

- Depression is due deficiency of monoamines: serotonin, dopamine or norepinephrine

Serotonin $C_{10}H_{12}N_2O$

Serotonin is thought to be a contributor of feelings of well-being and happiness. It helps regulate sleep cycles alongside melatonin and also regulates Intestinal movement. Low levels o serotonin have been linked to depression, anxiety, and mental illness. Many antidepressants work by increasing levels.

Exercise and light levels can also have a positive effect on the levels of serotonin.

Dopamine $C_8H_{11}NO_2$

Dopamine is associated with feelings of pleasure and satisfaction. It is associated with addiction, movement and motivation. The feelings of satisfaction caused by dopamine can become desired, and to satisfy this the person will repeat behaviours that lead to release of dopamine. These behaviours can be natural, like eating and sex, or unnatural as in drug addiction.

Norepinephrine $C_8H_{11}NO_3$

Norepinephrine is a neurotransmitter that affects attention and reactionary responses in the brain. Alonsgside adrenaline, it is also involved in the fight or flight response. Its effect in the body is to contract blood vessels to increase blood flow velocity.. Patients diagnosed with ADHD are often prescribd drugs that help increase or stabilize fluctuationsin in, norepinephrine levels.

Adrenaline/Epinephrine $C_9H_{13}NO_3$

Adrenalin is a hormone produced in response to high stress or exciting situations. It stimulates an increase in heart rate, constriction of blood vessels, dilation of airways, an increase in blood flow into muscles and lungs. Provides a physical boost, heightened awareness and anxiety.

Fight or Flight

Gamma-AminoButyric Acid $C_4H_9NO_2$

GABA is the major inhibitory neurotransmitter in the brain, it slows and calms the firing of nerves in the central nervous system. Increased levels can improve mental focus and relaxation, deficiency can be a contributor to anxiety and epilepsy. Most anti-seizure drugs are GABA-ergic and act by increasing GABA or improving its action.

Acetylcholine $C_7H_{16}NO_2+$

Acetylcholine is the principle neurotransmitter involved in thought, learning and memory. It is heavily involved in neurologic processing of Information. In the body, it is involved in activating muscle activity. Damage to the acetylcholine producing areas of the brain has been linked to memory deficits associated with Alzheimer's disease. Acetylcholine is also associated with Attention, problem solving, and enhancement of sensory perception.

Glutamate $C_5H_9NO_4$

Glutamate is the most common neurotransmitter in the brain. It is involved in cognitive functions such as learning and memory. It also plays a regulatory role in neurological development and the formation of nerve synapses Glutamate is an excitotoxin in larger amounts, and can contribute to brain damage after traumatic injury or stroke.

Endorphins
Euphoria producers

Endorphins are a family of compounds formed from long chains of amino acids. They are released in the brain during exercise, excitement, pain and sexual activity, and produce a feeling of well-being and euphoria. At least 20 different types of endorphins have been identified in humans. Chocolate and spicy foods are also stimulators of endorphin release.

Relevant Neuro-Endocrinology

Cortisol
Estrogen
Testosterone
Progesterone
Insulin

CORTISOL IS CONSIDERED THE "STRESS HORMONE"

- The wave of neurotransmitters activates the hypothalamus. The hypothalamus activates the adrenal cortex, which secretes cortisol.
- Cortisol can directly reduce the functioning of the prefrontal cortex by blocking transporters that clear norepinephrine and dopamine, therefore increasing the levels of neurotransmitters (Grundaman et al., 1998).
- Brief exposure to cortisol during 10 days was found to result in marked reduction of the neuronal complexity in the prefrontal cortex, causing less efficient information transmission

---

Clinical Strategies for Modulating Stress Response

Improve the receptor sensitivity of cortisol receptors—
    botanical adaptogens
        Eleutherococcus, Rhodiola, Cissus, Schisandra…
Decrease the absolute amount of cortisol being released
        Behavioral changes-Objectification, Meditation
        Phosphatidylserine
Inhibit the enzyme that breaks cortisol down, effectively extending its biological
Lifespan
        Licorice-Glycyrrhizic Acid

Adaptogens

A category of herbs that help to restore and modulate the body's ability to maintain a calm, balanced and sustained energy and focus, while strengthening the body's resistance to internal and external stress and anxiety conditions

---

Stress **Recovery**

Leonurus cardiaca-Motherwort
Leonotis—Wild Dagga
Mitrogyna-Kratom
Piper Methysticum-Kava
Humulus lupulus-Hops
Pedicularis spp.
Piscidia erythrina-Jamaican Dogwood
Pedicularis spp.-Cobra's head, elephant's head

Phosphatidyl-Serine

Facilitates dopamine release and acetylcholine production
Augments the function of Nerve GrowthFactor (NGF) reduces seizure frequency
Dosage 100 mg 3 times a day

Improvement and stabilization of mood
Involved in Myelin Sheath repair, maintenance of membrane fluidity
Phosphatidylserine prevents the decline in learning capacity that occurs with age, trauma and long term cortisol exposure
Prevents the decline in the number of brain dendrites that occur as a result of inflammatory Processes
Improves the durability of neurotransmitter receptor sites

Inositol

Direct architectural precursor to the phospholipids which comprise neural cell membranes.

Helps to maintain proper electrical energy and nutrient transfer across the neuronal cell membrane.

Establishes healthy, stable, neuronal cell membranes, which facilitate
predictable and self-reflective nervous impulses.

1500-2000 mg/day

Albizia julibrissin

Albizia Flower supports a relaxed state of mind without causing drowsiness

Mimosa flowers have been used for two thousand years to support a peaceful state of mind.

It helps mitigate restlessness and anxiety and can relieve tense frustration.

Albizia can help with nervous irritability and nervousness due to common everyday overwork and fatigue.

It provides excellent mood support

Mitrogyna speciosa-Kratom

Kratom is a tropical tree in the Rubiace family Native to Southeast Asia, its foliage has been used for the treatment of diarrhea, the improvement of mood and affect and as a pain reliever. There are more than 40 compounds in kratom leaves, including Raubasine, an anxiety relieving alkaloid also found in Rauwolfia serpentina and corynantheidine, also found in Corynanthe yohimbe.

The chemical structure of the mitragynine alkaloids, mitragynine, mitraphylline, 7-hydroxymitragynine and mitragynine pseudoindoxyl. Incorporate a tryptamine nucleus which is likely responsible for their effect on the serotonin and adrenergic systems. In mitragynine, the phenolic methyl ether is considered to be a strong analgesic.

Sceletium Tortuosum--Kanna

Sceletium has been used in South Africa since prehistoric times as a social lubricant, mood elevator, and as a means to reduce anxiety, stress and tension, and times, as an appetite suppressant. In intoxicating doses it can cause euphoria, initially with stimulation and later with sedation. Long-term use in the local context followed by abstinence has not been reported to result in a withdrawal state. The plant is not hallucinogenic, and no severe adverse effects have been documented.

Sceletium tortuosum-Kanna

Historically Sceletium was chewed, smoked or used as snuff producing euphoria and alertness which gently fade into relaxation. If chewed in sufficient quantity Sceletium has a mild anaesthetic effect in the mouthand is used by the San tribes for dental concerns and teething babies. Sceletium tea has a tradition of use for treating alcoholism.

Fermenting Kanna makes it more potent.

Sceletium is rich in "mesembrine-type alkaloids" (mesembrine, mesembrenone, mesembrenol and tortuosamine) which are considered to be responsible for the psychoactive properties of the plant. The ability of these alkaloids to remedy CNS related disorders is assumed to be, at least, related to their role in serotonin re-uptake inhibition and phosphodiesterase 4 (PDE4) inhibition. Mesembrine has been demonstrated to be a potent serotonin-reuptake inhibitor.

Leonurus cardiaca- Motherwort

Mildly sedative, decreases anxiety and muscle spasms and tends to lower blood pressure

A predictable agent for the treatment of heart palpitations and rapid heartbeat
Improves fertility and reduce anxiety associated with childbirth, postpartum depression, and menopausal symptoms
If used in early labor it will ease labor pains and helps calm Nervous parents after childbirth.
Motherwort helps bring on a delayed or suppressed menstrual flow, e specially when someone is anxious and tense.

Leonotis leonurus-Wild Dagga

Wild Dagga shares the anxiety reducing alkaloid, leonurine, with Leonurus, but has about 10 times the amount, and is severa times more effective, even mildly narcotic. Its leaves enjoy a folkloric history of being smoked for partial paralysis and epilepsy and are believed to modulate the dopaminergic/noradrenergic system. Effective dosage/ historic corroboration suggests a dosage of 1 tablespoonful of chopped dried leaf and flower, added to 3 cupfuls of boiling water, boil for 10 minutes, allow to cool, strain and use clear liquid for both internal and external use. The flowers are the most potent product of the plant, often, we just eat them.

Acorus calamus-Vacha

The common Sweet Flag grows wild on the edges of swamps throughout the world and has a long history of use as a medicine. In Ayurveda, it is primarily applied to open the mind, improve concentration, clarity and speech. It is useful in treating mental depression and sluggishness. It is said that it actually scrapes away the stagnation from the subtle channels of the mind. It has a long history of use in exhaustion recovery. Vacha specifically nourishes the Sadhaka pitta, strengthening the ability of the mind to receive information and recall from memory. Small amounts of root powder are easily added to other teas or herbs, dosage is 1-3 grams per day. The essential oil diffused into the environment is also helpful.

Mucuna pruriens-Kappi Kacchu

Traditionally used to treat tremors and spasms
Contains L-Dopa—in some cases up to 60%
Classically combined with Tribulus terrestris, intestinal MAO breaks L-Dopa down before it can be properly absorbed, Tribulus contains a number of harmala alkaloids that act as MAO inhibitors, improving L-Dopa effectiveness
Dosage: 60 mg-300 mg L-Dopa
The pharmaceutical carbidopa at 75 mg/day augments central nervous system L-Dopa effectiveness by inhibiting peripheral decarboxylation

Bacopa monniere--Brahmi

Brahman is the Hindu name given to Universal Consciousness, the name, Brahmi, is derived from the fact that this botanical can lead us to its understanding

Traditionally used to improve memory, learning ability and concentration. It has been used in Ayurveda for the treatment of mental illness, epilepsy, mania and hysteria. It is also a tonic and aid to recovery from exhaustion, stress and debility.

Often combined with milk or ghee to enhance its tonifying, nerve nourishing and cooling effects.

Combines well with Mucuna, Shankapushpi, and Ashwagandha for nerve regeneration.

Dosage is 2-6 gms per day

Tribulus terrestris-Gokshura

Ayurvedic medicine regards the roots and fruits as cooling, demulcent and strengthening to the digestive and reproductive system—a source of beta-sitosterol
Traditionally used as a diuretic, anthelmintic, and expecto rant, heart disease and impotence.
Modern research suggests that it is effective for lowering li pids, reducing hypertension, lowering blood sugar, lowering
Hyperuricemia in patients with gout.
Rich in saponins, and harmane/norharmane alkaloids MAO inhibition

Glycine

Inhibitory neurotransmitter for the locus ceruleus release of norepinephrine

Smallest amino acid…life would never have occurred if not for glycine

Deeply calming

Stabilizes seizure conditions lessens intensity and frequency of seizures

Looks like sugar, tastes like sugar

Dosage: ½ tsp. 3 times a day 1 tsp before bed

Theanine

Water soluble amino acid derived from black and green Teas-Camellia sinensis

Non-sedating reducer of anxiety

Dosage 50 -200 mg 1-3 times per day

Improves the restorative quality of sleep

Improves focus and retention of information

Phenibut

B-Phenyl-Gamma Amino Butyric Acid

Phenyl derivative of GABA

Non-sedating Anxiolytic

The pharmacological effects of phenibut are similar to but less potent than the antispasmodic drug baclofen

Phenibut exerts its effects by being an agonist at the metabotropic $GABA_B$ receptor and at higher doses also the ionotropic $GABA_A$ receptor.

Some studies suggest that phenibut can antagonize the effects of Phenethylamine (PEA)

Phenibut has been shown to increase dopamine levels.

Dosage is 250-300 mg daily…can be addictive, can cause rebound anxiety

Selegiline

MAO, type B inhibitor

Dextro-amphetamine (Phenethylamine derived)

Developed in 1964-65 by Dr. Joseph Knoll as a "psychic energizer," designed to integrate some amphetamine-like brain effects with antidepressant activity

Profoundly neuro-protective from a wide range of chemical and physical assaults

Useful in Parkinson's Disease and drug resistant depression

Available as a transdermal patch--Emsam

Sulbutiamine/ Benfotiamine

Fat soluble forms of Thiamine (B1)

Lipophilicity allows for better neurological uptake and utilization

Sulbutiamine has CNS effect reduces mental fatigue

Benfotiamine has more effect in peripheral nervous system neuropathy neuralgias

Dosage of either is 100-200 mg/day

Schisandra chinensis-Five Flavor Berry

- *In China it is called "wu-wei-zi", which means five taste fruit due to its sour, sweet, bitter, warm, and salty taste.*
- *Chinese folklore holds that Schisandra can "calm the heart and quiet the spirit" and is considered an "astringent" to one's mind and spirit.*
- *An ornamental plant found throughout the world, Schisandra is a woody vine with oval pink leaves and bright red berries.*
- *The most deeply historical use can be recorded in China and Russia where it has been consumed for centuries as a tea to help with fatigue.*
- *We often mix it 50% in Glycine and dose it in 1 tsp doses*

Oneiromancy

The use of botanical preparations in order to produce or to enhance the divinatory nature of dreams.

The dream state is recognized as a way to understand the mystery of life, it is on that dream level that waking consciousness and the consciousness of your own being meet, it is an accepted method of contacting that realm of suprasensory reality and, therefore, capable of conveying messages and information otherwise unavailable.

There are several plants used by indigenous communities to obtain divinatory messages from dreams. Several puffball mushrooms (Lycoperdon spp.) are eaten fresh when they are very small and still solid by the Mixtec people before going to bed in order to facilitate prophetic or healing dreams, Calea zacatechichi and Salvia divinorum also fall into this category.

Silene capensis-African Dream Root

Indigenous to South Africa, this herb is regarded by Xhosa diviners as a sacred plant with the ability to induce remarkably vivid and prophetic dreamsThere exists very little to no documentation of the pharmacology of Silene capensis. It is suspected that its oneirongenic or dream-inducing activity is likely due to triterpenoid saponins contained within its roots.

Diviners prepare the root by powdering it, and adding about 1 heaping tbsp of it to about 1.5 liters of water and then briskly churning the mixture with a forked mixing-stick to produce a head of foam (the mixture will be reused over the next several days). Mouthfuls of the foam are swallowed until the diviner feels bloated or burps up some of the foam. Initiates will usually participate in ubulawu drinking sessions over the course of three consecutive days at the full moon.

We most often dose it at 200-300 mg before bed

Entada Rheedii-African Dream Herb

Used in South Africato commune with the spirit world by inducing vivid and prophetic lucid dreams. The inner meat of the seed is consumed, even smoked, just before bedtime.

Several active compounds, essential oils, saponins, fatty oils and psychoactive alkaloids have been discovered and cited in the literature.

Entada rheedii-African Dream Herb

The seed is considered to increases one's ability to fall asleep and stay asleep, as well as producing longer lasting, more vivid and memorable dreams. Other reports describe the seed's effect as an entry into the dream world, stating that the seeds promote increased awareness during REM sleep, making it easier for the sleeper to realize that they are dreaming and thus giving them an edge in achieving lucidity. Entada rheedii has a world-wide reputation for being a dream herb par excellence, comparable only to **Calea zacatechichi.**

Calea zacatechichi

Calea is a plant that is relatively well known and used medicinally in Oaxaca, Mexico. An infusion of the plant (roots, leaves and stem) is employed against gastrointestinal disorders, as an appetite stimulant, cholagogue, cathartic, antiparasitic, and also as a febrifuge.

In 1968, a Chontal native reported that the leaves of the plant were to be either smoked or drunk as an infusion to obtain divinatory messages. Whenever it is desired to know the cause of an illness or the location of a distant or lost person or item, dry leaves of the plant are smoked, drunk and put under the pillow before going to sleep. Reportedly, the answer to the question comes in a dream.

Calea zacatechichi

Zacatechichi is a Chontal name that means "bitter grass"

A favorite method of administration is by extraction with peppermint schnapps, it can be made 3:1 and dose it at ½-1 tsp. before bedI have also employed capsules with people, dosed at 3-5 capsules before bed, with mixed results.

The taste of the plant seems to arouse a more primal area of the psyche through the dream state.

The Troubled Trail of Testosterone:
Social Expectation and the Search for Meaning along the Edge of Libido

Dr. Kenneth Proefrock

Testosterone

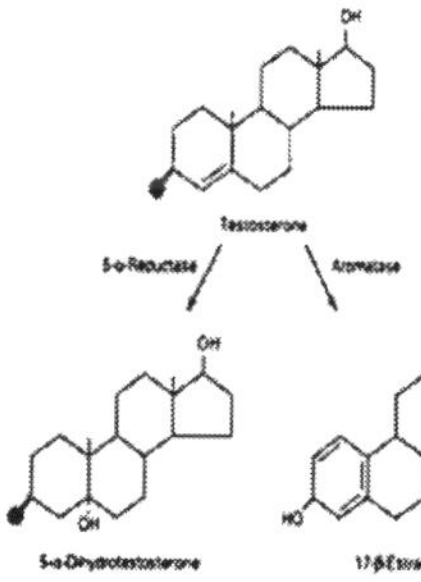

Testosterone is the prohormone for dihydrotestosterone and estradiol

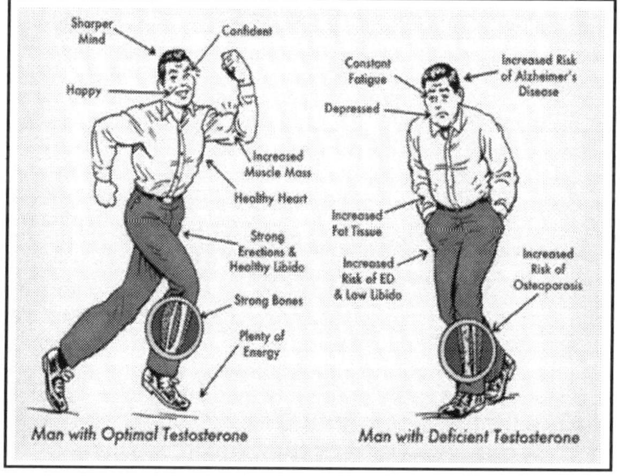

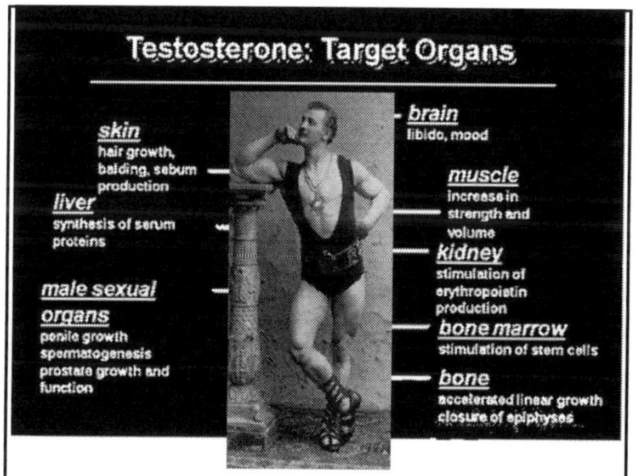

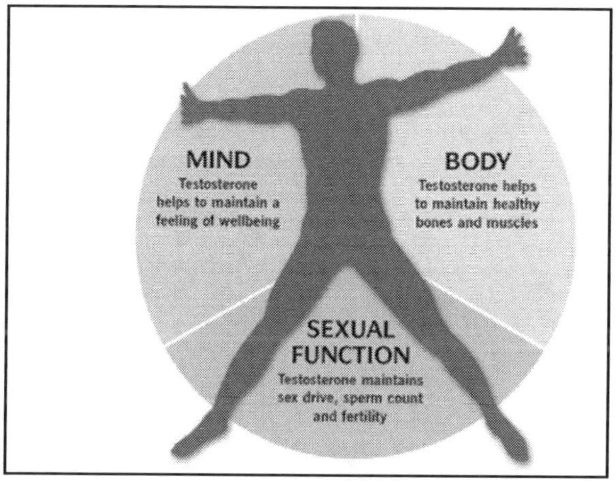

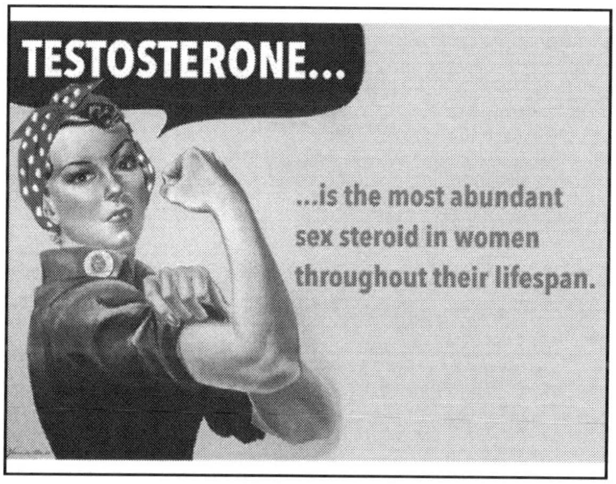

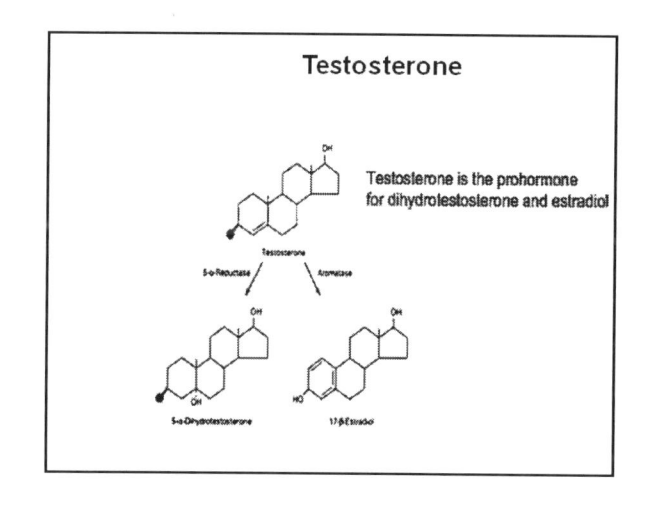

Testosterone in Males and Females

Testosterone increases endurance and strength in males and females

The average adult male testosterone levels are 20 times greater than the normal female levels

Men exposed to ovulating women maintain a consistently higher testosterone level than men exposed to non-ovulating women

At various times during the menstrual cycle, female testosterone levels may be 10-20 times higher than her estrogen levels

Same city partnered women have lower testosterone than women in long distance relationships

After watching a sexually explicit movie, men can experience a 35% increase in circulating testosterone

Testosterone in Males and Females

Men who have random sexual encounters or multiple partners experience large spikes of testosterone the morning after

Men with lower testosterone levels are more likely to get married than men with higher levels

Men who father children experience decreased testosterone and increased estrogen levels while their children are infants

Falling in love decreases a males testosterone levels and increases female testosterone levels

REM sleep increases nocturnal testosterone production

Low Testosterone Effects in Women

- Poor tolerance for exercise
- Dry skin
- Thinning skin
- Loss of motivation
- Loss of muscle tone in legs and arms
- Loss of bone density
- Weight gain around the abdomen
- Depression and/or anxiety

Elevated Androgen Levels In Women Are Linked To:

1. Acne
2. Obesity
3. Aggression
4. Temporal Balding
5. Menstrual Cramps
6. Uneven & Oily Skin
7. Excess Hair Growth
8. Deepening Of The Voice
9. Heavier Menstrual Cycles
10. Increased Risk For Chronic Illnesses

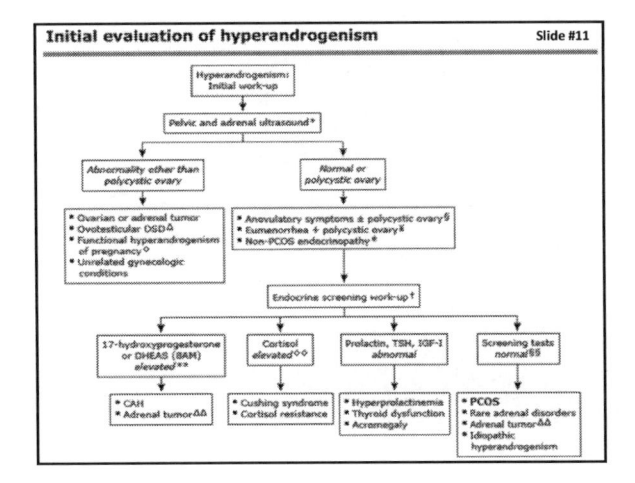

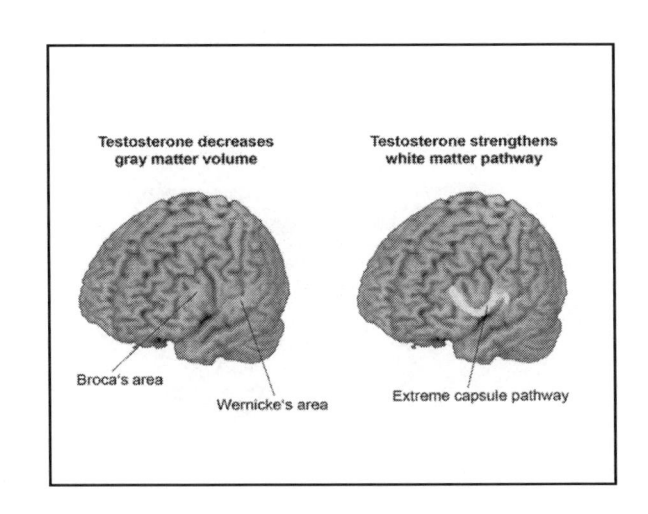

Initial evaluation of hyperandrogenism — Slide #11

Hyperandrogenism: Initial work-up → Pelvic and adrenal ultrasound*

- Abnormality other than polycystic ovary:
  - Ovarian or adrenal tumor
  - Ovotesticular DSD
  - Functional hyperandrogenism of pregnancy
  - Unrelated gynecologic conditions
- Normal or polycystic ovary:
  - Anovulatory symptoms ± polycystic ovary
  - Eumenorrhea ± polycystic ovary
  - Non-PCOS endocrinopathy

Endocrine screening work-up:

- 17-hydroxyprogesterone or DHEAS (8AM) elevated**
  - CAH
  - Adrenal tumor
- Cortisol elevated
  - Cushing syndrome
  - Cortisol resistance
- Prolactin, TSH, IGF-I abnormal
  - Hyperprolactinemia
  - Thyroid dysfunction
  - Acromegaly
- Screening tests normal
  - PCOS
  - Rare adrenal disorders
  - Adrenal tumor
  - Idiopathic hyperandrogenism

Testosterone decreases gray matter volume
Broca's area, Wernicke's area

Testosterone strengthens white matter pathway
Extreme capsule pathway

Normal Prenatal Development: The Brain

- Sexual differentiation:
  - Male:
    - Testosterone secreted into the blood reaches the brain
    - testosterone converted to estradiol and dihydrotestosterone in the brain
    - estradiol masculinizes the brain
  - Female:
    - alpha-fetoprotein binds to estradiol
    - prevents estradiol from entering the brain
    - protects female brains from being masculinized by estradiol

Prenatal Testosterone

- Presence of testosterone during critical period will cause rudimentary genitals of fetus to develop into male structures
- Testosterone acts in brain to promote development of neural systems for male sex drive and inhibit systems for female drive
- Absence causes development of female structures
- Stressful events experienced by pregnant rats reduce level of prenatal testosterone

Real Impact of Testosterone

Testosterone is not responsible for the masculinization of the male brain

- Estrogen, binding to estradiol sites, results in masculinization of a developing fetus
- Females do not produce surges of estrogen early in development and so miss the stage.
- Testosterone organizes masculinization early on and is needed again to trigger puberty
- Testosterone becomes estrogen within the nervous system

Developmental effects

- Prenatal development
  - Testosterone stimulates male pattern of development or reproductive system ducts and descent of testes
  - DHT stimulates development of external genitalia
- Development of male sexual characteristics
  - At puberty, they bring about development of male sex organs and development of male secondary sexual characteristics
- Development of sexual function
  - Androgens contribute to male sexual behavior, spermatogenesis and sex drive (libido)
- Stimulation of anabolism
  - Stimulate protein synthesis – heavier muscle and bone mass in men

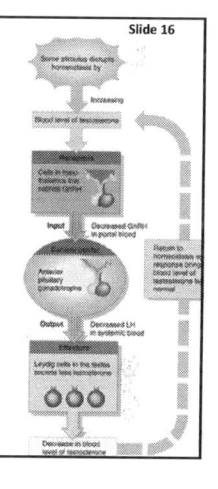

The Nature of Gender

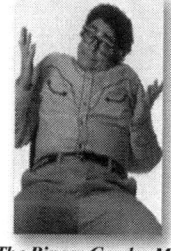

- The 23rd Pair
  - XX- Female
  - XY- Male
- The Prenatal Brain
  - More Testosterone for boys
  - Females exposed to more testosterone in the womb have more masculine features & are frequently treated more like boys
- Brain Development
  - Females have larger area for language
  - Males have larger area for spatial reasoning

The Binary Gender Myth
  heterosexuality = the only 'natural' tendency
  male=man
  female=woman

Reality: There is a Continuum of Gender LGBTI-neither Adam nor Eve

In fact, males are altered females....
  Everybody is a variation on the female theme!!
    Default gender is female
    Fully altered gender is male
    Partly altered is intersex
Intersex individuals differ physically from the "standard" male or female
  There is a wide range of potential variability here-including:
    ambiguous genitalia
    brain structures

Sexual Identity and Orientation

Nature versus Nurture?

We don't choose our genitalia...
  What about our sexual behavior?

There is ample evidence for Organization-Activation Mechanisms in the Brain
  Nonhuman mammals
  David Reimer
  Sexual activities of intersex individuals
  Human Brain structures related to gender tendencies
    (LaVey)

Organization-Activation Theory of Sexual Development in Mammals

"Organization"
  Sexual organization of body prior to birth
  Genetic (XX or XY)
  Hormonal effects on architecture
    (Quantitative testosterone effects)

"Activation"
  Maturation/Functionality at puberty
  Hormonal effects from Ovaries, Testes, and Adrenals

Sexual Development in Mammals

Sexual Behavior and the Anterior Hypothalamus

Sexual Dimorphism in the Hypothalamic Nuclei

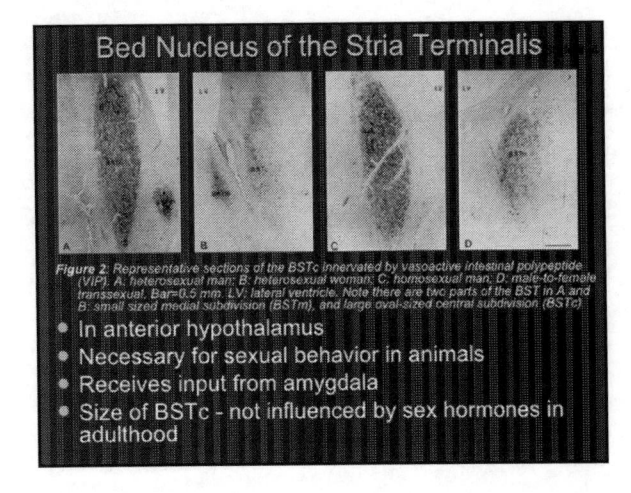

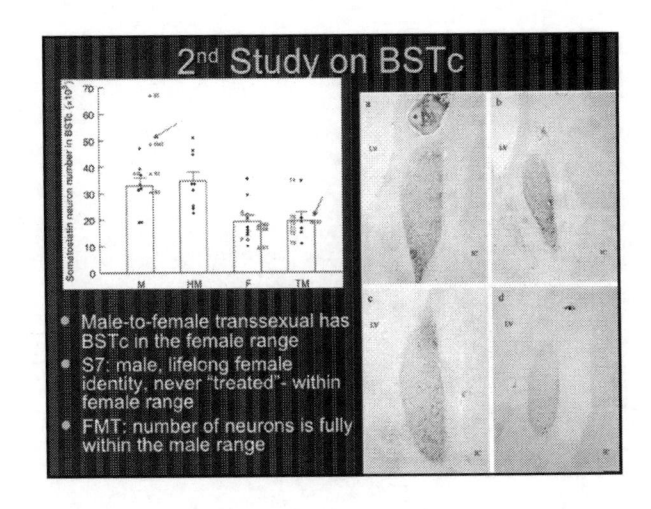

Bed Nucleus of the Stria Terminalis

Figure 2: Representative sections of the BSTc innervated by vasoactive intestinal polypeptide (VIP). A: heterosexual man; B: heterosexual woman; C: homosexual man; D: male-to-female transsexual. Bar=0.5 mm. LV: lateral ventricle. Note there are two parts of the BST in A and B: small sized medial subdivision (BSTm), and large oval-sized central subdivision (BSTc)

- In anterior hypothalamus
- Necessary for sexual behavior in animals
- Receives input from amygdala
- Size of BSTc - not influenced by sex hormones in adulthood

2nd Study on BSTc

- Male-to-female transsexual has BSTc in the female range
- S7: male, lifelong female identity, never "treated" - within female range
- FMT: number of neurons is fully within the male range

Genetics of Transexuality

Male to female-Linked with longer version of gene for androgen receptor that weakens testosterone effectiveness

Female to male-Linked with a gene variant that causes higher concentrations of androgens and estrogen in developing brain Structures

Biology of Sexual Orientation

Anthropology-Gay people everywhere, throughout history across the planet

Same sex behavior in nearly all animals

Simon LaVey-"The Sexual Brain"

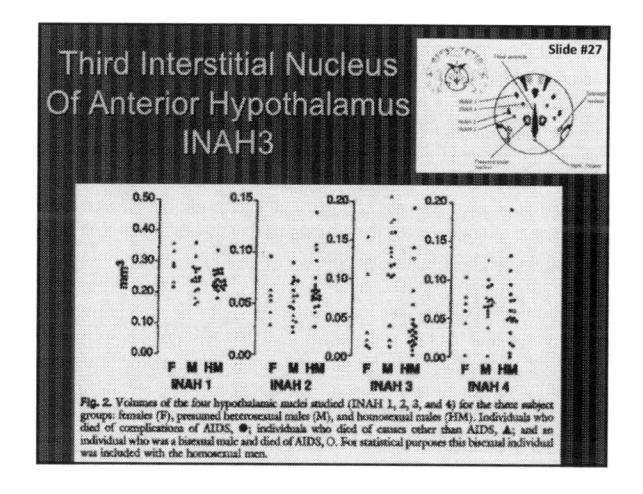

Third Interstitial Nucleus Of Anterior Hypothalamus INAH3

Slide #27

Fig. 2. Volumes of the four hypothalamic nuclei studied (INAH 1, 2, 3, and 4) for the three subject groups: females (F), presumed heterosexual males (M), and homosexual males (HM). Individuals who died of complications of AIDS, ●; individuals who died of causes other than AIDS, ▲; and an individual who was a bisexual male and died of AIDS, ○. For statistical purposes this bisexual individual was included with the homosexual men.

- 2nd human study confirmed INAH3 finding
- Gay sheep brains
  - About 8% of rams are exclusively homosexual
  - "Duplicated" human INAH3 work
- Sex pheromone effects in anterior hypothalamus correlate with sexual orientation
- Genetic components – gayness, lesbianism

Summation of Gender Science

- "...gender identity and sexual orientation are programmed or organized into our brain structures when we are still in the womb"
- "...since sexual differentiation of the genitals takes place in the first two months of pregnancy and sexual differentiation of the brain starts in the second half of pregnancy, these two processes can be influenced independently, which may result in extreme cases in transsexuality."
- "This also means that in the event of ambiguous sex at birth, the degree of masculinization of the genitals may not reflect the degree of masculinization of the brain."
- "There is no indication that social environment after birth has an effect on gender identity or sexual orientation"

Testosterone literally organizes neural circuits during adolescence that will stay with them throughout adulthood (Somerville & Jones, 2010). The effect of testosterone on the maturing brain predicts agnostic behaviors as an adult (Schulz & Sisk). Agnostic means aggressive, defensive, or combative. Higher than average levels of testosterone correspond to an **increased volume** in the amygdala (Cunningham et al., 2007; NuFeng et al., 2009).

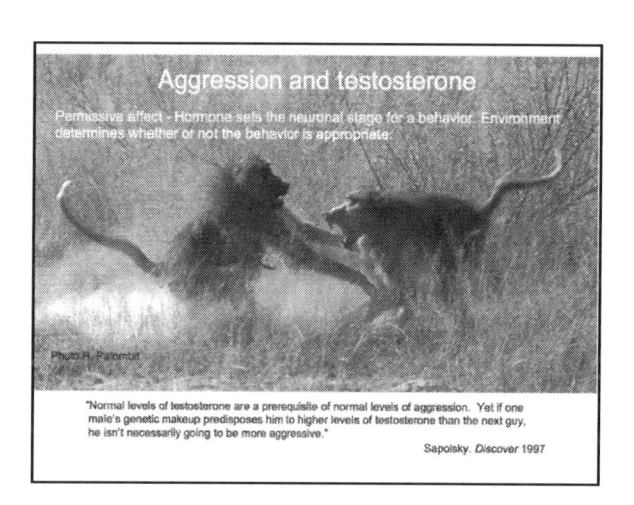

Aggression and testosterone

Permissive effect - Hormone sets the neuronal stage for a behavior. Environment determines whether or not the behavior is appropriate.

"Normal levels of testosterone are a prerequisite of normal levels of aggression. Yet if one male's genetic makeup predisposes him to higher levels of testosterone than the next guy, he isn't necessarily going to be more aggressive."

Sapolsky, *Discover* 1997

Aggression and testosterone

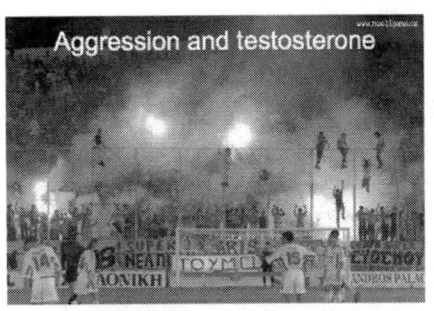

For one or two hours after the match, T levels of winners are high relative to those of losers (Mazur and Lamb 1980; Elias 1981; Campbell et al. 1988; Booth et al. 1989; also see Johnsen and Zuk 1995, for the same effect in male red jungle fowl).

T levels of winners are high relative to those of losers following chess matches (Mazur et al. 1992) and contests of reaction time, (Gladue et al. 1989; McCaul et al. 1992). Similar effects occur among sports fans who are not themselves participants in the physical competition. Following the 1994 World Cup soccer tournament in which Brazil beat Italy, T increased significantly in Brazilian fans who had watched the match on television, and decreased in Italian fans (Fielden et al. 1994).

NEUROCHEMISTRY OF AGGRESSION

☐ **TESTOSTERONE:** Influence of testosterone on overt aggression depends both on fetal and pubertal brain exposure.
- Rough correlations are found between testosterone levels and aggression, high testosterone is probably more predictive of dominance seeking and dominance winning than of violence.
- Finally, testosterone hardly acts in isolation. We are just beginning to uncover neurochemical interactions that help to explain the role of this hormone in inappropriate aggression.

☐ **CORTISOL:** Chronically low salivary cortisol levels are associated with disruptive, aggressive behavior in boys.
- Decreased cortisol levels have also been reported in adolescent girls with conduct disorder.
- Yet not all findings are consistent with this low-cortisol–aggression association

Libido

The energy of the sexual drive as a component of the life instinct

Humans are sexual beings

We have spiritual, relational and sexual aspects to our psyche, whether we are engaging in sexual activity or not

The brain is the primary sexual organ—sex begins and ends in the brain

Your sexual beingness impacts every aspect of your life, personal and professional

Hormones and Sexual Behaviour

- **Testosterone** increases libido in both men and women
- **Estrogen** is a key factor in the lubrication involved in female arousal and may increase sensitivity in the woman to stimulation.
- **Progesterone** mildly depresses desire in men and women as do excessive **prolactin** and **cortisol**.
- **Oxytocin** is involved in pleasurable sensations during sex and is found in higher levels in men and women following orgasm. It reinforces pleasurable activities

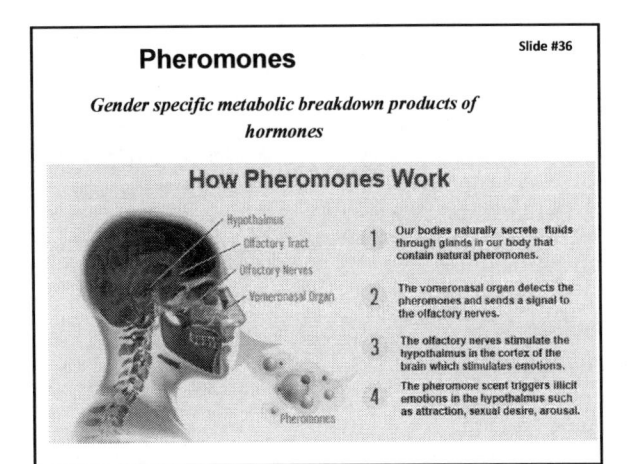

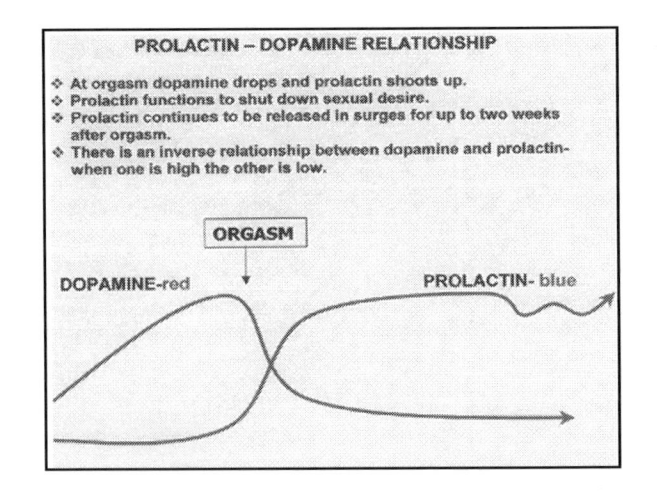

Pheromones

Gender specific metabolic breakdown products of hormones

How Pheromones Work

1. Our bodies naturally secrete fluids through glands in our body that contain natural pheromones.
2. The vomeronasal organ detects the pheromones and sends a signal to the olfactory nerves.
3. The olfactory nerves stimulate the hypothalmus in the cortex of the brain which stimulates emotions.
4. The pheromone scent triggers illicit emotions in the hypothalmus such as attraction, sexual desire, arousal.

PROLACTIN – DOPAMINE RELATIONSHIP

❖ At orgasm dopamine drops and prolactin shoots up.
❖ Prolactin functions to shut down sexual desire.
❖ Prolactin continues to be released in surges for up to two weeks after orgasm.
❖ There is an inverse relationship between dopamine and prolactin- when one is high the other is low.

DOPAMINE-red   ORGASM   PROLACTIN- blue

Oxytocin

- A posterior pituitary hormone
- Some refer to it as the "love hormone" because it plays an essential role in reproduction, feelings of attraction and interpersonal bonding
- Big surges of Oxytocin are involved in uterine contractions during orgasm and childbirth as well as in breast tissue during breast feeding
- It plays emotional roles in decreasing fear and promoting feelings of trust
- Oxytocin means "quick birth" and was the first endogenous polypeptide to be synthesized—"pitocin" is commonly used to stimulate contractions during childbirth—in super-physiologic doses
- Oxytocin release can be stimulated through sex, nipple stimulation, cuddling/being held in safety, chocolate, soft music, human touch/massage

---

When it comes to love

The story increases in complexity

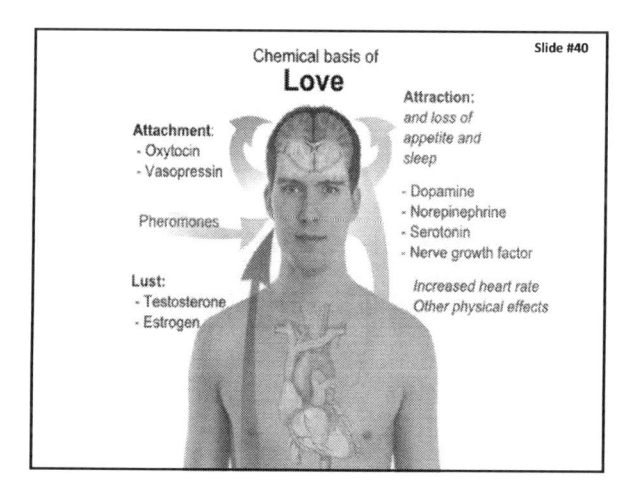

Chemical basis of Love — Slide #40

Attachment:
- Oxytocin
- Vasopressin

Pheromones

Lust:
- Testosterone
- Estrogen

Attraction:
and loss of appetite and sleep
- Dopamine
- Norepinephrine
- Serotonin
- Nerve growth factor

Increased heart rate
Other physical effects

Sexual Shame

- Sexual toxic soup: sex is all around us & we still don't have the language to talk about it » we internalize the message that...
- Man's number of sex partners is equal to his value as a male, that man must "perform", that "manhood" is constantly tested in bed...
- Pick up and take on the embarrassment or shame of the adults around them when something sexual is said or done
- Sex = a powerful and all-pervasive force in human life » most of shame triggers are associated with sex

---

Shame/humiliation about sexual feelings often come from religious moral imperatives

---

Arguably outdated social hierarchies affect libido for all genders

Hot terms in the current social order like rape culture, virginity, slut shaming, and sex workers create an atmosphere that is oppressive to half the population who have been historically treated as 'property' by the other half

The Search For Meaning

A new ethic is emerging, emphasizing such values as openness in personal relationships, hospitality, cooperation, tolerance, involvement, creativity, experimentation, spontaneity, participation, self-esteem, self-determination, self-transcendence, awareness of one's feelings and honesty in expressing them, consciousness, and self-responsibility in searching for a meaningful life.

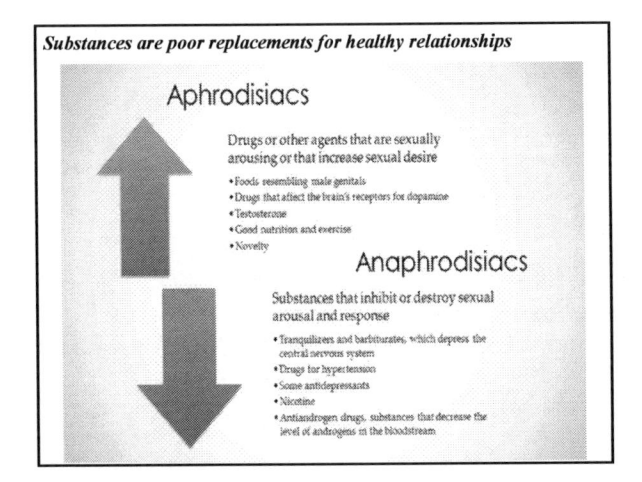

Substances are poor replacements for healthy relationships

Aphrodisiacs

Drugs or other agents that are sexually arousing or that increase sexual desire
- Foods resembling male genitals
- Drugs that affect the brain's receptors for dopamine
- Testosterone
- Good nutrition and exercise
- Novelty

Anaphrodisiacs

Substances that inhibit or destroy sexual arousal and response
- Tranquilizers and barbiturates, which depress the central nervous system
- Drugs for hypertension
- Some antidepressants
- Nicotine
- Antiandrogen drugs, substances that decrease the level of androgens in the bloodstream

---

Saw Palmetto-Serenoa repens

King's American Dispensatory (1898) says of the extract:
It is also an expectorant, and controls irritation of mucous tissues. It has proved useful in irritative cough, chronic bronchial coughs, whooping-cough, laryngitis, acute and chronic, acute catarrh, asthma, tubercular laryngitis, and in the cough of phthisis Pulmonalis. Upon the digestive organs it acts kindly, improving the appetite, digestion and assimilation. However, its most pronounced effects appear to be those exerted upon the urogenital tracts of both male and female, and upon all the organs concerned in reproduction. It is said to enlarge wasted organs, as the breasts, ovaries, and testicle, while the paradoxical claim is also made that it reduces the hypertrophy of the prostate

---

Serenoa repens-Saw Palmetto

Saw palmetto is used in several forms of traditional herbal medicine. Native American people used the fruit for food and as a treatment for urinary and reproductive issues. The Mayans drank it as a tonic and the Seminoles used the berries as an expectorant and antiseptic.

Inhibits conversion of Testosterone to DHT, decreasing severity of acne and hair loss, in males and females.

Increases conversion of Testosterone to Estrogen

Dosage is typically 320 mg/day

Cissus Quadrangularis

Cissus quadrangularis is sometimes referred to as Veldt Grape, Devil's Backbone, or Hadjori. Most sources suggest that the plant is native to Sri Lanka or India, but it can also be found throughout Southeast Asia, Africa and Arabia.

Cissus quadrangularis

Cissus quadrangularis is an ancient medicinal plant that was prescribed in the ancient Ayurvedic texts as a general tonic and analgesic, with specific bone fracture healing properties.

Modern research has shown it to have a glucocorticoid antagonistic effect. It is anabolic in its ability to offset cortisol effects, it helps preserve muscle mass as well as bone mass.

It has a relaxing effect and promotes deeper more restful sleep

Dosage is 100-500 mg 3 times a day
Some Ayurvedic texts recommend 3-6 grams per day in acute cases

Hemidesmus indicus
Anantamul, Indian Sarsparilla

Indian Sarsaparilla is regarded as a bitter, blood purifier, astringent, depurative, carminative, tonic, anti-syphilitic, anti-leucorrhoeic, antiviral, antifungal, antibacterial, anti-inflammatory, anti-diarrhoeal, anti-rheumatic, febrifuge and alterative.

This herb is useful in autoimmune/rheumatic conditions, chronic skin disorders (esp psoriasis), leucoderma, gonorrhoea, asthma, bronchitis, hemorrhoidss, jaundice and dysentery.

Clinically effective at helping people maintain an anabolic state.

Dosage is 1-4 grams/day

It is a pleasant smelling powder

Catuaba
A Guarani word that means "What gives strength"

Catuaba is not a distinct herb, although, most commonly it refers to Erythroxylum vaccinifolium or Trichilia catigua, and, less frequently, Anemapegma. A tea made from the bark of any of these trees is used in traditional Brazilian medicine as a central nervous system stimulant

It was believed that the original catuaba was Erythroxylum catuaba, but this tree has been described only once, in 1904, and it is not known today to what tree this name referred. E. catuaba is therefore not a recognised species (Kletter et al.; 2004).

Local synonyms are Chuchuhuasha, Tatuaba, Pau de Reposta, Piratancara and Caramuru. A commercial liquid preparation, Catuama, contains multiple ingredients, one of these being catuaba from Trichilia catigua.

300-600 mg 2-3 times a day

Pedicularis spp

Members of the Pedicularis genus are varyingly called "Lousewort" or "Wood Betony". The genus name, "Pedicularis", was established in 1753 by Linnaeus, and is derived from the Latin "pediculus", or "louse". The belief of the time had it that the plant was a treatment for or a source of infestation of lice in both people and cattle. "Wort" is from the Old English, "wyrt", meaning "plant" (Figwort, Spiderwort, Spleenwort).

Pedicularis species are used medicinally as a skeletal muscle relaxer and general sedative.

The flowers are often made into a tea or smoked.

Extracts of the flowers have a strong relaxing effect when smoked. When used in a smoking blend, they add a nice flavor and relaxing effect.

Oral Dasage: 100-300 mg 3-4 times a day

Tincture—10-30 drops four times a day

Sceletium Tortuosum--Kanna

Sceletium has been used in South Africa since prehistoric times as a social lubricant, mood elevator, and as a means to reduce anxiety, stress and tension, and times, as an appetite suppressant. In intoxicating doses it can cause euphoria, initially with stimulation and later with sedation. Long-term use in the local context followed by abstinence has not been reported to result in a withdrawal state. The plant is not hallucinogenic, and no severe adverse effects have been documented.

Historically *Sceletium* was chewed, smoked or used as snuff producing euphoria and alertness which gently fade into relaxation. If chewed in sufficient quantity *Sceletium* has a mild anaesthetic effect in the mouth, and is used by the San tribes for dental concerns and teething babies. Sceletium tea has a tradition of use for weaning alcoholics from alcohol. Fermenting Kanna makes it more potent.

Sceletium is rich in "mesembrine-type alkaloids" (mesembrine, mesembrenone, mesembrenol and tortuosamine) which are considered to be responsible for the psychoactive properties of the plant. The ability of these alkaloids to remedy CNS-related disorders isassumed to be, at least, related to their role in serotonin re-uptake inhibition and phosphodiesterase 4 (PDE4) inhibition. Mesembrine has been demonstrated to be a potent serotonin-reuptake inhibitor.

Glycine

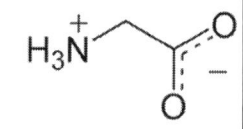

Inhibits release of norepinephrine from the locus ceruleus

Smallest amino acid...life would never have occurred if not for glycine

Deeply calming

Stabilizes seizure conditions lessens intensity and frequency of seizures

Looks like sugar, tastes like sugar

Dosage: ½ tsp. 3 times a day 1 tsp before bed

Schisandra chinensis-Five Flavor Berry

- *In China it is called "wu-wei-zi", which means five taste fruit due to its sour, sweet, bitter, warm, and salty taste.*
- *Chinese folklore holds that Schisandra can "calm the heart and quiet the spirit" and is considered an "astringent" to one's mind and spirit.*
- *An ornamental plant found throughout the world, Schisandra is a woody vine with oval pink leaves and bright red berries.*
- *The most deeply historical use can be recorded in China and Russia where it has been consumed for centuries as a tea to help with fatigue.*
- *Up to 19% of the fruits weight consists of lignans.*
- *Take 1 teaspoon a day as an infusion in fruit juice...up to ½ cup Schisandra in a 1-gallon pitcher of a dark fruit juice and allow it tosoak.*
- *We often mix it 50% in Glycine and dose it in 1 tsp doses*

Tribulus terrestris-Gokshura

Ayurvedic medicine regards the roots and fruits as cooling, demulcent and strengthening to the digestive and reproductive systems —a source of beta-sitosterol

Traditionally used as a diuretic, anthelmintic, and expectorant, for heart disease and impotence.

Modern research suggests that it is effective for lowering lipids, reducing hypertension, lowering bloodsugar, lowering uric acid in patients with gout.

Rich in saponins, and harmane/norharmane alkaloids—MAO inhibition

Dosage is 150-300 mg 3-4 times a day

Cimicifuga racemosa-Black Cohosh

Traditional Native American Botanical Medicine with a reputation for helping with female hormonal balance.

Also helpful in males for sexual function

Improves tone and relative health of reproductive organs

Black cohosh contains numerous chemical constituents, among them isoflavones which may mimic hormonal activity. It is useful for hot flashes, vaginal dryness, and some forms of depression

Dosage 1000-1500 mg/day

Piper methysticum-Kava Kava

Mild acting botanical hypnotic that reduces anxiety. This is a root that puts one's mind in a non-sedated place and makes it easier to be with other people, interestingly, the mind remains fully conscious even with fatal doses. It acts like a social lubricant, reduces inhibitions and facilitates deep connection between people.

I recommend an open fire and sharing a bowl of kava tea

300-1000 mg doses 1-2 times per day

"NATURE IS ALIVE AND TALKING TO US.

THIS IS NOT A METAPHOR."

-TERRENCE MCKENNA

Slide References

Slide #11
Mary Gayle Sweet, MD; Tarin A. Schmidt-Dalton, MD; and Patrice M. Weiss, MD, Virginia Tech Carilion School of Medicine and Research Institute, Roanoke, Virginia and Keith P. Madsen, MD, Joint Base McGuire-Dix-Lakehurst, New Jersey Am Fam Physician. 2012 Jan 1;85(1):35-43.

Slides #24 & 25
Dr. Veronica Drantz, PhD entitled "The Gender Binary and LGBTI People: Religious Myth and Medical Malpractice" that was given on April 9th 2015 at Northern Illinois University. the images Chapter 12 of "Christianity Is Not Great: How Faith Fails" John W. Loftus (editor), Prometheus Books, 2014

Slide #16
Tortora's Anatomy and Physiology, published Dec 2013 by John Wiley and Sons. Unit 5, chapter 28, The Reproductive System.

Slide #27
Simon LeVay, "The Sexual Brain" published by Bradford books in 1993.

Slide #40
Wikipedia's "Biological Basis of Love" entry

Three Ayurvedic Wonders — Ashwagandha, Brahmi and Holy Basil

Presentation & edits by JoAnn Sanchez
Research & writing by Sankar Jayavelu

Ashwagandha *(Withania somnifera)*

Introduction: Ashwagandha is a highly revered herb in the Indian Ayurvedic system of medicine. It is referred to as "Indian ginseng" and is used to calm the mind, relieve weakness, nervous exhaustion, build sexual energy and promote healthy sleep. It is considered as an important tonic because, rather than being over-stimulating, Ashwagandha has a sedative aspect. Therefore, it is very good for people who are "stressed-out". It is classified as an adaptogen, meaning that it assists the body's immune and other defense mechanisms and in coping with stress factors. It is known as the "promoter of learning and memory retrieval". The common name - Ashwagandha, means "strong as a horse," while the botanical species name, somnifera, means "restful sleep.

Family: Solanaceae

Common Names: Winter cherry, asgandh (Hindi), Indian ginseng

Description: Stout shrub, 1.5 m, with oval leaves, greenish to yellow flowers and scarlet berries.

Parts Used: Root

Ethnobotanical and historical uses: In Ayurvedic practice, Ashwagandha is considered as a rasayana, which means that it acts as a tonic to promote physical, mental health, longevity. This herb provides defense against diseases and adverse environmental factors. It is helpful for people with debility, nervous exhaustion especially due to stress, emaciation especially in children, convalescence after acute illness or extreme stress, chronic disease especially if inflammatory in nature like connective tissue disease and impotence due to devitalization.

Traditionally Ashwagandha has been used as an aphrodisiac, a liver tonic, an anti-inflammatory agent, an astringent, to treat bronchitis, asthma, ulcers, insomnia and senile dementia. Ayurvedic practitioners have used the roots of this plant for centuries to treat health conditions as diverse as tumors and arthritis.

Ashwagandha is believed to infuse fresh energy and vigor in a system worn out due to any constitutional disease like syphilis, rheumatic fever etc., or from over work and thus prevents premature decay. In India it was used frequently for low back pain. The decoction of dried root boiled down with milk and ghee is recommended for curing the sterility of women. It is to be taken for a few days soon after the menstrual period. In Africa the decoction of the root for is used for chills and colds and as a uterine tonic for women who habitually miscarry.

Body/mind energy: Ashwagandha is primarily sharp and pungent. This indicates that it is warming, raises the metabolism, stimulates digestion, clears mucus, and improves circulation. It decreases Vata and Kapha. It balances Vata and Kapha disorders.

Major plant constituents: The major components include alkaloids (isopelletierine and anaferine), steroidal lactones (withanolides, withaferins), saponins (including sitoindoside VII and VIII), and iron.

Therapeutic actions: Ashwagandha possesses adaptogenic, antitumor, tonic, immunomodulation, anti-inflammatory, increases hemoglobin, white blood cells and neutrophils. It is also used as a sedative, antiepileptic, hypotensive and enhances cognition.

Therapeutic applications: Ashwagandha is a calming adaptogen. It has been found to provide potent anti-oxidant protection, stimulate the activation of immune system cells such as lymphocytes and phagocytes and also counteract the effects of stress and generally promote wellness. Ashwagandha root was found to stimulate the thyroid, making it useful for hypothyroidism. It also can be useful for neck and back pain, restless legs syndrome (when taken with magnesium), and arthritis.

Combinations
1. For insomnia - Ashwagandha can be mixed with valerian root and oyster shell. As a general nerve tonic, especially for hypoglycemia or low blood pressure, Ashwagandha is combined with Goksura.
2. For chronic fatigue - Ashwagandha may be combined with Shatavari, Licorice, Amla or minerals especially calcium and magnesium.
3. In treating impotence - Ashwagandha can be used alone or combined with fried mucuna seeds. For weak lungs, Ashwagandha may be combined with Sida cordifolia(Bala)
4. To stimulate milk production in nursing mothers, Ashwagandha may be combined with Shatavari along with Licorice taken three times daily.
5. Ashwagandha is often combined with Long Pepper to increase its tonic effects.

Therapeutic dosing range:
1. Crude herb (Dried root and leaves): 3 to 10 grams
2. Fluid extract – Dried root (1:1): 2 to 8 ml
3. Standardized extract – Dried root (4.5 percent withanolides): 100 to 1,000 mg

Toxicology/potential adverse reactions: Ashwagandha is classified as a nontoxic herb contraindicated in pregnancy.
1. Very large doses, however, have been shown to cause gastrointestinal upset, diarrhea, and vomiting, such quantities may possess abortifacient properties as well, so caution should be taken during pregnancy.
2. The powder of Ashwagandha roots should not be used internally in cases of hemochromatosis (excess iron).
3. This herb is contraindicated for hyperthyroidism.

Safety Class: 2b – Not to be used during pregnancy.

Herb/Drug Interactions
1. Ashwagandha can enhance or increase the effect of barbiturates (any of a class of sedative and sleep-inducing drugs).
2. Prevents myelosuppressive activity of cyclophosphamide (cancer medication), azathioprine and prednisolone (mice).
3. Enhances antiepileptic effects of diazepam and clonazepam.
4. Used as adjuvant for benzodiazepine and opiate withdrawal (both empirical).

Contra indications: Not for use in pregnancy except under the supervision of a qualified health care practitioner.

Pregnancy and Lactation: In ethnobotanical literature, there are references of Ashwagandha uses as both an "abortifacient" and a "pregnancy tonic" The strength and accuracy of this information is difficult to assess given the lack of detail regarding dose, duration and plant part used. In a review of scientific literature, an animal study failed to detect any decreased number of pregnancies, change in litter size or fetal loss in rats when administered 100 mg/kg/day of an aqueous root extract for 8 months. Based upon this data, it may be that low doses of Ashwagandha pose little danger however clinicians should discuss the strengths and limitations of the evidence when counseling about its use in pregnancy.

In Ayurvedic medicine, Ashwagandha is traditionally used to promote lactation.

Review of scientific literature:

	Anti-Stress Activity
Study	GABA like activity in Withania somnifera
Results	Research conducted at the Department of Pharmacology, University of Texas Health Science Center indicated that extracts of Ashwagandha produce GABA-like activity which may account for the herbs anti-anxiety effects. GABA (Gamma Amino-Butyric Acid) is an inhibitory neurotransmitter in the brain. It function is to decrease neuron activity and inhibit nerve cells from over-firing. This action produces a calming effect. Excessive neuronal activity can lead to restlessness and insomnia, but GABA inhibits the number of nerve cells that fire in the brain and helps to induce sleep, uplift mood and reduce anxiety.

	Anti-inflammatory activity
Study	Research has explored the capacity of Ashwagandha to ease the symptoms of arthritis and other inflammatory conditions.
Results	Rats given powdered root of Withania somnifera orally one hour before being given injects of an inflammatory agent over a 3-day period showed that Withania produced anti-inflammatory responses comparable to that of a hydrocortisone sodium succinate.

	Anti- aging activity
Study	Ashwagandha was tested for its anti-aging properties in a double-blind clinical trial. A group of 101 healthy males, 50-59 years old, were given the herb at a dosage of 3 grams daily for one year.
Results	The subjects experienced significant improvement in hemoglobin, red blood cell count, hair melanin and seated stature. Their serum cholesterol decreased and nail calcium was preserved. Of the research subjects, 70% reported improvement in sexual performance and seated posture.

	Cardio protective activity
Study	Ashwagandha was evaluated with human subjects for its diuretic, hypoglycemic and hypocholesterolemic effects. Six type 2 diabetes mellitus subjects and six mildly hypercholesterolemic subjects were treated with a powder extract of the herb for 30 days
Results	A decrease in blood glucose comparable to that of a hypoglycemic drug was observed. Significant increases in urine sodium, urine volume and decreases in serum cholesterol, triglycerides and low-density lipoproteins were also seen.

	Thyroid-Stimulating activity
Study	An aqueous extract of dried Withania root was given to mice daily for 20 days.
Results	Significant increases in serum T4 were observed, indicating that the plant has a stimulating effect at the glandular level. Withania somnifera also may stimulate thyroid activity indirectly via its effect on cellular anti-oxidant systems. Ashwagandha may be a useful botanical in treating hypothyroidism

Brahmi (*Bacopa monniera*)

Introduction: Bacopa, also referred to as water hyssop and "Brahmi", has been used in the Ayurvedic system of medicine for centuries. Traditionally it was used as a brain tonic to enhance memory development, learning and concentration. Bacopa also provides relief to patients with anxiety or epileptic disorders. The plant has also been used in India and Pakistan as a cardio tonic, digestive aid and to improve respiratory function in case of bronchoconstriction.

Family: Scrophulariaceae (Figwort family)

Related species: There is a controversy about the identity of Brahmi and Gotu Kola. These two herbs possess similar properties (though Gotu Kola is a stronger diuretic and a weaker nervine). Bacopa is Brahmi in Kerala (South India) and Mandukaparani in North and West India. Centella asiatica is called as Brahmi in North and West India and Mandukaparani in Kerala (South India).

Description of the herb: Bacopa is a creeping perennial that grows in a wet soil, shallow water and marshy area. The fresh leaves are succulent and fleshy. They are "opposite" to each other on the stems. The beautiful tender white or purple flowers have 5 petals.

Parts used: Herb (Ariel portion) or whole plant.

Ethnobotanical and historical uses: Bacopa is an important ingredient in several Ayurvedic preparations, and is considered a Rasayana herb, which is believed to prevent aging, re-establish youth, prevent disease, promote healthy longevity, and strengthen life, brain, and mind.
In Nepal, the fresh juice is used to treat burns.
1. Leaves fried in clarified butter are taken for hoarseness.
2. Juice of the leaves is given in children who have diarrhea.
3. Ancient Sanskrit writing: - A powder composed of equal parts of Brahmi, Acorus calamus, Chebulic myroblan, root of Justica adhatoda and long pepper is given with honey in the hoarseness of pulmonary tuberculosis or a similar progressive systemic disease.
4. Oil is also prepared with this crude drug which is used in habitual headaches and to relieve brain fog.

Body/mind energy: Bacopa is strongly bitter, astringent and cooling in its energy.

Major plant constituents: Compounds responsible for the pharmacological effects of Bacopa include alkaloids, saponins and sterols. The memory enhancing effects of Bacopa extracts have been attributed to 2 saponins: Bacoside A and B. Bacopa's constituents are lipophilic and thus have the ability to cross the blood brain barrier. This explains the ability to affect the brain.

Therapeutic actions: The triterpenoid saponins and their bacosides are responsible for Bacopa's ability to enhance nerve impulse transmission. The bacosides aid in repair of damaged neurons by enhancing kinase(an enzyme that catalyzes the transfer of a phosphate group from ATP to a specified molecule) activity, neuronal synthesis and restoration of synaptic activity and ultimately nerve impulse transmission. Bacopa also increases the level of serotonin, a brain chemical known to promote, relaxation. Bacopa is used as a nervine tonic, mild sedative, mild anticonvulsant, cardiac tonic , respiratory system tonic, astringent, diuretic, anti-Inflammatory, antispasmodic effects on intestinal smooth muscle and can prevent or enhance healing of gastric ulcers. Bacopa also functions as antioxidant.

Therapeutic applications: Brahmi is wondrous Ayurvedic herb for the improvement of intelligence and memory as well as revitalization of sense organs. It is capable of imparting youthful vitality, longevity, clears hoarseness and improves digestion. Brahmi is indicated against dermatosis, anemia, diabetes, cough, arthritis, anorexia, dyspepsia, emaciation and insanity. This important herb assists in epilepsy mental illness, depression and helps with mental retardation by enriching intelligence.

Combinations:
1. A cup of Brahmi tea taken with honey before meditation is a great aid in the practice.
2. As a milk decoction the herb is a good brain tonic particularly if combined with Ashwagandha.
3. Taken with basil and a little black pepper, Brahmi acts as a febrifuge.
4. As a rejuvenate, it is traditionally prepared in ghee. Brahmi ghee is an important medicine for the mind and heart.
5. Bacopa can be paired with Gotu kola (Centella asiatica) for improving cognitive functions.
6. Improved neuroprotective effects were observed by combining Bacopa and Rosmarinus officinalis supercritical CO2 extracts.

Therapeutic dosing range:
1. 2 to 6 g/day of the dried herb
2. 4 to 12 ml/day of the 1:2 extract.
3. Leaf juice - 2 teaspoonful

Toxicology/potential adverse reactions: Human dose escalation and safety studies have indicated that bacopa is generally well tolerated with only minor and transient adverse events, primarily gastrointestinal discomfort reported.

Drug and supplement interactions: No case reports of suspected drug or supplement interactions were identified.

Precautions: An animal study with large doses (250mg/kg) of Bacopa demonstrated a decrease in sperm count and viability. All parameters were shown to return to normal several weeks after cessation of treatment.

Contraindications: No case of contraindications was identified.

Pregnancy and lactation: No information on the safety of bacopa in pregnancy or lactation is identified in the scientific or traditional literature.

Review of scientific literature:
Recent researches have focused primarily on Bacopa's cognitive-enhancing effects, specifically memory, learning and concentration and results support the traditional Ayurvedic claims.

Cognitive effects in Adults	
Study	Healthy subjects (aged 18-60 years) were treated with 300 mg/day Bacopa for 12 weeks.
Results	Significant improvements in learning rate, speed of information processing, and anxiety reduction were evident at 12 weeks but not at 5 weeks.

Cognitive effects in Children	
Study	40 children from rural India(ages 6-8) were divided into treatment and placebo groups of 20 children each Children in the treatment group received 1 Tsp Bacopa syrup (350 mg Bacopa powder/teaspoon) 3 times daily for 3 months. The placebo group received Syrup Simplex.
Results	A series of test measuring visual motor and perceptual abilities and memory span were administered at baseline and end of treatment. Significant improvements were noted in perceptual organization and reasoning ability.

ADHD in children	
Study	A double blind, randomized, placebo controlled trial of 36 children with diagnosed attention defict/hyperactive disorder was conducted over a period of several weeks. Dosage was 50 mg twice daily of standardized 20% bacosides), 17 subjects were given placebo.
Results	Evaluations were done at 4,8,12 and 16 weeks. A significant benefit was observed in Bacopa treated subjects at 12 weeks as evidenced on sentence repetition, logical memory and paired associated learning tasks.

Anxiety and Depression	
Study	Research using a rat model of clinical anxiety demonstrated a Bacopa extract of 25% bacoside A exerted anxiolytic activity compared to Lorazepam, a common benzodiazapene anxiolytic drug.
Results	Importantly the Bacopa extract did not induce amnesia, side effects associated with Lorzepam, but instead had memory-enhancing effect. Same effects were observed in a clinical trial of 35 patients with diagnosed anxiety.

Epilepsy	
Study	Research in animals shows anticonvulsant activity only at high doses over extended periods of time.
Results	Researchers determined that intraperitoneal injections of high doses of Bacopa extract (close to 50% LD50) given for 15 days demonstrated anticonvulsant activity. When administered acutely at lower doses (approaching 25% LD50), anticonvulsant activity was not observed.

	Gastro intestinal Disorders
Study	In vitro, animal and human studies have investigated the effects of Bacopa extracts on the gastrointestinal tract. In vitro studies have demonstrated direct spasmolytic activity on intestinal smooth muscle, via inhibition of calcium influx across cell membrane channels.
Results	This study suggests Bacopa extracts may be of benefit in conditions characterized by intestinal spasm such as irritable bowel syndrome (IBS). A recent in vitro study also demonstrated Bacopa extract's specific anti-microbial activity against Heliobacter pylori, a bacteria associated with chronic gastric ulcers. When the extract was incubated with human colonic mucosal cells and H. pylori it resulted in accumulation of prostaglandin E and prostacycline, prostaglandins known to be protective for gastric mucosa.

Holy Basil (*Ocimum sanctum*)

Introduction: Holy basil or Tulsi is one of the principal herbs used in the Ayurvedic medicine system, in which it is known alternately as "The Queen of Herbs," "The Incomparable One," and "The Mother Medicine of Nature." In the Ayurvedic tradition, Holy basil is revered as a "Rasayana," or an herb that, on its own nourishes a person's growth to perfect health and enlightenment. Today, Tulsi enjoys its well-deserved reputation as an adaptogen, herbs that to balance different bodily processes and assist in the body's response to stress. It holds a supreme place in the ancient Vedic scriptures and is integrated into daily life by Hindus through religious worship.

Common names: Holy basil, Tulsi, sacred basil, Tulasi

Latin name: Ocimum sanctum L., Ocimum tenuiflorum L.

Family: Lamiaceae/Labiateae (Mint Family)

Different species: There are at least 3 different types Holy basil. (1) Tulsi plant with green leaves is known as 'Rama Tulsi' (Ocimum sanctum) and is most commonly cultivated (2) Tulsi plants with purple leaves are known as 'Krishna Tulsi' (Ocimum sanctum) (3) Vana Tulsi (Ocimum gratissimum) is a perennial that is difficult to find in commerce. In India it grows in the wild.

Parts used: Leaves are generally used for medicinal purposes.

Ethnobotanical and historical uses: Tulsi is esteemed as the most sacred plant in the Hindu religion. This native and deeply revered mint of India has a history of use that dates back over two thousand years. It is said to be found in or near almost every Hindu house and temple throughout India. The plant is believed to offer protection from harm and it represents purity, serenity, harmony, fortune, happiness, and health. Traditionally, the plant's leaves and flowers are added to bath water or a bowl of water at the entrance of a home for guests to clean their hands in when they arrive.

Several stories surround the Tulsi plant in Hindu mythology. One tells of the plant as the transformed nymph Tulasi, the beloved of the Hindu deity Krishna. Another says that it represents the embodiment of the goddess

Lakshmi, who was the spouse of Vishnu. Many Hindu ceremonies, including weddings, poojas and funerals, involve Holy basil leaves.

A Holy basil plant often occupies a central location in the home, and many Indian women are said to begin the day by offering blessed water to the plant to promote the well-being of the household. Even now, virtually every traditional home has a Tulsi-plot right in front of it and people usually start their daily chores after worshipping it. Holy basil is known for treating skin conditions and deterring insects, including malaria carrying mosquitoes. The plant drives away mosquitoes.

A primary action of Holy basil is its ability to bring down fevers. A folk remedy for fever is to cook onion and Tulsi in coconut oil and apply this to the head of the person after the oil cools. Traditionally, Holy basil is used to strengthen the respiratory system. It is one of the main herbs for coughs and colds, especially asthma and bronchitis. Leaf juice is a domestic remedy for infantile cough, cold, bronchitis, catarrh, dysentery and diarrhea. Infusion of leaves is given in malaria, as a stomachic in gastric disease of children and in hepatic circumstance and also as a vermifuge.

Drinking the juice of Tulsi helps affections of skin disease, such as itches, ringworm, leprosy. Dried plant in decoction is a domestic remedy for catarrh, bronchitis and diarrhea. Leaf juice poured into the ear is considered first-rate remedy for earache.

Body/mind energy: Holy basil is pungent, sweet, and warm. It is useful in kapha-vata disorders.

Major plant constituents: The compounds in Holy basil leaf include eugenol (a volatile oil that is the main compound in clove), ursolic acid (a triterpenoid), rosmarinic acid (a phenylpropanoid), ocimumoside A and B, and ocimarin. Ursolic acid is one of the cosmetic industry's latest favorites because it quickly heals the skin, returns elasticity and removes wrinkles. Ursolic acid is also antimicrobial, and antiviral. Tulsi contains Vitamin A and C, calcium, zinc and iron.

Therapeutic actions: Tulsi is an adaptogen, expectorant, demulcent, aromatic, carminative, antipyretic, diaphoretic, antiemetic, hypolipidemic and antistress.

Therapeutic applications of Holy basil:

External uses: Holy basil has insecticidal, deodorant and stimulant actions. The paste of the leaves is useful in chronic ulcers, edema and pain. Scrubbing of the juice on the skin improves the intradermal circulation.
Respiratory system: Tulsi has a main action on respiratory system. It helps to mobilize mucus in bronchitis and asthma thus is very beneficial for maintenance of a healthy respiratory tissue. Water boiled with Tulsi leaves is taken in case of sore throat. This water can also be used for the purpose of gargles.

Adaptogen - Antistress effects: Research has repeatedly shown that, Holy basil helps to lower cortisol production in the adrenal glands and as such, helps reduce fat around the lower abdomen. Tulsi helps cope with the stress and other sensory stimulation.

Eye (Ocular Disorders): The leaf juice of Ocimum sanctum L. along with Triphala is used in Ayurvedic eye drop preparations. It is recommended for glaucoma, cataract, chronic conjunctivitis and other eye disease with pain.

Diabetes Mellitus: The essential oil in Tulsi improves pancreatic beta cell function and thus enhancing the insulin secretion for patients suffering by diabetes.

Oral Infections and toothache: A few leaves chewed helps in maintaining oral hygiene. Tulsi can act as COX-2 inhibitor, like modern analgesics due to its significant amount of Eugenol. Ocimum sanctum leaves contain 0.7% volatile oil comprising about 71% eugenol and 20% methyl eugenol. Tulsi leaves dried in sun and powdered can be used for brushing teeth. It can be mixed with mustard oil to make a paste and used as toothpaste.

Combinations:
1. Decoction of leaves with cardamom powder makes a nourishing and aphrodisiac drink.
2. Holy basil is often combined with other cardio tonic herbs like Arjuna to address heart issues.
3. Tulsi can be combined with other cerebral stimulants such as Rosemary, Bacopa, and Ginkgo to help people with menopausal cloudy thinking, poor memory, attention deficit disorder (ADD) and attention deficit hyperactivity disorder (ADHD), and to speed up recovery from head trauma.
4. Taking Tulsi as a tea with dried ginger is a common treatment for indigestion.
5. Holy basil leaf juice mixed with a little ginger is given for colic in children.
6. Holy basil is mixed with black pepper is given in catarrhal fever and in cold stages of intermittent fever.
7. With honey, ginger and onion juice it forms a good expectorant remedy, useful in cough, bronchitis and children's fever.
8. Leaves sweetened with honey can be given to children in chronic cough and are good expectorant.
9. A mix of four parts Holy basil with one part black pepper can be used for a fever with stuffiness.
10. A honey preparation offers tasty support for issues such as vomiting, skin disorders.

Therapeutic dosing range:
1. Standardized extract (ursolic acid >2.50 percent): 200 to 500 mg daily
2. 1:1 fluid extract: 3 to 5 mL daily
3. Infusion: 2 to 4 cups daily

Toxicology/potential adverse reactions: No case of adverse events was identified.

Drug and supplement interactions: No clinical trials of drug or supplement interactions were identified.

Precautions:
Safety Class: 1
Animal studies have indicated that Holy basil may temporarily reduce sperm count and sperm mortality. A reduction in serum levels of thyroxine (t4) was observed in an animal study with relatively high dose (500mg/kg) of Holy basil. Serum levels of T3 and the T3/T4 ratio were unaffected.

Contraindications: None known

Pregnancy and Lactation: In animal studies with relatively large doses of Holy basil (4gm/kg), reductions in embryo implantation and in litter size were observed. No information on the safety of Holy basil during lactation was identified in the scientific or traditional literature.

Review of scientific literature:

	Anti-Diabetic Activity
Study	Human and animal studies have demonstrated that Holy basil may modify glucose regulation. In a randomized, placebo-controlled, crossover single-blind trial with type 2 diabetes volunteers, patients were administered 2.5 g of Holy basil daily for 60 days.
Results	The postprandial blood glucose levels in those taking the Holy basil leaves fell by 7.3% (15.8 mg/dl) in contrast to those taking the placebo.

Immuno-modulatory activity	
Study	Tea prepared from Ocimum sanctum, Withania somnifera, Glycyrrhzia glabra, Zingiber officinale and Elettaria cardamomum was studied for immune enhancing natural killer (NK) cell activity in comparison to regular tea.
Results	This study was done with healthy 55 years and older who had relatively low baseline NK cell activity and a history of recurrent coughs and colds. This herbal tea significantly improved the NK cell activity when compared to a population consuming regular tea.

Anti-Fungal activity	
Study	Researchers in New Delhi set out to assess the antifungal activity of the essential oil of this plant and its synergy with fluconazole and ketoconazole. The oil was prepared by hydro distillation and then analyzed. It was found to be made up of 53 compounds, predominantly methychavicol (45%), linalool, carvone and D-limonene.
Results	Essential oil of Ocimum sanctum was found to be active against all 84 tested strains of Candida. The two highest ingredients, linalool and ethychavicol were also the herbs most powerful when isolated. Holy basil essential oil displayed significant synergism with the two antifungal drugs tested.

Generalized anxiety disorder (GAD)	
Study	Holy basil was investigated for its effect on generalized anxiety disorder (GAD) in a 2008 study. The study was conducted on 35 patients suffering from GAD from the outpatient clinics of the J. B. Roy State Ayurvedic Medical College and Hospital in Calcutta, India. Each subject was given 500 mg Holy basil orally twice daily after a meal for 60 days.
Results	Baseline score index and stress index score was noted at the beginning of the test. At the end of 60 days the scores were measured again and showed decrease in GAD, depression and stress levels.

Chemo preventive and Radio protective effects	
Study	Preclinical studies carried out in the past two decades have clearly shown that Tulsi possess chemo preventive and radio protective effects.
Results	Several mechanisms are likely to be responsible for the observed effects, the most important being the free radical scavenging, antioxidant, anti-mutagenic activities, anti-inflammatory, increase in the antioxidant enzymes, modulation of Phase I and II enzymes, induction of apoptosis of neoplastic cells and immunomodulatory effects.

Resource List:

Dr.K.M. Nadkarni's - Indian Materia Medica - Volume 1. with Ayurvedic, Unani-Tibb, Siddha, Allopathic, homeopathic, naturopathic and home remedies, Appendicies and indexes, Popular prakasan Pvt Ltd, 1976

Adaptogens in Medical Herbalism, Elite Herbs and Natural Compounds for Mastering Stress, Aging and Chronic Disease – by Donald R. Yance, CN, MH, RH(AHG), Healing Arts Press, 2013.

Adaptogens for Stamina and stress relief- by David Winston and Steven Maimes, Healing Arts Press, 2007.

Ayurvedic Herbs – The Comprehensive Resource for Ayurvedic Healing Solutions, by Dr Virender Sodhi MD (Ayurved) ND, Book Publishers network, 2014

The Yoga of Herbs, by Dr David Frawley and Dr Vasant Lad, Lotus Press, 2008

Breaking ground, by JoAnn Castigliego Sanchez, 2014

Seed Sowing, by JoAnn Castigliego Sanchez, 2013

AHPA - Botanical Safety handbook, by Zoë Gardner (Editor), Michael McGuffin (Editor), CRC Press, Second edition.

Principles and Practices of Naturopathic Botanical Medicine – Volume I: Botanical Medicine Monographs, by Dr Anthony Godfrey, ND, PhD & Dr Paul Richard Saunders, PhD, ND, DHANP, CCH with Dr Kerry Barlow ND, Dr Cyndi Gilbert, ND, Institue of Naturopathic Education and research, CCNM Press, 2010

Clinical Applications of Ayurvedic and Chinese herbs, Monographs for the western herbal practioner, By Kerry Bone with technical and research assistance from Michelle Morgan, Photherapy press, 1996 Edition

Ayurvedic pharmagology and theraputic uses of medicinal plants (Dravyagunavignyan), Vaida V.M. Gogte, English edition - October 2000.

Ayurvedic drugs and their plant sources, V.V. Sivarajan, Indira Balachandran, International Science Publisher, USA, A division of independent scholars associated, 1994 edition

The Encyclopedia for Herbal Medicine, by Andrew Chevallier, DK Publishing, 2000

The Complete Book of Ayurvedic Home Remedies, by Vasant Lad, Three rivers press, NY,1999

http://cms.herbalgram.org/herbalgram/issue91/HERBPRO_Bacopa.html - Herbalgram - American Botanical Council, 2011

http://cms.herbalgram.org/herbclip/430/041157-430.html - Herbalgram research paper related to central nervous system – American Botanical Council, 2011

http://cms.herbalgram.org/herbclip/403/review021015-403.html - Herbalgram research paper – Cognitive enhancing effects of Bacopa on healthy adults, 2010

http://cms.herbalgram.org/herbclip/293/review44313.html - Herbalgram research paper – Overview of Bacopa monniera and its potential to enhance brain function, 2005.

Bacopa monniera - Monograph - Alternative medicine reivew journal, Pg 79-85, Volume 9, Number 1, 2004

Bacopa - HerbalGram. Aug-Oct2011, Issue 91, p1-4. 4p.

Improve memory with Bacopa, by Ellis, Libby, Natural Health. Jul2002, Vol. 32 Issue 5, p29. 1p. 1

Improved neuroprotective effects by combining Bacopa monnieri and Rosmarinus officinalis supercritical CO2 extracts by Ramachandran C; Dharma Biomedical LLC, Miami, FL, USA, Journal Of Evidence-Based Complementary & Alternative Medicine [J Evid Based Complementary Altern Med] 2014 Apr; Vol. 19 (2), pp. 119-27. Date of Electronic Publication: 2014 Feb 25.

Theapeutic benefits of Holy Basil(Tulsi) in general and oral medicine: A Review : Bhateja Summit, Arora Geetika.. Int. J. Res Ayur. Pharm. 2012. 3(6):761-764

Herb Profile - Holy Basil - HerbalGram. May-Jul2013, Issue 98, p1-5. 5p.

Ocimum Sanctum L (Holy Basil or Tulsi) and Its Phytochemicals in the Prevention and Treatment of Cancer - Nutrition and Cancer, 65(S1), 26–35 by Manjeshwar Shrinath Baliga, Rosmy Jimmy, Karadka Ramdas Thilakchand, Venkatesh Sunitha, and Neeta Raghavendra Bhat - Research and Development, Father Muller Medical College, Kankanady, Mangalore, Karnataka, India

Reviews of articles on medicinal herbs - Australian Journal of Medical Herbalism 2010

Health benefits of Tulsi – http://www.herbalremediesadvice.org/health-benefits-of-tulsi.html - Herbs with Rosalee

Multiphasic Dosing During a Woman's Cycle
© Katie Stage, ND, RH (AHG), 2016
Southwest Conference of Botanical Medicine

A woman's monthly cycle can be understood to occur as an overlapping progression of four distinct phases. By convention, day 1 of the menstrual cycle is the day menstruation starts, so the first phase is menstruation. At this point, the endometrium is thick with fluids and nutrients designed to nourish an embryo. If no egg has been fertilized, estrogen and progesterone levels are low, which causes the top layers of the endometrium to shed[27]. This typically lasts about 4 days.

Overlapping and including menstruation is the follicular phase, which takes place day 1 until ovulation (typically around day 14). During this phase, the anterior pituitary secretes FSH (follicle stimulating hormone), which induces the maturation of ovarian follicles. Estrogen levels slowly rise during this period, stimulating the growth of the endometrium and myometrium. This is called the proliferative phase of the endometrium. The increasing estrogen also stimulates luteinizing hormone (LH) release[27].

The next phase is ovulation, which is induced by a surge of LH. LH stimulates the dominant follicle to emerge from the surface of the ovary, releasing the egg. This phase lasts between 16 and 32 hours, and ends when the egg is released. The egg travels through the fallopian tubes to the uterus, and if fertilized (~12 hour window), will implant[27]. Ovulation typically occurs around day 14, or in the middle of the cycle (which is typically around 28 days long).

The last phase is the luteal phase. This phase takes place from day 15 (or after ovulation) until the next cycle starts, typically day 28. The unfertilized follicle transforms into the corpus luteum, which produces progesterone and some estrogen. The progesterone stimulates the endometrium to thicken, filling with fluids and nutrients to nourish a potential embryo. This is called the secretory phase of the endometrium. Progesterone also causes the mucus in the cervix to thicken, so that sperm or bacteria are less likely to enter the uterus, and body temperature to increase slightly. This cycle is dominated by progesterone, although estrogen levels can contribute to symptoms during this phase. If the egg is not fertilized or implanted, the corpus luteum degenerates, dropping estrogen and progesterone levels and stimulating menstruation[27].

A healthy menstrual cycle occurs regularly, approximately every every 28 days. If the cycles are longer, more than every 35 days, it is called oligomenorrhagia. This is usually due to a prolonged follicular phase. If there has been no menstruation for 6 months, or 9 months in a female with irregular cycles, it is called amenorrhea. If cycles occur too frequently, less than every 21 days, it is called polymenorrhea. This is often due to a shortened luteal phase[27].

In a healthy menstrual cycle, menstrual bleeding is not excessive, meaning duration does not exceed 7 days, blood loss does not exceed 80ml, and clots are not larger than a quarter (this is not a criteria for a diagnosis of menorrhagia, but something I consider as part of the overall symptom picture). There should not be bleeding between cycles, often called spotting. Finally, there should not be severe or disabling premenstrual changes, or pain with menstruation or ovulation.

Symptoms of hormone imbalances are common[1], and include irregular cycles, long or short menstrual cycles, spotting, pain with ovulation, heavy menstrual bleeding (or large clots), severe pain with menstruation, and premenstrual symptoms, which may include mood changes, bloating, breakouts, cravings, fatigue, headaches, and breast tenderness or enlargement. All of these symptoms can be addressed with a multiphasic formula. Infertility has many causes, and some of these, particularly those relating to poor follicle count or development, or lower than optimal progesterone, may be addressed with a multiphasic formula.

It is often unclear whether or not testing is required in order to treat the patient. I feel that *symptoms* are very meaningful, and that hormone testing is often unnecessary. Ask about cycle frequency, duration of menses, amount of menstrual bleeding (number and type of pads or tampons on heaviest day), symptoms before, during, and after menstruation, symptoms that occur at other times, and importantly, how her symptoms affect her life. Many women will endure significant symptoms, but feel that these symptoms are normal, or dismiss them because they are not life threatening. Please reassure them that this is not the case. Objective signs, such as tracking basal body temperature, are also useful.

There are a few types of situations where blood tests to assess hormone levels are helpful. First, if there is amenorrhea, you must rule out pregnancy, and then certain hormones should be tested (see reference 26 for a nice overview). If the patient has heavy menstrual bleeding, you must check for anemia and should consider a pelvic and transvaginal ultrasound to assess for fibroids. Some patients really need to see lab results because it helps them to understand the big picture. Occasionally, confirmation of imbalance can aid with compliance. Finally, testing hormone levels can be very helpful when a woman is in her mid- to late 30's or 40's, when relative hormone *deficiency* is suspected. If she is cycling, estrogen(s), FSH, and LH should be tested on days 2-3 of the cycle, and progesterone in day 21. Testosterone should be tested in the morning before 10am, when levels are at their highest. Other labs that may be of interest, such as TSH, PRL, and DHEA-S, can be tested at any time of the month.

Multiphasic dosing has been utilized in many different medical traditions, such as TCM, Ayurveda, and western herbalism. While not well represented in the literature, this type of approach makes intuitive sense. Research studies are limited but indicate efficacy and safety. Eric Yarnell, ND, RH (AHG) and Kathy Abascal, BS, JD, Herbalist RH (AHG) have published a paper describing their experience with multiphasic dosing (reference 22). There is also research on the use of two Japanese formulas, Shakuyaku-kanzo-to and Toki-shakuyaku-san, which were dosed in a cyclic manner. This approach showed efficacy for dysmenorrhea in endometriotic and adenomyotic patients who desired pregnancy.[23]

The benefits of multiphasic dosing include the ability use herbs to support the body's natural hormonal rhythms, as well as the ability to customize herbs to particular symptoms that occur throughout the cycle. It also allows many women to be in better touch with their natural rhythms, which can be very empowering. Multiphasic dosing is beneficial when relative hormone *deficiency*, particularly progesterone deficiency, is an issue. Fertility challenges can have many etiologies, but if due to a follicular issue, then support during this phase of the cycle is indicated (likewise, if due to low progesterone levels in the luteal phase). Multiphasic dosing may also facilitate faster results in reduction of symptoms.

Drawbacks to multiphasic dosing include the need for several formulas to support a woman through her cycle. Sometimes this can feel financially overwhelming or confusing, since conventional treatments typically do not vary in a cyclic manner. It does require a woman to be aware of her cycle so that she knows when to change formulas, and can feel confusing at first if she isn't cycling regularly. However, with good education these concerns can usually be overcome.

The simplest way to dose a multiphasic formula is to have one formula for the follicular phase (this can be dosed from days 1-14, or started after menstruation and dosed until day 14). The second formula, for the luteal phase, is given days 15-28 (stopped when menses starts). Sometimes a third formula is added to support menstruation itself. This is dosed during the menstrual period only. If cycles are irregular, patients should follow the dosing regimen as if their cycle *were* regular. If there hasn't been a cycle for some time, she can choose the start date for a 28-day cycle (starting on a weekend day, perhaps, or link to the moon cycle).[22]

Menstrual Formula

The most common concerns during menstruation itself are menorrhagia, or heavy bleeding, and dysmenorrhea, or painful periods. Sometimes is it necessary to treat these symptoms during menstruation, because the symptoms are very severe. However, my goal is always to modulate hormones so this step is no longer needed in the future. Other symptoms (irregular cycles, lack of menstrual cycles, and premenstrual symptoms) are best treated throughout the cycle.

For menorrhagia, give herbs that are astringent and/or styptic. They can be given during menstruation itself, and are sometimes also given during the luteal phase to help prevent heavy bleeding for the next cycle. Herbs to consider include *Capsella bursa-pastoris* (shephard's purse herba), *Achillea millefolium* (yarrow leaf, flower), *Cinnamomum verum* (cinnamon inner bark), *Trillium grandiflorum* (beth root), *Rosa spp* (rose flower), *Hibiscus sabdariffa* (hibiscus flower), *Rubus idaeus* (raspberry leaf), *Plantago lanceolata / major* (plantain leaf), *Vinca major / minor* (periwinkle herba, root), and *Geranium maculatum* (cranesbill root, herba).

The other major concern during menstruation is dysmenorrhea, or painful periods. Herbal actions include spasmolytics and anodynes. If menses are very painful, I prefer to have my patients start taking a formula before the pain starts. All of the herbs in this list are spasmolytics; some are also anodynes (marked with ❖). Several are lower dose herbs so please make sure your dose is safe. Consider *Viburnum opulus / prunifolium* (crampbark / black haw bark), *Zingiber officinale* (ginger rhizome[21]), *Dioscorea villosa* (wild yam root/rhizome), *Angelica sinensis* (dong quai root), *Actaea racemosa*❖ (black cohosh root), *Valeriana officinalis / sitchensis*❖ (valerian root), *Piscidia piscipula*❖ (Jamaican dogwood bark), *Corydalis spp*❖ (corydalis root), *Piper methysticum*❖ (kava kava root), *Passiflora incarnata* (passionflower flower and leaf), *Leonurus cardiaca* (motherwort herba), *Anemone pulsatilla / Pulsatilla vulgaris*❖ (pulsatilla / pasque flower herba), *Verbena officinalis / hastata* (vervain / blue vervain herba), *Lavandula spp* (lavender flower and leaf), and *Mitchella repens* (partridge berry herba).

Inflammation modulators are another important consideration. High levels of prostaglandins are associated with heavy menstrual bleeding and dysmenorrhea[2,3,4]. The conventional treatment approach to this is to use NSAIDS, but these drugs can be hard on the stomach. Herbs are much safer, and have similar effects at both decreasing pain and heavy bleeding. These can be dosed during menses, or started in the luteal phase to prepare for menstruation. Herbs to consider include *Achillea millefolium* (yarrow leaf, flower), *Cinnamomum verum* (inner bark), *Zingiber officinale* (ginger rhizome), *Curcuma longa* (turmeric rhizome), *Scutallaria baicalensis* (baikal skullcap root), and *Tanacetum parthenium* (feverfew herba), as well as any herb or food rich in bioflavonoids.

If a women's menses is late, or there is oligomenorrhea / amenorrhea, first rule out pregnancy!! Emmenagogues can bring on late menses. I most often use *Leonurus cardiaca* (motherwort herba), but may also consider *Actaea racemosa* (black cohosh root / rhizome) or *Caulophyllum thalictroides* (blue cohosh root).

Herbs to Support Follicular Phase

The follicular phase occurs days 1-14; follicular formulas may be started day 1 or after menses is completed. The follicular phase, as one might guess, is when follicle selection and development happens. Estrogen reaches its peak levels, and the endometrium proliferates. Herbs dosed during this time support these physiologic actions.

Angelica sinensis root, also called Dong quai, Chinese angelica, or "female ginseng", is an excellent spasmolytic, uterine tonic, inflammation modulator, and pelvic decongestant. It is traditionally used to nourish the blood, an action that can help regulate cycles and decrease dysmenorrhea,[5] and is often combined with *Paeonia lactiflora* and *Rehmannia glutinosa* for these actions. It is used to decrease Qi and blood stagnation, which can address fibroids, endometriosis, and PCOS.[5] Consider combining with *Paeonia lactiflora*, *Glycyrrhiza glabra*, *Curcuma longa*,

Salvia milthiorrhiza, Corydalis spp, or *Rehmannia glutinosa.* It is also used to treat infertility and menopause as part of a formula.[5] *Angelica sinensis* root can increase menstrual bleeding, as both a blood thinner and pelvic decongestant, so continuous use during menses should be avoided in women with menorrhagia. It should be avoided in the first trimester of pregnancy and is traditionally avoided in those with a tendency to spontaneous abortions. It is compatible with lactation.

Glycyrrhiza glabra / uralensis root, licorice or Gan Cao, has many actions, the most relevant to this topic being phytoestrogen, adaptogen, anti-inflammatory, and hepatoprotective. *Glycyrrhiza* modulates estrogen levels[6,7], acting as an agonist and antagonist to ER-α and also selectively binding to ER-β[7]. *Glycyrrhiza* may be used in moderate doses to help regulate a cycle, to address estrogen imbalance (the cause of many menstrual symptoms, including fibrocystic breasts, cyclic breast tenderness, some types of PMS, dysmenorrhea, and menorrhagia), and for menopausal symptoms. As an adaptogen it helps modulate the stress response, which plays a large role in hormone imbalance. *Glycyrrhiza* is also used in low doses as a synergist and a corrigent. *Glycyrrhiza* should be avoided in pregnancy as glycyrrhizin potently inhibits 11β-hydroxysteroid dehydrogenase type 2, the feto-placental barrier to higher maternal cortisol levels[8]. It is compatible with lactation. Chronic high doses can increases blood pressure and water retention and also have the potential to decrease testosterone. Use caution in hypertension, CHF, and kidney disease.

Paeonia lactiflora root, or Chinese peony, white (peeled) peony, or Bai Shao, is an excellent analgesic, spasmolytic, inflammation modulator, immune modulator, antioxidant, and astringent[10]. It is traditionally used to nourish the blood, relieve spasm, nourish the liver, and move blood in the pelvis. These actions help address endometriosis, chronic pelvic pain, fibroids, and PCOS[5]. It also tonifies yin[11]. *Paeonia lactiflora* should be avoided in pregnancy; there is a lack of data on safety in lactation. It has blood-thinning activity so use caution in those on anti-coagulents.

Actaea (Cimicifuga) racemosa rhizome and root is also known as black cohosh or black snakeroot. Famous now for menopause, it was traditionally used as a spasmolytic and analgesic, and also acts as a hormone modulator, emmenagogue, uterine tonic, inflammation modulator, and nervine. It improves the coordination of uterine contractions, decreasing pain. Its mechanism of action is not well understood; *Actaea* is thought to be a type of SERM (selective estrogen receptor modulator)[13] with most activity at ER-β receptors. Thus it may strengthen bone, but do not seem to cause endometrial proliferation. I use it for hormonal imbalance, especially if there are signs of congestion, aching pain, or amenorrhea. It is often used for menopause – and works, not so much, in my opinion because of its "estrogenic" effects, but because it has some action as a serotonin agonist (likely mechanism for alleviating hot flashes. This action is also proven effective as a treatment for PMS, dysmenorrhea, and menstrual migraines[21.] *Actaea* can be used throughout the cycle, but I feel it has an affinity for the follicular phase. Use should be avoided in the first trimester of pregnancy; and use in pregnancy should be limited to short term. Avoid in lactation. Use caution in those with ER+ cancer, celiac disease, or malabsorption. Some people, especially those who carry a lot of heat in their head, can get a headache from *Actaea*.

Chamaelirium luteum root and rhizome, also known as false unicorn or helonias root, is a uterine tonic and hormone modulator. Consider in cases of irregular menses due to uterine atony or ovarian insufficiency, when there is a sense of uterine weakness and it feels as of the contents of pelvis are falling out, and when infertility is due to insufficient cervical mucous, poor follicle development, or amenorrhea. *Chamaelirium* is pregnancy category B2; often in partus preparatory formulas as a uterine tonic. It is compatible with lactation. Use caution in Celiac disease and those with malabsorption due to its saponins. More sustainable alternatives are preferred, but I mention it here because it is in most follicular formulas on the market.

Asparagus racemosus root, shatavari or "female ashwaghanda" is an excellent herb for almost any phase of a women's life. It modulates hormones, is a galactagogue, anxiolytic, aphrodisiac, fertility enhancer, and memory enhancer. The mechanism of its hormone modulating action isn't understood, but it does contain isoflavones (phytoestrogens), steroidal saponins, which have hormone modulating effect, and is nutritive and moistening. I find *Asparagus* useful for irregular menstrual cycles, dysmenorrhea, infertility, threatened abortion, low libido, and vaginal dryness. It balances vata and pitta (or you could call it a yin tonic), and is my replacement in many cases for *Chamaelirium luteum*. *Asparagus* is traditionally used in pregnancy and lactation; use should be avoided in states of excess kapha (damp/mucous). There are some reports of overharvesting so ensure ethical sourcing.

Tribulus terrestris fruit and leaf is also known as puncture vine or gokshura. It is a genitourinary tonic, hormone modulator, aphrodisiac, adaptogen, nervine, and analgesic. *Tribulus* increases FSH and β-estradiol in women and is thus most indicated in the follicular phase. Research on this plant for infertility due to anovulation indicates use on cycle days 5-14. *Tribulus* also increases production of red blood cells, increasing oxygen availability and thus overall health. Besides infertility, consider for menopausal symptoms, low libido, anxiety, and fatigue. This is another possible replacement for *Chamaelirium luteum*. *Tribulus* is contraindicated in pregnancy in Ayurveda and TCM; category B3. Lactation CC (compatible, use caution). Avoid use in those with significant kidney disease or CVD, and use caution in those with bradycardia. Watch for supplement quality – there have been reports of adulteration with anabolic steroids of *Tribulus* products marketed for energy and stamina.

Phytoestrogens are often used in follicular phase, as estrogen levels are highest then. Phytoestrogens modulate estrogen activity, and are thought to be ER-β selective agonists. Consider *Trifolium pratense* (red clover) flower, *Medicago sativa* (alfalfa) herba, *Foeniculum vulgare* (fennel) fruit, *Pimpinella anisum* (anise) fruit, and *Pueraria montana var. lobata* (kudzu) root. You can also have patients increase dietary intake of *Punica granatum* (pomegranate) seed, organic *Glycine max* (soy), *linum usitatissimum* (flax) seed, and legumes.

Herbs to Support Luteal Phase

The luteal formula should be dosed days 15-28, or after ovulation to the last day before menses. Progesterone produced from the corpus luteum is at its highest in this phase, so the focus here is to support progesterone production. Also, overt "follicular enhancing herbs" are removed from the formula[22]. Also consider inflammation modulators, astringent/styptics, spasmolytics, "cleansing" herbs (including hepatics, alteratives, and lymphagogues), adaptogens, and phytoestrogens.

Vitex agnus-castus fruit, or chaste tree or monk's pepper, is perhaps our best-known hormone modulator that supports progesterone. It does this through several mechanisms: (1) by binding dopamine receptors on the anterior pituitary, decreasing PRL, which indirectly affects progesterone and estrogen, (2) by binding opiate receptors, which decrease GnRH, thus decreasing LH and FSH from the anterior pituitary and modulating estrogen and progesterone levels, and (3) by the constituent apigenin directly binding to progesterone receptors[28,29]. *Vitex* can be used during entire cycle, but has an affinity for luteal phase due to these actions. Use *Vitex* for any symptom due to estrogen dominance (cyclic mastalgia, acne, short cycles, menorrhagia, etc); it is also useful for any symptom that is cyclical or worse premenstrually. *Vitex* is sometimes used in pregnancy to support low progesterone levels (discontinued by week 20), but is not typically dosed throughout pregnancy. It is compatible with lactation, although higher doses inhibit PRL, thus decreasing breast milk production. It interacts with dopamine receptor antagonists so use caution in those on drugs with this action.

Smilax spp root or root bark, sarsaparilla or Tu Fu Ling (*Smilax glabra*), is an excellent inflammation modulator, alterative, hormone modulator, adaptogen, pelvic tonic, and anti-rheumatic. Its mechanism is not well understood, but hormonal action is thought to be due to steroidal saponins, which are structurally similar to hormones. *Smilax* has been used to direct energy to the pelvis, increasing libido and restoring strength and vitality to the entire body. Its alterative action is useful in the luteal phase for helping decrease premenstrual symptoms. *Smilax* is often added to formulas as a synergist due to its saponins. There is no data on the safety of this herb in pregnancy or lactation.

Dioscorea villosa root and rhizome, or wild yam, colic root, or rheumatism root, has an incorrect reputation as containing progesterone. Its steroidal saponin diosgenin was the original source material used for the production of progesterone for OCPs and other steroid hormones, but the plant does not contain progesterone or estrogen. It is beneficial as a spasmolytic and inflammation modulator – which, when taken before menses, decreases pain and heavy bleeding – and as a cholagogue, which can enhance removal of the estrogen that can contribute to premenstrual symptoms. It also increases SHBG[14], thus binding bioavailable estrogen and androgens, thus modulating premenstrual symptoms such as breast tenderness, bloating, and acne. Its spasmolytic and inflammation modulating actions may also be useful in follicular phase, particularly if spasm of the fallopian tubes is contributing to infertility[24]. There is lack of data on safety in pregnancy and lactation, but it has been used acutely in pregnancy and for afterbirth pains.

Cinnamomum verum inner bark, cinnamon, is an excellent styptic that can be used during menstruation to decrease bleeding. Starting styptics in the luteal phase can be helpful in cases of significant menorrhagia. Spasmolytic and circulatory stimulant actions are also useful. One study showed that *Cinnamomum* provided equal pain relief to mefenamic acid (NSAID), and decreased pain intensity in subsequent cycles, even after cessation of treatment[20]. It should also be considered for the luteal phase because one of its essential oils, cinnamaldehyde, selectively stimulates production of progesterone in *adrenocorticoid* cells (ovaries/gonaldal cells were not addressed in this particular study)[20]. This action would be beneficial in the luteal phase, as we have seen. It also decreased testosterone and DHEA levels[20] which may decrease premenstrual breakouts. *Cinnamomum* is an emmenagogue so use should be avoided in pregnancy and lactation (it is safe for culinary use). Long-term use (high doses) may cause GI irritation due to tannins. Avoid if there is a known hypersensitivity to cinnamaldehyde.

Other useful actions in the luteal phase include hepatics (some favorites are *Cnicus benedictus*, blessed thistle, *Silybum marianum*, milk thistle, and *Taraxicum officinale*, dandelion root/leaf), alteratives, and phytosterogens to help break down higher than optimal estrogen levels. Lymphagogues, to move stagnant lymph in the pelvic area, inflammation modulators to decrease menstrual and premenstrual symptoms, and adaptogens, to modulate stress and increase vitality, should also be considered. If symptoms indicate, use astringent / styptics to decrease menorrhagia, spasmolytic herbs to decrease dysmenorrhea, diuretics to decrease symptoms such as bloating and breast tenderness, and anxiolytics and/ or antidepressants.

In closing, multiphasic formulas are an excellent way to regulate abnormal menstrual cycles and to decrease heavy menstrual bleeding, painful menstrual periods, and premenstrual symptoms. They can also be used for some forms of infertility. By helping to enhance the body's natural rhythms, they can work quickly and effectively. I hope more people will consider this type of dosing for hormone imbalance. Other cyclic activities that support hormonal balance include seed cycling, eating according to cycle phase, and adjusting activity levels to cycle stage.

References available in the downloadable version of this book, for purchase at www.botanicalmedicine.org

PLANT INTELLIGENCE
A GARDEN CHAT
Dr jillian stansbury

"A system is cognitive if and only if sensory inputs serve to trigger actions in a specific way...."
From an article on Artificial Life, Polytechnic Institute, Massachussets

Meanderings on Phytophenomenology

Higher plants represent about 99% of the eukaryotic biomass of the planet. Plants are certainly successful as a life form, which itself is evidence that they have "skills". Some believe that the phytophemonological skills that plants display is evidence of "intelligence". The standing green nation, as some native peoples referred to our photosynthetic brethren, are increasingly being realized to map their environments in order to locate and utilize resources, suggesting that they are aware. More anthropomorphic terms for describing this mapping – such as *consciousness* or *intelligence* - are argued against by the scientific community, but none the less, appeal to me personally, given my extensive study of *Plant Spirit Medicine* in the Amazon. I would like to weave together my studies on *Plantas Maestras*, and my own metaphysical musings, with the following ideas and studies emerging from the scientific community.

What is "Intelligence"?

Intelligence is defined in various ways, but generally includes the ability of an organism to respond to environmental stimuli and challenges with appropriate responses, given the situation. The biological functions that enable this in living systems include sensation and interpretation of sensation, learning and memory that allow for motor or other responses to information received, and all allowing for informed decision-making and creative problem solving.

The evolutionary perspective is that intelligence involves pattern recognition in its simplest form, and that more information, and more complex patterns are processed as life forms have evolved to be more and more complex themselves. Further, different life forms have evolved as they have become specialists in solving problems in specific ways.

Plant Neurobiology

Plants are sensitive organisms. It is odd how rarely it is discussed, but plants possess a nervous system of sorts, albeit different than that of animals. In mammals, brains, nerves, and neural nets enable memory and learning. Even though plants have no such discernable equivalent organs or tissues, they still appear to display behaviors in response to environmental clues, and can even be said to "remember". Rather than under the direction of a neural net, plant tissues appear to act in coordinated holographic ways - throughout the entire organism. The integrated signals and responses include electrical signals, vesicle-mediated transport of auxin, and production of diverse chemicals, including compounds identical to mammalian neurotransmittors. In fact, almost all of the known neurotransmitters are also found in plants. As with animals, genes may be up or down regulated in response to stresses such as dehydration, over hydration, cold temperature, hot temperature, tactile stimuli, environmental ques, etc.

Luigi Galvani first demonstrated that electrical stimulation would cause frogs' legs to twitch, leading to the earliest nerve research, and early concepts of action potentials, furthering the understanding of the mechanisms of nerve conduction. Some of the obviously "sensitive plants" were tested, such as *Mimosa pudica,* and it was realized that they too, reacted to electrical stimuli. It has since been established that all plants are electrically active. The field of neurobiology is still rather new to plant research, despite these early realizations. Plants may be able to respond to a variety of stimuli via subtle and holographic electromagnetically active molecules. Plant may hold water and molecules in a semi-crystalline array, rather than in discrete organs akin the central and peripheral nervous system of animals. Through flickers and waves through this ordered molecular network, plants may be every bit as electrically, tactilely, and chemically sensitive as animals.

There are many similarities between plant cells and neurons, such as polarity where electric signals enter through one pole, travel through the cell and flow out of the opposite pole, and cells arrange themselves in along electromagnetic gridworks. As with neuronal end-bulbs and synapses in animal neurons, plant cells secrete signaling molecules and generate action potentials. Instead of the action potentials traveling down neural axons, the xylem and phloem channels in plants, with their regular linear arrangements, may serve similar functions and allow for water, electrolytes and other molecules to become ordered with the chambers and plant cells, with each cell to cell arrangement behaving like a synapse. Some researchers have termed this "neuroid conduction", meaning neuron-like electrical conduction. Plants are able to monitor for the various nutrients, chiefly minerals, in their surroundings with complex sensing and signaling mechanisms. Once ingested, minerals influence phytohormone biosynthesis, and as with animals, complex K+ and Ca2+ signaling cascades have been identified to move minerals across a wide spectrum of concentration gradients, all helping to establish electrically active tissues. Endocytotic vesicles also transmit sensory input through the cell, and plant cells can integrate multiple sensory inputs at once, recognize patterns, and act on the information.

The Root Brain
Roots are particularly electronically active and sensitive where the transition zone interpolates between the apical meristem and elongation region. Darwin reported plants to have a "root brain", noting that the growing tip has brain-like properties, sensing the soil and choosing where and how to grow. Roots discern humidity, mineral gradients, and encroachment of competition from other plants. Charles Darwin wrote several books on plants, including The Power of Movement of Plants, in which the final summary sentence concludes, "*It is hardly an exaggeration to say that the tip of the radicle thus endowed [with sensitivity] and having the power of directing the movements of the adjoining parts, acts like the brain of one of the lower animals; the brain being seated within the anterior end of the body, receiving impressions from the sense-organs, and directing the several movements.*"

Auxin as a Neurotransmitter-Like Substance
Auxin was first noticed early in the 20th century due to the role is plays in allowing plants to respond to the directionality of available light. Auxin has since been noted to play an important role in plant growth, and also acts like a plant neurotransmitter, playing numerous roles in responding to various environmental stimuli in addition to light.

Technically, auxin is considered to be a phytohormone that moves with the help of polarized influx and efflux carriers in plant cell plasma membranes, creating a direction flow and flow gradients plant tissue. Plants secrete auxin at presynaptic poles of transition zone cells of the root tips and elicit electrical responses and signaling cascades. The xylem and phloem transport steams in plants then move nutrients from the tips of roots to new shoots. Auxin is asymmetrically distributed in plant tissues and auxin gradients are established, and may change dynamically in response to various stimuli, stressors, development processes. Auxin helps to establish polarity and patterning in plant tissues.

Auxin is also involved in the diverse regulation of various plant developmental processes, including embryogenesis, organogenesis, vascular tissue formation and tropisms. Auxin controls division, elongation, and differentiation as well as the polarity of the cell. Numerous other complex mechanisms help modulate auxin's signaling and contribute to extensive roles the phytohormone plays plant growth, sensation, defense, and neurobiology.

Minimal Cognition
Awareness or Cognition is a self-organizing phenomenon usually attributed to animals. The term *minimal cognition* has emerged to acknowledge that plants display consciousness of their surroundings, but so many scientists seem uncomfortable with saying so, the term minimal cognition is preferred. Whatever term is used, the fact is that plants ARE sentient and attentive. Plants respond actively to the environment thus philosophers have said that plant attention is active. It is difficult to say if they are contemplative. Plants integrate many different signals including light, humidity, gravity, tactile sensation, molecular sensation, and various signals that correspond to the presence of allies and predators, in real time. In animals, cognition is considered to be

embedded in the body, and the fact that it is decentralized in plants, should not necessarily make it less sophisticated. Plants process information and may therefore be argued to be cognizant.

Individual versus Group Wills
Nietzsche contended that plants' search for nutrients was a manifestation of its will. My own studies, and overlap with concepts from Plant Spirit Medicine, help me to recognize that all plants exert their "will" to survive in creative ways. Plants overcome the challenges of drought, salt marshes, insect predation, wind storms, and a myriad of other issues, in unique ways. The ways and methods that plants have evolved, or expressed their will to find a way to survive, has given them skills, and dare I say, personalities. There are strong plants and weak plants, shy plants and aggressive plants, stoic plants and dramatic plants, and so on. However, unlike humans, each *individual* plant specimen does not have its own personality, but rather, each *species* of plants shares the same personality.

Plant Intelligence – More than Darwinian Survival of the Fittest?
Intelligence is generally defined to include the phenomena of retaining memories and learning from those memories. And the concept of memory itself is the ability to store and access specific events, actions, and consequences of actions. Do plants remember that a certain insect is a harmful predator? Do plants remember the consequences of inundated riverbanks and take measures to limit water uptake? Does an individual "store and access" that information? Does the collective plant species have the capacity to share the experiences, memories, and information with members of its species?

Plant Intelligence – Something Different than Free Will
In some philosophy circles, judgement of the degree of intelligence in animals has been equated with freedom of choice, or free will – the ability to discern the outcomes of various choices and make a judgement as to which course of action will bring the most desirable life, make a choice, and act on it. For example, turkeys are known to drown in a heavy downpour as they stare at the sky with their mouths agape. Their intelligence is not sufficient to act on the sensory input in order to survive. They could choose to get out of the rain but apparently lack the intelligence to do so. They have some basic survival instincts sufficient to eat and roost, but no higher or rational thought capacity to recognize patterns and discern suitable choices.

Are plants "mindless" and the seeming behaviors only a manifestation of rote survival mechanisms? Can plants display intelligent behavior superior to that of a turkey? Plants receive numerous complex signals, interpret, and act upon them and these responses are not automatic, but rather intelligent, and aware. Various signals compete for the plants' "attention" and those given the highest priority can contribute to the plant's behavior.

An interesting question remains, that if there are choices being made by plants, where in the body of the plant is the discerning and judging taking place? It there a local choice happening, a non-local quantum collective, something science has not yet identified?

The "Parsimony principle' and Plant Intelligence
Parsimony is the concept that the simplest ideas, and the least number of assumptions needed to propose plausible explanations of scientific phenomena, are the ideas most likely to be true. So what is the simplest explanation of how plants appear to be purposeful and willful? The simply explanation may be that they have a will! We can observe that plants display complex mechanisms of signaling, communication, patterning, and organization, making the underlying idea that they do this to survive and thrive, both simple and reasonable. This explains *how* they appear to have a will. Making the more spiritual leap to ask *why* plants "want" to survive, *why* they have the "will" to survive is more difficult. If a lifeform displays a *will to survive*, what is it that sparks or motivates that will? The very notion that something has a will, begs a bit of selfhood, does it not?

Aristotle thought that plants had a vegetative soul, and that animals had the additional quality of sensation, and humans the further additional quality of rational thought. But some botanists and environmental philosophers argue that plants, too, display some higher rational capacities – displaying decision-making, and thereby a type of rational intelligence in the acts of rejecting pollen sharing the same alleles, and of roots preferring a certain patch of soil over another. Plants may actually be more aware of, and more sensitive to their immediate surroundings than animals. Being rooted to a particular space may have driven plants to develop a greater degree of sensitivity to their environments than animals. The bio-attention of plants, may be more present and more attentive than that of animals. Being rooted to a particular location may also lead to a need to have creative ways of accessing information from the non-local environment.

Non-Passivity of Plants
Although Aristotle granted plants a vegetative soul, he has stated them to be "deficient animals", a perspective perpetuated for millennia. Plants were seen as inferior, lacking selfhood, and only having existence in relation to the sun and minerals, wholly subordinate to animals, and passively bound to the inorganic world. This view of plants has been found to be erroneous. Plants produce toxins in response to herbivory, for example. Plants can communicate with other individuals of the same species, as well as different species, and perhaps even to highly different species, such as insects and animals, with volatile compounds that can travel in the air significant distances. Plants may even anticipate coming threats, and begin producing more alkaloids, or bitter compounds, when they receive information and signals that a herd of elk is coming their way. Plants may communicate via chemical messengers to attract or repel different pollinators and predators, and likely serve other purposes we have yet to discover.

A Darwinian Mechanism for Phenotypic Plasticity
The phenotype of a plant, that is to say its outward appearance or morphology, is plastic and malleable given environmental situations. For example, one can take ordinary pumpkin seeds and grow ordinary pumpkins or extraordinarily large pumpkins given different soil, water, and environmental parameters, yet with the same underlying genetic make-up. *Nasturtiums* grown in rich soil will produce abundant vegetation and few flowers, while in dry poor soils, will produce few leaves and many flowers. The plants express themselves differently, even though the genetic makeup is identical. Plants may display "intention" when they express various phenotypes, making "choices" based on the information and resources they are given. Plants may have a small, but none the less significant, degree of control to how they move and grow, to best help them to survive. Part of the *phytophenomena* driving the divergence of plant species appears to be co-evolutionary phenomena, whereby plants are aware of their surroundings, and of the other life forms with which they coexist. Due to this awareness, plants may have *intended* or *willed* to offer nectar to beneficial insects, domiciles to insect work crews, and beautifully patterned landing platforms for pollinators. The plants' response to sensory information contributes to its shape, form, and phenotypic expression, and thereby plants evolve in part, in response to their wills and creativity.

Living systems embody their memories and store their knowledge in their tissues. The experiences and sensory input received in living systems affect the genome, i.e. gene expression, but can affect non-genomic, "plastic" phenotypic expressions as well. The phenotype is shaped structurally by experience, and experience is mediated via neural process that receive the sensory input. The accumulation and storage of sensory-mediated experiences in sensory cells changes the structure of the cell. As with human brain plasticity, so too are plant sensory cells and neurobiological tissues "plastic." This in turn affects the evolution, development, behavior, "personality", shape and form of the plant. Due to their life "experiences", like all sensory and neuronal tissues, the shape and structures of the tissue can morph accordingly. In this way, the shape and form of a plant is a reflection of its experiences, choices, will, and creativity.

The Doctrine of Signatures
Part of the ancient ideas on the *Doctrine of Signatures*, whereby the shape, color, pattern, and form of a plant has significance, and can hint at its medicinal and nutritional qualities, may itself be a phytophenomena. Plants may grow and hold their leaves in a manner that benefits certain plants, protectors, or symbionts, who then defer them a survival advantage. This trait is shared with all species, and specific insects co-evolve over millennia to only survive with the aid of their companion plant (Figs and Fig moths, Milkweeds and Monarch,

etc.) Insects may "read" the signature of plants, animals can of course taste the sugar and see the beauty, and highly aware humans may receive information from the plant by its very appearance. Plants may evolve to willfully and creatively express color, number, habit, shape, form, and personality, even though they lack the sense organs to which those traits have evolved to appeal. Plant display beauty that seems intended for animal eyes, aroma that seems intended for olfactory apparati, and all manner of creative seed dispersal and propagation methods that involve insects and animals to do their bidding. Clever that.

Plants are Aware of Their Surroundings
Plants are known to map their surroundings, and move their bodies in intentional ways in 3-dimensional space. Plants orient themselves and respond dynamically to the gravitational field, with respect to the arc and rays of the sun, with respect to available nutrients and water, and with respect to other plants, fungi, microorganisms, and in some cases other life forms. Researchers are starting to say that plants "forage" for resources, just like animals do. Plants can interpret numerous chemical signals from other plants, and likely other animals and insects as well. Furthermore, plants not only sense these things, plants communicate and interact with these surroundings, releasing volatile oils into the air, and chemical signals underground.

This is an example of *intention* or *will* in plants – growing in desired directions due to an awareness of 3 dimensional space. Plants are aware of other plants that may compete for resources, and may take measures to prevent further growth and encroachment. Plants' willfulness can include control over directional growth vectors toward heat, light, open space, and kin, away from unsuitable environments, predators, and undesirable neighbors.

Don't be so Hasty – Differences in Time Scale Between Plants and Animals
Human time frame is much faster than plants. Although some bamboos species can grow a centimeter per hour, and some seaweed many feet in a single day, in general, human beings operate in second and minute-based time scales, while plants usually operate in weeks and months, or even year-based time scales. Only through time lapse photography are humans able to appreciate the movements, responsiveness, and intentionality or willfullness of plants. It may be that we miss other plant phenomena as we lack research techniques that operate on their time-frames, and look hastily for physiology with which we are familiar. Indeed, it takes time for herbalists to "see" the personalities of plants and develop familiarity with the unique behavior of various species. But most gardeners learn, over years' time, the plants that are rather annoying (*Dulcamara, Rununculus*), the plants that are rather charming (*Johnny Jump Ups*), and the plants that are touchy drama queens (*Begonias*). Those who don't "get" that last sentence, have probably never slowed down to observe plants and their behaviors on their own time-scales.

Plants have Group Souls
Now I am really treading in taboo waters for a scientist, but I am nearing retirement, and emboldened to share my honest observations and opinions. If anything has a soul at all, something more than the sum total of its chemical parts, than I don't see why humans would be anymore soulful than other animals, nor why animals would be any more soulful than plants. All religious ideation aside, who can say why the universe goes to all the bother of existing? And if the most basic laws of thermodynamics dictate that order decays away into disorder, and that all organized life breaks down into a steady state of homogeneity with its surroundings - that is to say reach entropy – then why has there been a slow and patient evolutionary timeline heading towards more and more order, and increasingly complex organisms? If the "arrow of time" points toward chaos and disorder sooner or later, then why has life evolved to be increasingly ordered and complex? One commonly overlooked "given" hidden in the laws of thermodynamics is, ...wait for it......**that there can be order.** If the law is for all matter to reach a steady state of disorder, then why is there any order at all?

Rudolph Steiner used the term *negentropy* to refer to the force that opposes entropy. I believe that negentropy is akin to, if not the same thing as, the "vital force", that innate healing wisdom that causes minerals to accrete, plants to exert their will in creative ways, and animals to become more and more complex, to the point of contemplating their navels. It is negentropy that drives minerals to accrete into the highly ordered living crystals of our bones, drives our wounds to repair themselves, and our organs to continually regenerate. It is this healing, negentropic, vital force with which true healers work.

I was taught in Naturopathic medical school that a large part of helping people to heal, no matter how fancy and biochemical our evidence-based research evolved, was to simply remove the obstacles to cure and stimulate the vital force. There is an innate wisdom and impetus in the body to continually repair and regenerate itself, oppose entropy, and keep the order, the body heat, and the "aliveness" going. Plants too, exert their will, and maintain their order and biochemical systems sufficient to sustain their aliveness. Plants appear to do this collectively among their own kind – that is to say, among their own species. While humans have individual wills, plants appear to have group wills. There are some animals, the animals which are most linked to humans such as dogs and cats, that seem to have individual personalities, but many animals, and all plants, seem to have identical wills and personalities within the species. For example, while there may be aggressive dogs and lazy dogs, or skittish cats and social cats, one sparrow is more less the same, personality-wise, as another sparrow, and one gold fish more or less identical to the next. In the same way, one plantain is identical to another plantain growing on another continent. Ditto that a lotus blossom, a yarrow, a tomato, or a coconut tree. Plants do not have individual wills or souls, if you believe in souls, but rather, a group personality or spirit that is shared collectively among the species. So rather than search for the seat of the soul, the brain behind the will, or the ghost in the machine in the tissues of any one individual plant, perhaps we should look a little wider. Could there be collective consciousness shared among all species in a non-local way? Could there be microrrhizal communication networks? Could there be volatilized communication networks, or other yet to be discovered systems of intelligence in plants?

Examples of Plant Intelligence
Plants can sense reflective infrared and red light, and note its movement, and respond to coming shade ahead of time. *Taraxacum*, Dandelions, can realize that they are being repeatedly mowed down in the lawn, and begin flowering at the level of the ground, rather than on a 6 inch or loner stem. Plants may have a memory of winter in that seeds may not be fooled into breaking dormancy during an unusual February warm spell, because they "know" that the real spring may not be until April.

Many plant leaves, such as the laminas of *Lavatera cretica*, will track the trajectory of the sun, moving across the sky and maximize the photosynthetic surfaces. Researchers have shown that you can place such plants in a darkened box, and the plants will still display the movement for a number of days. Thus, the plant anticipates the sun, rather than just responding to it. It displays an action based on a memory, and the memory appears to be stored in the collective of plant cells, rather than a centralized organ.

Cuscuta species, Dodder, responds to touch stimuli and coiling around other host plants to parasitize their cholorphyll, have given up producing their own. *Cuscuta* will touch various plants and discern plants that are rich nutrient sources. *Cuscata* will invest more energy in coiling around a plant and usurping its nutrients then it anticipates gaining as a reward for the expenditure.

The "Sandbox Tree" *Euphorbia hirta*, releases chemical toxins from its roots that prevent other trees, vines, and herbaceous plants from sprouting in the vicinity of its trunk. Thus this jungle tree always has a lot of space around it.

Many jungle trees possess ant domatia, living quarters for specific ant species that protect the tree and prune any vines or parasites that would otherwise grow on the trees. For example, Palo Santo, a *Triplaris* species houses ants that will come pouring out by the millions anytime the tree is touched. They will prune away vines and epiphytes, but will also inflict highly painful bites on animals who disturb the trees.

The Stilt Palms, *Geonoma* species have tall adventitial roots that can "walk". When conditions are difficult, or the other plants encroach upon its territory, the plant can grow new roots in the desired direction, and allow others to die off, effectively taking a step.

Syngonium is tropical climbing plant that has scale-like leaves on the ground, and then changes its form entirely as it grows into the canopy, and to spread to other trees, can by seeking darkness and growing an extension back down to the ground and start the process over again.

Glechoma and *Hydrocotyle*, choose patches of soil to colonize, and then grow just the right number and vigor of leaves to match the resources that the particular patch has to offer.

Pisum sativum, peas, are able to communicate environmental stress or hardship to other peas through chemical signaling from root to root.

Lycopersicon, tomato, can communicate mechanical trauma from a wounded leaf, to adjacent leaves via chemical signals.

The Venus flytrap, *Dionaea muscipula*, will not close its trap when rain drops or leaf matter strike its surface, but will only spend the energy for choice insects. It does this by having a memory of the precise sensory hair stimulated, and if another nearby sensory hair is stimulated within a short time frame, will invest the energy to obtain a valuable return. It can discern between rain and other disturbances and insects with sophisticated judgements based on both time frame and spatial arrangements of sensory input.

Potentilla reptans will decrease the length between internodes when in nutrient-rich soil. When cuttings are made of these ramets and allowed to grow new ramets, that information from the older cells was passed on. Information from a different time and space was house, like a memory in the new clones. These data suggest that the decision to grow a stolon or to root a ramet at a given distance from the older ramet results from the integration of the past and present information about the richness and the variability of the environment.

What are some of the plants which you have observed display a personality, an intelligence, an intentionality?

ANDROGENETIC ALOPECIA
Dr Jillian Stansbury

Male Pattern Baldness is referred to medically as *Androgenetic Alopecia* (AGA), defined as a hereditary and androgen-dependent, progressive thinning of the scalp hair that follows a defined pattern. The accumulation of 5α-dihydrotestosterone (DHT) in dermal papilla cells is implicated in androgenetic alopecia. DHT decreases cell growth by inducing cell death and increasing the production of reactive oxygen species.[1,2] Hair loss can involve changes to hair fiber caliber, density per unit area, and/or the duration of anagen and telogen in the hair growth cycle. Scalp dermoscopy is used routinely in patients with androgenetic alopecia, as it facilitates the diagnosis and differential diagnosis with other diseases, allows staging of severity, and helps monitor the progress of the disease, and response to treatment.[3] Since the condition progresses over time, the most success in halting hair loss is seen with early intervention.[4] Leading pharmaceutical therapies for AGA include oral finasteride (especially for men) and topical minoxidil (for men and women).[5] This paper will introduce herbal medicines used traditionally for hair loss, that may work via similar mechanisms as the pharmaceutical options.

ADROGENETIC ALOPECIA

Androgenetic alopecia affects both men and women. In men it produces male pattern hair loss with bitemporal recession and vertex baldness. In women it produces "female pattern hair loss" (FPHL) with diffuse alopecia over the mid-frontal scalp, as hair follicles become miniaturized. As with men, the most common cause of alopecia in women is androgenetic, and affects approximately one-third of adult caucasian women[6]. Male pattern baldness, may be associated with an increased risk of prostate cancer, as both may involve increased sensitivity to testosterone, and resulting oxidative stress in the tissues.[7] However one study following over 35,000 men did not find a correlation between baldness and prostate cancer.[8]

In addition to genetic predisposition to androgenic alopecia, poor nutrition, poor circulatory health, and stress may exacerbate the process. Acute stress causes hair loss in animals and humans. One investigation of serum cortisol level and glucocorticoid receptor expression in patients with severe alopecia areata, showed a lower expression of glucocorticoid receptors compared to controls[9], and researchers believe this contributes to pathological changes in the scalp and contributes to alopecia. Therefore, adaptogenic and nervine herbs are logical to include in formulas for patients with hair loss where stress and adrenal activation is suspected to play a role, although research is lacking.

The Androgen Paradox
Androgens stimulate beard growth but suppress head hair growth in androgenetic alopecia, and in women, promote hirsuitism, but thinning of head hair. Those with androgenetic alopecia may have increased expression of androgen receptors, making them more susceptible to body hair growth, concomitant with head hair loss.

HAIR LOSS AND HORMONES

Hair disorders may be triggered by inflammation, genetics, the environment, and very commonly hormones.[10] Androgenic alopecia is associated with the androgens testosterone and 5α-dihydrotestosterone, both of which bind androgen receptors and induce androgen-sensitive genes within the human hair dermal papilla cells. 5α-DHT exhibits much higher binding affinity and potency than does testosterone, and therefore, inhibiting 5α-DHT is one possible method of treating androgenic alopecia.

One study investigated routine TSH testing of over 16,000 patients found that the hair loss correlated to low TSH levels.[11] PCOS may be associated with androgenic alopecia due to elevated androgens that are the hallmark of the condition.[12] Men may more susceptible to hair loss when some degree of insulin resistance exists, or when there is PCOS in women of the lineage.[13] Prolactin secretion is controlled by prolactin inhibitor factor that is secreted from hypothalamus; factors like vasoactive inhibitory peptide (VIP) and thyroid releasing hormone (TRH) lead to increase in prolactin secretion. Hyperprolactinemia is a common condition that can result from a number of causes including hypothyroidism.[14] SHBG levels are lower in women with hyperandrogenic disorders than in normal women, even in the absence of hyperadrogenemia. Investigators propose that SHGB levels may be a more sensitive laboratory indicator than androgens.[15] Several studies have showed that topical melatonin may support hair regrowth.[16] Steroidogenic acute regulatory proteins (StAR) also play a role in the skin and positively correlate with testosterone concentration, such that increased StAR expression is association with significantly fewer hair follicles.[17] Studies suggest that combination therapies may be more effective that any one therapy alone.[18]

TOPICAL PROGESTERONE
Progesterone is a natural precursor to estrogen and cortisone, as well as inhibits 5-alpha-reductase. Progesterone oral medication for women, as well topically on the scalp for both men[19] and women, can help deter testosterone-driven damage to the hair follicles. Progesterone is one of the first steroids synthesized and can be shunted into both reproductive hormone pathways, as well as mineralocorticoid pathways. Progesterone may be transformed into aldosterone, then hydroxyprogesterone, and ultimately cortisol and androstenedione. Androstenedione can be further transformed into testosterone, estrone, and estradiol. Stress can "steal" all of the progesterone to make corticoids, leaving little left over to make reproductive hormones. The use of adaptogenic herbs may help maintain optimal levels of progesterone in the body by supporting the adrenal glands and helping to treat stress and activation of the Hypothalamus-Pituitary-Adrenal axis. Consider using adaptogenic herbs in all cases of low progesterone. Topical progesterone solutions

5α-REDUCTASE INHIBITORS TO SLOW HAIR LOSS - OVERVIEW
Dihydrotestosterone (DHT) is the most influential androgen and plays a very important role in the pathogenesis of androgenetic alopecia. Some individuals appear to have a genetically-determined sensitivity of hair follicles to DHT, and therapies that reduce androgen load in the scalp can therefore be helpful. One such molecular target is the 5 α-reductase enzyme, which converts testosterone to DHT. Inhibiting DHT has therapeutic value for treating benign prostatic hyperplasia, alopecia, hirsutism in women, and prostate cancer.

5 alpha-reductase is a steroid metabolizing enzyme that reduces the double bonds of some steroids, including testosterone, reducing its conversion to DHT. 5α-reductase inhibitors are considered to be among the most effective treatments of androgenetic alopecia, and Finasteride is a leading pharmaceutical 5α-reductase inhibitor, however even this therapy has very limited success. The side-effects of pharmaceutical 5α-reductase inhibitors are usually minimal with short term use, but prolonged use may have significant adverse effects on sexual function such as erectile dysfunction and diminished libido[20]. Thus far, such side effects have not been reported from herbal 5α-reductase inhibitors.

Many herbs and their constituents have been shown to be natural 5 alpha-reductase inhibitors, such as the green tea catechin, epigallocatechin gallate[21], and a more complete list is found in the accompanying side bar. Other flavonoids that potently inhibit type 1 5 alpha-reductase include myricetin, quercitin, and baicalein, while biochanin, daidzein, genistein, and kaempferol inhibits type 2 5alpha-reductase.[22] Many legume family herbs such as *Trifolium* and *Pueraria* are 5α-reductase inhibitors due to the genistein and daidzein they contain. The topical application *Trifolium pratense* has been found to retard hair loss in human subjects experiencing a receding hair line.[23] Topical *Trifolium* also reduces inflammatory reactions and stimulated extracellular matrix protein synthesis in the vicinity of hair follicles. Formononetin, a well-studied isoflavone found in Red Clover and other leguminous foods and herbs may promote hair regrowth when topically applied. Formononetin induces hair follicles to recover normal size and induces inhibits apoptosis of the follicle stimulate regrowth of lost hair.[24] Procyanidin oligomers, the red, blue, and purple pigment common in blueberries, pomegranates and other berries, may promote hair growth via selective inhibition of protein kinase C[25], when orally consumed. One study showed procyanidins to have the greatest effect on hair growth compared to other flavonoids.[26] The Materia Medica section of this document details the research on numerous other 5 alpha reductase inhibitors, flavones, circulatory enhancing herbs, and traditional herbal hair tonics.

IMPROVING SCALP CIRCULATION TO ALLAY HAIR LOSS
Minoxidil is a vasodilating pharmaceutical that improves circulation to the follicles and may slow or stop hair loss, and promote hair regrowth when applied topically, and is further discussed below. Natural agents that have vasodilating effects, from topical arginine, to counter irritants such as *Capsicum*, and warming volatile oils

may have therapeutic activity. Scalp massage and hydrotherapy to the head may be other natural means of improving circulation to the hair follicles. The turmeric relative *Curcuma aeruginosa* inhibits 5α-reductase and one multicenter, randomized, double-blind, placebo-controlled study showed the herb combined with minoxidil boosted the efficacy of the pharmaceutical in slowing hair loss and stimulating hair regrowth.[27]

NUTRIENTS
Some trace elements may play a role in alopecia, including androgenetic alopecia, which may associate with low levels Cu and Zn content in the frontal areas compared to the occipital area, and increased levels of Cu and decreased Mn, Se, Zn contents in the occipital area of scalp.[28] Depleted iron stores and suboptimal intake of the essential amino acid l-lysine may correlated with hair loss in women, but not men.[29] Niacin and nicotinic acid derivatives such as octyl nicotinate and tetradecyl nicotinate, may promote hair fullness in female alopecia.[30] Biotin levels may also correlate with hair loss and supplementation may be beneficial.[31]

ANTI-ANDROGENS
Alpha-5 reductase inhibitors: Finasteride, *Serenoa, Urtica*
Androgen receptor antagonists: spironolactone and cyproterone acetate
Aromatase promoters: *Peonia* – Chinese Peony
Prolactin Inhibitors: *Vitex*
Flutamide
Dutasteride
Prostaglandin analogs: bimatoprost, latanoprost
Ketoconazole

AGENTS THAT SUPPRESS OVARIAN AND ADRENAL PRODUCTION OF ADROGENS[32,33]
Oral Contraceptive
Glucocorticoids
Adaptogens?

ALPHA-5 REDUCTASE INHIBITORS
Spironolactone Rx
Finasteride Rx (Proscar), Oral 5 mg daily for 12 months

Botanical 5α-reductase inhibitors
Avicennia marina [34]
Benincasa hispida
Camellia sinensis – Green Tea
Carthamus tinctorius
Chrysanthamum
Citrullus colocynthis[35]
Curcuma aeruginosa
Cuscuta reflexa[36]
Ganoderma lucidum - Reishi
Glycyrrhiza - Licorice
Lepidium meyenii – may protect from testosterone-induced hyperplasia of the prostate.
Magnolia - Honokiol
Mangifera - Mango
Mentha spicata - Spearmint
Panax ginseng ginsenosides
Phyllanthus emblica, niruri – Stone Breaker[37]

Polygonum multiflorum – Fo Ti
Pueraria lobata, spp
Serenoa repens– Saw Palmetto[38]
Sphaeranthus indicus
Thuja occidentalis - Cedar
Urtica dioica– Nettle Root

AROMATASE EFFECTORS
Aromatase inhibitors in the skin markedly decreases estrogen synthesis, and increase testosterone, which may be detrimental for AGA. When aromatase is higher in the skin, thicker elastic fibers result, which may be beneficial to the skin and hair.
Aromatase inhibitors – honokiol[39], indole-3-carbinol[40], Eurycoma longifolia (Tongat Ali)[41], Grape Seed Extract[42], and many others, are NOT desirable for AGA, or at least not desirable topically.
Aromatase Promotor – *Peonia* and *Glycyrrhiza* are both shown to inhibit testosterone synthesis and stimulate aromatase activity. Both may considered as ingredients in teas, tinctures, and topical formulas for AGA. Paeoniflorin, glycyrrhetic acid and glycyrrhizin are all shown to significantly decrease testosterone without significant effects on androstenedione or estradiol.[43] *Epimedium brevicornum* and the Icariin it contains may promote aromatase and be one of the mechanisms where by the plant promotes bone growth in osteoporosis.[44] *Styrax perinsiae* contains egonol gentiobioside and egonol gentiotrioside credited with promoting aromatase.[45]

LASER THERAPY[46]
Low level laser therapy may improve male and female pattern hair low and appear safe. Laser therapy may also speed recovery following chemotherapy-induced hair loss.[47]

PHARMACEUTICALS FOR ANDROGENETIC ALOPECIA

FINASTERIDE
Finasteride is the leading pharmaceutical used to reduce dihydrotestosterone to treat both androgenetic alopecia and benign prostatic hypertrophy. Finasteride, is a type II 5alpha reductase inhibitor and may regrow a noticeable amount of hair in about 40% of balding men. Further drug developments have led to the development of a dual type I and type II inhibitors where 90% of those treated regrow a noticeable amount of hair. However, Finasteride is commonly associated with side effects, so sometimes used topically, rather than orally. Finasteride is so commonly associated with adverse side effects in men, that a condition referred to as *"Post-finasteride Syndrome"* may result, and includes erectile and orgasmic dysfunction, ejaculatory irregularities such as reduced force, decreased penile sensitivity, reduced concentration, and anhedonia.[48] The topical use of finasteride may help treat alopecia while avoiding these side effects. Human clinical trials show oral finasteride to reduce serum DHT by 60-70%, while topically applied finasteride, roughly by one quarter as much.[49]

Finasteride is less commonly used in women, but one study showed 81% to improve hair density and thickness, however, most of them only slightly or moderately. Side effects included headache, menstrual irregularity, dizziness and increased body hair growth, all mild, and that subsided with continued therapy.[50] Oral finasteride, 5 mg/day, may be an effective and safe treatment for normoandrogenic women with female pattern baldness[51]. Women of childbearing potential must adhere to reliable contraception while receiving finasteride, and treatment is contraindicated in pregnancy, due to known teratogenicity.

MINOXIDIL
Minoxidil is an ATP sensitive potassium channel opener believed to stimulate vascular endothelial growth factor[52], and may exert direct effects on ATP-sensitive potassium channels and support hair growth[53] when topically applied as a 1 to 3% solution. Although minoxidil is one of the main therapies for andogenetic alopecia, only 30-40% of patients experiences any success.[54] Minoxidil appears more effective for arresting further loss of

hair than in regrowing hair.[55] Minoxidil is converted to minoxidil sulfate in the scalp by sulfotransferase enzymes, and the presence of this enzyme in hair follicles may correlate with the best treatment outcomes.[56] Some researchers are developing nanoparticle micelles to more effectively deliver minoxidil through the scalp.[57] Complexing minoxidil with antibodies that target follicles and dermal papilla may help deliver the medicine directly to the follicles and improve the limited success of the therapy.

Although Minoxidil has been for more than two decades to treat androgenetic alopecia and thought to work, in part, via K channels, the precise mechanisms of action are uncertain. A number of in vitro effects of minoxidil have been described in monocultures of various skin and hair follicle cell types including stimulation of cell proliferation, inhibition of collagen synthesis, and stimulation of vascular endothelial growth factor and prostaglandin synthesis. Some or all of these effects may be relevant to hair growth.[58] One study suggested that minoxidil may directly suppress androgen receptors and/or otherwise inhibit downstream signaling, and affect the expression of proteins involved with signal transduction including peptides and co-regulators.[59]

Minoxidil requires 12 or even 24 months to see results.[60,61] Minoxidil 5% foam once a day or 2% foam 2 times daily[62,63], are the dosages used in publishedstudies, and as long as well tolerated, most users prefer the once daily option.[64]

ADENOSINE
Adenosine is reported to increase the growth of fibroblasts. Adenosine is used topically in Japan for androgenetic alopecia[65] and one study on Caucasian men reported use to significantly increase hair thickness.[66] One study investigated the effects of a topical preparation containing minoxidil (5%) with adenosine (0.75%) on androgenetic alopecia, and reported minor benefits at 3 and 6 months' time, slowing further loss of hair, and re-growing new fine hairs, however, no one experienced significant regrowth of hair.[67]

SPIRONOLACTONE
Spironolactone has been used for 30 years as a potassium-sparing diuretic, and has been used "off label" for female androgenic alopecia for over 20 years. Spironolactone is a synthetic steroid structurally related to aldosterone. Since the serendipitous discovery 20 years ago that spironolactone given to women for polycystic ovary syndrome (PCOS) related hypertension, also improved hirsutism, it has become a primary medical treatment for female hirsutism.

Spironolactone both reduces adrenal androgen production and exerts competitive blockade on androgen receptors in target tissues. It has been shown to arrest hair loss progression with a long-term safety profile. A significant percentage of women also achieve partial hair regrowth. Spironolactone is not used in male androgenetic alopecia because of the risk of feminization.[68]

HAIR TRANSPLANTATION
Follicular unit transplantation is the gold standard for surgical management. There are 2 types of graft harvest technique: donor strip and follicular unit extraction. Each technique has its own advantages and disadvantages and should be tailored to the individual patient. Understanding of the anterior hairline design is essential to achieving a natural-appearing and long lasting result.[69]

INDIVIDUALIZED MATERIA MEDICA FOR ANDROGENETIC ALOPECIA

ADIANTUM CAPILLUS VENERIS – Maidenhair Fern
Adiantum Capillus veneris is shown to promote hair grown in animal models of testosterone-induced alopecia.[70]

ANGELICA SINENSIS – Dong Quai
Angelica applied topically is shown to promote hair growth and enhance the size of hair follicles, and length of hair shaft in animal models of androgenic alopecia.[71] Hair loss is accompanied by keratinocyte apoptosis-regression during catagen and prolonged telogen. *Angelica sinensis* may promote hair growth, notably decreasing apoptotic cells during catagen phase. Molecular studies suggest that this is accomplished due to

inhibition of NF-κB and the phosphorylation of three mitogen-activated protein (MAP) kinases, and the activation of c-Jun with decreased TNF-α.[72]

CAMELLIA SINENSIS - Green Tea
Green Tea polyphenols may promote hair growth.[73,74,75] The Green tea catechin, epigallocatechin-3-gallate, may promote hair growth when consumed orally and/or topically applied.[76] Topical application of epigallocatechin-3-gallate (EGCG) reduces testosterone-induced apoptosis of hair follicles [77]

CHRYSANTHEMUM ZAWADSKII - Chrysanthemum
Flavinoids in *Chrysanthemum zawadskii* promote hair growth with topical application, stimulating the differentiation and proliferation of pluripotent epidermal matrix cells in the matrix region and epithelial stem cells in the basal layer of the epidermis. [78]

COFFEA INDICA – COFFEE[79]
Caffeine has potent antioxidant properties. It helps protect cells against the UV radiation and slows down the process of photo-aging of the skin. Caffeine is being increasingly used in cosmetics due to its high biological activity and ability to penetrate the skin barrier. The commercially available topical formulations of caffeine normally contain 3% caffeine. When used topically, caffeine may exert anti-cellulite activity, preventing excessive accumulation of fat in cells below the dermis, and stimulating lipolysis through inhibition of the phosphodiesterase activity. [80] Caffeine may also improve the penetration of other drugs into the skin and scalp and improve delivery and efficacy.[81]

Caffeine reportedly counteracts the suppression of hair shaft production by testosterone in organ-cultured male human hair follicles, and one human tissue culture study showed caffeine to enhance hair shaft elongation, prolonged anagen duration and stimulated hair matrix keratinocyte proliferation. Female hair follicles have shown higher sensitivity to caffeine than male HFs. Caffeine counteracted testosterone-enhanced TGF-β2 protein expression in male HFs. In female HFs, testosterone failed to induce TGF-β2 expression, while caffeine reduced it. In male and female HFs, caffeine enhanced IGF-1 protein expression. In ORSKs, caffeine stimulated cell proliferation, inhibited apoptosis/necrosis, and upregulated IGF-1 gene expression and protein secretion, while TGF-β2 protein secretion was downregulated.

ECLIPTA ALBA
Eclipta alba is a traditional herb used to promote hair growth, *Eclipta alba* may increase the number of follicular keratinocytes in the basal epidermal and matrix cells of the scalp, and reduce the levels of transforming growth factor-β1 (TGF-β1) expression during early anagen and anagen-catagen transition. [82] Topical application has been shown to significantly increase the growth in mice with genetically-induced abnormal keratinization.[83]

HURA CREPITANS – Catawa, Hura
Hura crepitans is used in the Amazon to prepare hair oil known as Hura oil. The Bora tribe with whom I have studied, prepares a hair wash from the plant and uses it several days in a row to make the hair thick and shiny prior to important community celebrations. A compound known as daphne factor is shown to induce catagen in the hair cycle via inhibiting inducing neurotrophin-4. Neurotrophin (NT)-4 is known to be an inducer of catagen in the hair cycle, [84] This oil is shown to balance ratios between neurotrophin, a naturally occurring compound, and androgens, in a manner that induces hair growth[85].

ILLICIUM – Star Anise
Illicium anisatum Star Anise contains shikimic acid shown to induce mRNA expression of insulin-like growth factor-1, keratinocyte growth factor, and vascular endothelial growth factor in the hair follicles.[86]

LYCOPERSICON ESCULENTUM - Tomato
Tomatoes contain the flavonoid lycopene. Lycopene is a carotenoid with strong anti-oxidant properties. Lycopene occurs in tomato-based food products primarily as an all-E isomer (80-97%), but its Z-isomers accounts for 79 to 88% of total lycopene in benign or malignant prostate tissues.[87] One study showed the topical application of tomatoes increased hair growth in mice in a manner similar to 3% minoxidil. *Lycopersicon esculentum* extracts significantly increased mRNA expression of vascular endothelial growth factor (VEGF), keratinocyte growth factor, and insulin-like growth factor-1 (IGF-1) was observed than PC, as well as the negative control (NC). [88]

MENTHA SPICATA – SPEARMINT
Mentha spicata, Spearmint has anti-androgenic properties, and in women, may reduce hirsuitism without significant effects on testosterone or DHEA.[89] One clinical study on women with PCOS compared spearmint tea to a placebo tea and reported that androgens and gonadotrophins were significantly reduced by spearmint. In the small study LH and FSH increased and both free and total testosterone decreased over a 30 day period. Women in the group receiving the verum noted subjective improvements in hirsuitism compared to the placebo group, which did not however, correlate to the researchers objective ratings.[90]

Mentha spicata may induce oxidative stress in the hypothalamus in a manner that decreases the synthesis of LH and FSH, and thereby down-regulate testosterone.[91],[92] Regular consumption of the tea in male rats is shown to reduce testicular 3beta-HSD and 17beta-HSD enzymes, and ultimately lead to decreased sperm density, and degeneration of testicular tissues. Peppermint, *Mentha piperita*, has not been shown to have the same detrimental effects on the testes. Due to the rather significant effects on the testes, spearmint is probably best reserved for women with androgenetic alopecia, or for topical use only in men.

ORYZA - RICE BRAN OIL
A "supercritical CO2" rice bran extract applied topically is shown to promote hair growth in patients with androgenic alopecia compared to placebo, increasing hair count, diameter of individual hairs, and follicle density.[93] Rice Bran oil contains linoleic acid, policosanol, γ-oryzanol, and γ-tocotrienol noted to support hair follicles when topically applied via mechanisms involving vascular endothelial growth factor, insulin-like growth factor-1, and keratinocyte growth factor were also significantly increased and that of transforming growth factor-β (TGF-β).[94]

PANAX GINSENG – Ginseng
Panax ginseng ginsenosides are credited with 5α-reductase inhibition[95] and may have a proliferative effect on human hair dermal papilla cells.[96] *Panax ginseng* promotes hair growth when applied topically in animal models of androgenic alopecia.

PIPER NIGRUM - BLACK PEPPER
Black pepper is a natural alpha–5 reductase inhibitor[97]. The plant is also noted to potently stimulate melanogenesis, an activity credited to cubebin compounds. *Piper nigrum* and *cubeba* are most noted to be the strongest reductase inhibitors of various species, credited to piperine, the major alkaloid amide.

POLYGONUM MULTIFLORUM – Fo Ti
Polygonum multiflorum root goes by the common names Fo-Ti and He Shou Wu, and is a traditional medicine in China for promoting hair growth and preventing the hair from turning gray, but little research has been done as to its mechanisms of action. The plant is generally considered safe, with low toxicity and few side effects. *Polygonum multiflorum* is widely distributed throughout the world and has been used as a traditional medicine for centuries in China. The ethnomedical uses of *Polygonum multiflorum* have been recorded in many provinces of China and Japan for this plant and related species.

More than 100 chemical compounds have been isolated from this plant, and the major components have been determined to be stilbenes, quinones, flavonoids and others. Crude extracts and pure compounds of this plant are used as effective agents in pre-clinical and clinical practice due to their anti-aging, anti-hyperlipidaemia, anti-cancer and anti-inflammatory effects and to promote immune modulation, neuroprotection, and the curing of other diseases. However, at high doses, some fractions, particularly the quinones, such as emodin and rhein, may lead to hepatotoxicity, nephrotoxicity and embryonic toxicity. [98] Pharmacokinetic studies have demonstrated that the main components of *Polygonum multiflorum,* such as 2,3,5,4'-tetrahydroxystilbene-2-O-β-d-glucopyranoside and emodin are distributed among many organs and tissues. Gallic acid esters of tetrahydroxystilbenes and other compounds may promote growth of dermal papilla cells, and in one study, to a greater degree than minoxidil.[99]

The therapeutic potential of *Polygonum multiflorum* has been demonstrated in the conditions like Alzheimer's disease, Parkinson's disease, hyperlipidaemia, inflammation and cancer, which is attributed to the presence of various stilbenes, quinones, flavonoids, phospholipids and other compounds in the herb. In Asia, *Polygonum multiflorum* has been used to prevent hair from turning grey, or even reverse grey hair, an action most likely involving effect on melanin, α-MSH, and melanocyte regulating pathways.[100] Animal studies suggest hair growth may also be promoted via increased expression of fibroblast growth factor.[101] *Polygonum multiflorum* is a 5alpha-reductase inhibitor[102], and is shown to promote hair growth by inducing the anagen phase in resting hair follicles by inducing the expression of β-catenin.[103]

POLYPORUS UMBELLATUS
Polyporus umbellatus – This polypore mushroom promotes telogen hair in mice.

PUERARIA SPECIES - Kudzu
Pueraria thomsonii flowers are reported to have a potent inhibitory effect on testosterone 5α-reductase, more potent that *Pueraria lobata* roots, an activity credited to the saponins soyasaponin I and kaikasaponin III. The flowers promoted hair growth when topically applied and is reported a possible therapy for treating androgenic alopecia.[104] One human randomized, double-blind clinical trial on women with greying of hair, reported that an extract from *Pueraria lobata* reduced the development of new grey hairs without any significant side effects.[105]

ROSMARINUS OFFICINALIS - Rosemary
Rosmarinus officinalis has traditionally been rubbed into hair for stimulating the hair bulbs to stimulate growth and to prevent premature baldness.[106],[107] *Rosmarinus officinalis* enhances microcapillary perfusion in the scalp, and one clinical investigation included the essential oil in a minoxidil topical preparation, and reported that its inclusion reduced the occurrence of scalp itching and irritation commonly caused by the pharmaceutical.[108] Inclusion of this and other essential oils in shampoos is also reported to treat a variety of fungal and scalp infections, in both humans and animals.[109] One mouse study reported *Rosmarinus* leaf extract to ameliorate hair loss induced by high levels of testosterone. Investigators reported that the antiandrogenic effect occurred via inhibition of testosterone 5α-reductase enzymes due to the constituent 12-methoxycarnosic acid.[110]

Several important constituents of rosemary are caffeic acid and its derivatives such as rosmarinic acid. These compounds have antioxidant effects. The phenolic compound, rosmarinic acid, obtains one of its phenolic rings from phenylalanine via caffeic acid and the other from tyrosine via dihydroxyphenyl-lactic acid. Relatively large-scale production of rosmarinic acid can be obtained from the cell culture of *Coleus blumei* when supplied exogenously with phenylalanine and tyrosine. Rosmarinic acid is well absorbed from gastrointestinal tract and from the skin. It increases the production of prostaglandin E2, reduces the production of leukotriene B4 in human polymorphonuclear leucocytes, and inhibits the complement system.

SCUTELLARIA BAICALENSIS - Scute
Scutellaria baicalensis is a long-standing anti-inflammatory medicinal herb in Asian herbal traditions, and its main component baicalin, may antagonize androgen-driven alopecia and support on proliferation of human scalp dermal papilla cells.[111] Baicalin can dissociate the androgen receptor-agonist complex, reduce androgen-driven cell proliferation, and inhibit nuclear translocation of the androgen receptor stimulated by dihydrotestosterone in human dermal papilla cells, supporting hair growth in the scalp.

SERENOA REPENS – Saw Palmetto
Serenoa repens is one of the most studied natural alph-5 reductase inhibitors, and shown to promote hair growth in human subjects with androgenetic alopecia.[112] Clinical trials on med with androgenetic alopecia have shown positive results in 60% of subjects using *Serenoa repens*.[113]

THUJA ORIENTALIS - Cedar
Thuja may induce the anagen phase of hair growth via induction of B-catenin and SHH proteins in the follicles.[114]

URTICA DIOCIA - Stinging Nettle Roots
Urtica dioica has 5α-reductase inhibitory effects credited to β-sitosterol and scopoletin

CLINICAL APPLICATIONS

NUTRITIONAL SUPPLEMENTS
Consider Copper, zinc, and biotin for 2-24 months. For women, also consider iron and L- lysine.

HERBAL HAIR WASHES TO PROMOTE HAIR GROWTH
Numerous studies have shown the topical application of the legume and other herbs to promote hair growth. Carnosic acid in *Rosmarinus* and other botanical 5α-reductase inhibitors,[115] may be use topically as a daily hair rinse. Green Tea and other anti-oxidant, anti-inflammatory botanicals may be used topically on the scalp may protect the hair follicles from normal skin aging that contributes to hair loss.[116] Herbs containing dadzein and formononetin such as *Medicago* and/or *Trifolium* are inexpensive enough to use topically in a large volume. The topical use of aromatase promotors such as *Peonia* and *Glycyrrhiza* may be added to the 5α-reductase inhibitors, as an additional method of deterring DHT in the scalp.

COMPOUNDING IDEAS
Minoxidil may be compounded with finasteride for men to use topically, and compounded with progesterone for women. This may be applied 1-2 times per day depending on the strength of the formulation, once or twice a day. Herbs such as rosemary oil may be added to these pharmaceutical formulations, and followed with a botanical hair rinse, as exemplified below. The addition of Castor Oil, *Angelica,* Adenosine, and other compounds may enhance the absorption of the pharmaceuticals into the scalp and improve the efficacy. Caffeine, as described above, may enhance the absorption of a wide variety of compounds into the scalp and hair follicle.

TEA TO SLOW HAIR LOSS
Urtica root
Glycyrrhiza root
Angelica root
Pueraria root
Thea sinensis
Trifolium pratense
Mentha spicata (women only)
This tea can be prepared to drink as well as used as a scalp wash.

TINCTURE FOR HAIR GROWTH
Angelica sinensis
Glycyrrhiza
Pueraria spp
Polygonum multiflorum

Salvia miltiorrhiza
Combine equal parts and take 1-2 droppers 2-4 times per day.

HAIR PLASTER TO PROMOTE HAIR GROWTH

Polygonum multiflorum powder	2 TBL
Pueraria multiflorum powder	2 TBL
Glycyrrhiza powder	2 TBL
Castor Oil	2 TBL
Strong Coffee	3-4 ounces
Rosemary Oil	20 drops
Copper and Zinc solution	1 tsp

Place all in a small bowl and blend vigorously with a fork into a thick paste. Apply to the freshly washed hair and cover with a plastic bag and a towel. Leave in place for 30-60 minutes. Rinse out by several washings with a gentle shampoo. Follow with finasteride/minoxidil/progesterone, if chosen. And a rinse with herbal teas as follows.

HAIR RINSE

Medicago	1 pound
Trifolium	1 pound
Rosmarinus	1 pound
Glycyrrhiza	1 pound

Blend a large volume of the dried herbs, and store in 5 or 6 large ziplock bags. Steep 2 heaping cup in the largest stock pot of the house, and strain into a big bowl or pitcher, and store in the bathroom tub or shower. At the close of each shower or bath, as well as to rinse hair following using the above hair plaster, use the stored tea to rinse out the hair. When used frequently for many months, the hormonal effects of the topical herbs may help improve hormonal balance in the scalp.

ENCAPSULATION FOR HAIR LOSS
Look for a product formulated for BPH that may contain:
Serenoa repens
Urtica dioica
Pumpkin seed lipsterols
Zinc
Consume 2 or 3 capsules at a time, 2 to 3 times a day.

THE LYMPHATIC SYSTEM
And its Role in Fibrocystic Breast Disease

The White Bloodstream
Our bodies are 60-70-% fluid, and the lymphatic system is largely responsible for grooming and maintaining that fluid. The lymphatic system is responsible for collecting interstitial fluids, circulating these fluids around the body, and filtering out the impurities. Other than checking for gross lymph node abnormalities and enlargements, modern medicine gives the lymphatic system little attention. However, the lymphatic channels are vital to fluid distribution, waste elimination, immune function, and metabolic regulation. As this discussion aims to point out, loss of proper lymphatic function can result in the accumulation of waste and stagnation of fluid in the tissues. Wastes generated from the metabolic functions of all cells are excreted into the extra-cellular spaces to be taken up by the lymph channels and carried to the lymphatic nodes and blood circulation for processing. For all these reasons the lymphatic system has sometimes been referred to as the *White Bloodstream*.

The Lymph System as Part of the Reticuloendothelial System
The lymphatic system includes lymph nodes and the extensive lymphatic channels that connect them. Macrophages within lymph nodes are considered part of the reticuloendothelial system. These scavenging white blood cells are also found in the spleen and lungs. The liver houses specialized Kupffer cells and the brain contains specialized microglial cells which are both considered part of the reticuloendothelial system as well. The spleen is also a lymphoid organ and part of the reticuloendothelial system. The spleen maintains and recycles red blood cells, clears bacteria and particulate from the blood, and generates immune response. The spleen also provides vascular adaptation to stress and reverts to its gestational role as a blood forming organ in times of need. *B*-adrenergic stress stimulates the spleen to release stored red blood cells. Galen thought that the spleen was the seat of "melancholy" and "Black Bile".

The Lymph System as Part of the Immune System
Lymph nodes themselves are web-like reticular networks rich in circulating tissue fluid and leukocytes, and are considered to part of the immune system. Immune cells migrate from the bone marrow by the billions via blood circulation, and onward to the secondary lymphoid organs: lymph nodes, spleen, mucosal tissues of the digestive, respiratory, urinary, and genital organs. Immune cells concentrate in these organs where antigenic material may be encountered. Lymphocytes can migrate in and out of lymphoid tissues and may circulate between different organs via lymphatic channels. Lymphocytes may reach every cell of the body as lymphatic channels surround every organ and tissue bathing them in fluid. The lymphatic circulation drains into the thoracic duct of the vascular system.

Lymphatic Circulation
Lymphatic "capillaries" are tubular channels of endothelium, fenestrated at the basement membrane to allow interstitial fluids, proteins and particles to infuse. These channels connect clusters of lymphatic nodes and provide drainage inward from the periphery of the body and extremities to the thoracic circulation. Lymph nodes are found in the highest concentrations in the neck, axilla, groin, behind the knees, and about the ankles. It is no coincidence that these groupings of body lymph nodes are located at some of the main flexural creases of the body. Unlike the blood's circulatory system that operates under pressure with the aid of a pump to move the fluid about the vessels, the lymph system is not under pressure and has no such pumping apparatus. Instead, the lymph requires the friction, motion and pressure of muscles to move it through its channels. One-way valves in the channels help prevent back flow of fluid. Motion of the arms, legs, head, and trunk serves to massage the lymph nodes and channels. If a person is sedentary or if the amount of interstitial fluids and wastes to filter is great, the lymphatic system may become burdened, backed up, and unable to clear the fluid from the tissues. Some medical personnel specialize in manually massaging and working the lymphatic channels to assist their circulation and efficiency. Exercise, massage, and weight loss can be supportive to lymphatic drainage.

Local infections can result in minor or significant swellings the lymph nodes and affected lymphatic channels. Infections of the channels can appear as hot, tender swollen skin, with red streaks in the region of the enlarged lymph nodes. When the lymphatic drainage of a body quadrant is impaired, the limb of the afflicted quadrant may develop lymphedema, and in the extreme case, lymphangitis and cellulitis. Capillary beds may become seeded with pathogenic material from the lymph channels resulting in "blood poisoning" or septicemia.

Lymphatic Stagnation
Lymphatic stagnation can occur when the amount of fluid, cells, and wastes present, exceeds the capacity of the excretory organs. Both anabolism and catabolism produce substances that require elimination. Inflammation, infection, and oxidation, produce metabolites and cellular debris that require elimination. Ingestion of dietary or airborne allergens and toxins produces wastes requiring excretion. The sheer volume of wastes to process may exceed the abilities of the liver and kidneys. Liver or kidney disease might contribute an increased amount of waste material in the lymphatic channels. Poor circulation might also

impair elimination of wastes due to deficient circulatory dynamics. Lymphatic stagnation may also result from obstruction of the lymphatic channels due to tumors, inflammations, infections, trauma, irradiation, and any other mechanical cause. Long-term fluid stagnation in the lymphatic channels will cause the valves to fail and compound the problem. Stasis of the protein and mineral-rich lymphatic fluid can eventually lead to fibrosis of the lymphatic channels and surrounding tissues. Failure to eliminate waste material forces the body to store the waste. Hypertrophy, cyst formation, inflammation, infection, and fibrosis of affected, dependant organs and tissues will result. Lymphatic pain occurs when lymph nodes become enlarged and the capsule is stretched.

> **The body's ability to eliminate waste material depends on:**
> ♥ The type and quantity of electrolytes present in the interstitial fluid or capillary blood affects the ability of chemical ions to diffuse across membranes
> ♥ The metabolic competence of all organs
> ♥ The excretory competence of the liver, kidneys, and bowels
> ♥ The excretory competence of the special organs of elimination – skin, sweat glands, lungs.

The Impact of the Liver on Lymphatic Health
When the liver is inundated with work to do, such as processing many hormones, emulsifying fats and cholesterol, removing toxins, pesticides, drugs, alcohol, or other substances from the blood, it may have a difficult job metabolizing wastes, toxins, hormones, and pathogens. When lymphatic flow is stagnant, there may be more wastes than usual in the blood for the body to remove, resulting in stagnation in both the liver and the lymph system. For these reasons, improving liver function and intestinal function may optimize hormonal metabolism, waste accumulation, and lymphatic flow and have a positive impact on appendicitis, renal cysts, tonsilar enlargement and chronic sore throats, and fibrocystic disease of the breast.

When the liver is not digesting the food it is presented with, not synthesizing quality bile, and not supporting a healthy intestinal environment, the appendix may suffer. Constipation and bowel toxemia is highly associated with the development of appendicitis.

When the liver and spleen are not purifying the blood, infections can result. Colds, influenza, bladder infections, and sore throats can sometimes be the result of altered blood and tissue fluids that readily support bacteria and viruses. Enlarged tonsils occur when the tonsils are working hard to clear unwanted substances from the upper respiratory tissues, without the support of the surrounding lymphatic channels to clear the wastes away. Chronic infections are seen when the tonsils and immune system are weakened, fluid and waste accumulates, and pathogens are allowed to flourish.

The Impact of the Kidneys of Lymphatic Health
When the lymphatic and hepatic routes of elimination are challenged, more work is handed to the kidneys. When fluid and waste accumulates in the body, renal routes of elimination will be needed to compensate and assist the liver and lymphatic channels in clearing the body of unwanted fluids and substances. Kidney and bladder infections may result from inundation with toxic substances to process. Renal cysts may be the result of the kidneys attempt to remove unwanted fluid from circulation but having little power other than simply walling off the offending substances.

Altered mineral composition of the collecting urine may allow crystals and acid wastes to accumulate. Kidney stones, gout, and other diseases may result. A deficiency in the alkali minerals including Na, Ca, Mg, Li, and K may result in acid accumulation (CO_2 or carbonic acid, oxalic acid, uric acid, etc.) The alkali minerals are needed to neutralize acidic compounds in the bloodstream. Calcium for example is needed to neutralize acids such as oxalic acid. A calcium deficiency or an oxalate excess will cause irritating acids to build up in the tissues.

Early American physicians upheld the traditions of their vitalistic forerunners and believed that proper mineral balance was essential to the prevention of "*scrophula*", meaning the tendency to develop infections involving enlarged lymph nodes.

Berries are reported to neutralize acids and assist the kidneys in eliminating wastes. Cherry juice, for example is credited with anti-inflammatory activity and in promoting the excretion of uric acid via the kidneys. Cranberries are an unusual acid berry used to acidify the urine, act as a renal depurant, and inhibit the adherence of microbes to urinary mucosa. Even though they may contain organic acids such as malic and tartaric acids, berries are generally alkalinizing due to the high content of alkali minerals, and the tendency for some organic acid to be metabolized into alkaline substances ("alkaline ash"). Rheumatism and arthritis has long been said to be acidic diseases in folk medicine. Ancient ideas on the doctrine of signatures purported berries to be beneficial in clearing enlarged lymph nodes, swellings, and growths from the body. Berries were advised for those with lymphatic or scrophular tendencies. Ground cherry pits were used for those with a history of kidney stones.

The Impact of the Blood on Lymphatic Health
Abnormal blood composition will result in abnormal lymph composition. The competence of the liver and kidneys, as discussed, will affect the ability of these organs to purify the blood. When the liver does not transmute, emulsify, metabolize, conjugate or detoxify the blood as it is required to do, the quality of the exiting blood will be affected. When the ability of

kidneys to usurp acids, salts, and electrolytes is altered, the quality of the blood is affected. Likewise, imbalanced intestinal flora will affect the nutrients and toxins absorbed into the blood via the intestinal mucosa. Poorly digestive foods, allergenic foods, excessive food intake can all produce harmful substances that may be absorbed directly into the blood stream.

Effects of Lymphatic Stagnation on the Tissues and Organs
Stagnation of fluid can cause swelling or puffiness in the tissues. But even worse, stagnation of fluid will cause cells and organs to be bathed in cellular waste products and cause abnormal osmotic balances and pressures. Organs in the vicinity of the lymphatic stagnation will have a more difficult time receiving nutrients and eliminating wastes and will likewise lead to stagnation in these organs. Lymphatic organs such as the tonsils and appendix may become enlarged and inflamed, as lymphatic flow becomes insufficient. The organs of elimination – liver, bowels, skin, and especially kidneys – may try to compensate for lymphatic insufficiency and assist the body in the waste and fluid removal process. The kidneys in particular may suffer, being an organ involved with fluid balance. The breasts, being surrounded by lymphatic nodes and channels may also develop abnormal fluid accumulation and suffer from stagnant circulation of fluid. As the kidneys and breasts are unable to eliminate and metabolize wastes efficiently, unwanted substances will accumulate in these organs. Since wastes and toxins can be so damaging to cells and tissues, the organs may do the next best thing short of excreting the wastes – wall them off. When the breasts or kidneys form cysts, they are in effect removing the excessive fluid and unwanted wastes and metabolites from their workspace. Forming cysts is like tidying up and placing unwanted items in an out of the way storage space where they won't clutter metabolic business.

CHRONIC TONSILITIS AND ENLARGED TONSILLS
The tonsils sit like sentries on either side or the oral cavity to guard against ingested or inhaled intruders. Chronic tonsillitis indicates lymphatic insufficiency, dampness in the tissues, and immune challenge. Tonsillar enlargement is a sign that the tonsils are busy and working hard. Lymphatic stagnation will often be noted in the surrounding cervical, aural, and/or submandibular nodes. Long-term support of the liver, kidneys, and immune system, along with measures to facilitate lymphatic drainage will often improve the situation.

APPENDICITIS
Bowel toxemia, liver burden, and constipation will often precede acute appendicitis. Enlargement of inguinal lymphatic nodes will often accompany. Though heroic measures such as emergency surgery are sometimes necessary, simply removing an inflamed appendix will not fix the underlying pathology. Anyone having suffered an episode of acute appendicitis should undergo follow-up therapy to improve liver and intestinal function, as well as abdominal lymphatic circulation

POLYCYSTIC KIDNEY DISEASE
Lymphatic, hepatic, and renal tonics may all be indicated depending on the situation. Aim to lighten the workload on the kidneys by improving lymphatic flow in the pelvis and abdomen. Assist the kidneys by improving the quality of the blood they are asked to filter. Note the quality of the diet especially where proteins, minerals, and electrolytes are concerned. Insuring that the liver is keeping up with its portion of the eliminatory workload and offer support, alteratives, fats and toxins as needed.

FIBROCYSTIC BREAST DISEASE
In naturopathic medicine, fibrocystic breast disease may be a sign of hyperestrogenism or poor hormonal metabolism. Clearly, hormones play a role in the disease, as the cyclical nature of the complaint attests. Individuals who take hormones, such as birth control pills, may develop fibrocystic breasts as a result of the increased estrogen in the body, compared to the liver's ability to conjugate and excrete it. Breast pain and cysts is a common side affect of post-menopausal hormone replacement therapy. Birth control pills, other hormones, and other pharmaceuticals are known to promote cholestasis within the liver. Since it is the liver's job to metabolize hormones in circulation, and remove wastes from the blood stream, liver disease can lead to the development of hyperestrogenism and fibrocystic breasts. The liver removes active estrogens from circulation, conjugating them and releasing them to the GI tract for elimination. People who consume a lot of meat, poultry, eggs, or dairy products may also ingest estrogens in small amounts due to hormonal residues in animal products. Animals are often fed estrogens to bring them to market weight more quickly, or to increase milk and egg production. Hormonal residues consumed on a regular basis (milk, meat, and eggs are often consumed on a regular basis) can also contribute to the hormonal load on the body. Animal products are also the source or urate metabolites requiring renal excretion.

 The formation of cysts in the body may be thought of the body's attempt to remove substances it finds offensive from the tissues and circulation. In the formation of cysts, the body performs the role of the liver, when the liver is unable to do so. Pharmaceutical estrogen therapy is not effective for fibrocystic breasts, may worsen the complaint, and in fact, cause the complaint. Ingestion of exogenous hormones will increase the workload on the liver and contribute to cholestasis. Treatment for fibrocystic lesions varies greatly between standard allopathic medicine and natural medicine. Allopathic medicine may offer hormonal therapies. Standard treatment for severe fibrocystic breasts has been oral androgen therapy, such as danazol to counteract the effect of endogenous estrogens. Danazol reduces the release of all gonadotrophins from the pituitary, and is another hormone requiring liver conjugation and excretion.

The Lymphatic Constitution and The Scrophular Miasm

The *Four Elements Theory* is an ancient philosophy on the nature of physical reality. The theory has taken on many twists, adaptations, and associations as it was adopted by many peoples, cultures, and belief systems over many millennia. The theory has been applied to medicine and healing in various ways.

In ancient Europe, Galen adopted the notion of the Four Elements and assigned each element to a specific temperament in human beings. He spoke of the "4 humours" that circulated throughout the body and associated them with the various, temperaments, elements, and disease tendencies.

The Major Acquired Taints or Miasms

Psora is said to be the mother of all diseases. It is the most external and affects primarily the skin. Psora is sometimes call "The Itch", but all manner of skin afflictions, not only pruritic ones are representative of psora. The so called psoriatic diseases may move the body toward greater health in that psora may facilitate the removal of toxins out through the skin, from the interior to the exterior of the body. Supression of psora, or a lowered vitality may move diseases deeper into the body resulting in the Syphillitic, Sycotic, or Tubercular miasms.

Tubercular or the *Scrofular* taints are characterized by the tendency toward diseases involving lymph node enlargement. Tuberculosis is one such lymphatic disease, as is a susceptibility to colds, catarrh, sore throats, and glandular diseases.

Sycosis is defined as the tendency toward ulceration, deep infections, and tissue breakdown, as with gonorrhea.

Syphilis is defined as the tendency to blood diseases, weakness, wasting

---

EVALUATING THE LYMPH SYSTEM
- Note fluid accumulation in the tissues –
    puffiness around the eyes, thick boggy skin, pitting in the lower limbs.
- Note "dampness in the tissues" –
    chronic post nasal drip, boils, coated tongue, fetid tonsils
- Note the eyes –
    Discolorations or rough textures on the conjunctiva,
    A whitish ring around the outer iris indicates lymphatic impurities.
- Note the lymph nodes themselves –
    Palpate the cervical chains, axillary, sternal region, groin, popliteal and ankle regions.
- When lymphadenopathy or tenderness is present, note also –
    Fever, night sweats, inflammation, weight loss, immune status, occupation, pets, sore throat
- Note the extremities
    Palpate the hands and feet to note the temperature
    Examine the nail beds and color, the health of the nails, the shape of the fingers
    Examine the health and presence of fine body hairs on the lower limbs
    Note any varicosities or pigmentary changes on the limbs.

Diseases associated with Lymphadenopthy
Infections: Viral, Bacterial, Chlamydial, Ricketsial
Immune Disease – Rheumatoid Arthritis, Systemic Lupus, Sjogren's , Connective Tissue Disease, Silicosis
Drugs: Allopurinol, Diphenylhydantoin, Hydralazine
Malignancies: Hodgkins and Non-Hodgkins Lymphoma, Leukemia, Amyloidosis

IMPROVING LYMPHATIC FLOW WITH LYMPHATIC BOTANICALS:
Botanicals that assist the lymphatic system in clearing congestion and accumulated fluids or wastes from the tissues, may reduce some infectious, inflammatory, cystic and glandular pathologies. By assisting in the removal of excessive fluids, lymphatics prevent stagnation and cyst formation in the breasts and kidneys, fluid in the limbs, and remove bloating in the abdomen.

IMPROVING LYMPHATIC FLOW WITH CIRCULATORY TONICS
General circulatory tonics such as *Capsicum* (Cayenne) may improve the activity of other botanicals. If there is evidence of varicose veins, hemorrhoids, or poor circulation, also consider *Gingko, Vaccinium* (Blueberries, Bilberries, Whortleberries), *Crataegus* (Hawthorne berries), or *Hammamelis* (Witch Hazel).

Massage of the entire body will promote circulation and support lymphatic flow. Exercise is known to improve both blood and lymphatic circulation. Saunas and other methods of hydrotherapy can also increase dynamic circulation through the blood vessel and lymphatic channels, as well as promote elimination via the skin. Since our skin houses over 60,000 miles of capillaries that can assist in the elimination of wastes as well as transport Vitamin D in the superficial regions of the skin back to the kidney where it may promote the retention of calcium and the excretion of acidic wastes. In moderation, sunlight is thought to promote health, stimulate peripheral circulation, and to be essential to proper lymphatic activity.

IMPROVING LYPHATIC FLOW WITH
ALTERATIVE AND LIVER SUPPORTIVE BOTANICALS:
Silybum marianum, **(Milk Thistle),**
Curcuma **(Turmeric),**
Ceanothus **(Red Root)**
Taraxicum officinalis **(Dandelion)**
Arctium **(Burdock)**

LIPOTROPIC NUTRIENTS
The **B Vitamins choline, inositol** and **methionine** also support liver function and are found in commercial "Lipotropic" formulas. Lipotropic literally means fat-mover and the term is used to refer to substances that are able to help the liver metabolize fats and remove them from the blood stream. Besides improving fat metabolism, Lipotropics will also aid in the metabolism of fat soluble nutrients and aid the liver in its other metabolic functions: such as the processing of hormones, estrogen, sulfa drugs, glucose and glycogen. Choline may be synthesized from methionine, glycine, or serine in the body. Choline is necessary to synthesize acetylcholine, a crucial neurotransmitter and cellular messenger. Choline is notably high in egg yolks, and *lecithin*. Soybeans and other legumes are high in lecithin which provides phosphotidlycholine needed to emulsify fats, breaking them down to be metabolized.

Choline is also found in **eggs,**
Leguminosea family **(legumes or beans, especially soybean,** *Glycine max*),
Beta vulgaris **(beets),**
Silybum marianum **(Milk Thistle)**,
Cynara species and related **Artichokes** and **Thistles,**
Some **dark green leafy vegetables,** and
wheat germ also contain smaller amounts of choline.

Choline and inositol may be synthesized by sulfur-metabolizing intestinal bacteria. Inositol is a B vitamin that acts as a lipotropic agent in a manner similar to choline. Since inositol can be synthesized from glucose, it is not thought to be essential as choline and methionine. Methionine is a sulfur-containing amino acid that is necessary to the synthesis of choline, cysteine, and taurine. When converted to cysteine, this sulfur compound acts as a liver antioxidant and detoxifier. Methionine is not abundantly available in vegetarian diet, but is found in dairy, eggs, fish, and meat, especially organ meats. Vegetarian sources are legumes such as soybeans, and nuts and seeds. Other food plants containing methionine include the cereal grains **wheat, corn,** and **rice.** Choline and methionine may be transformed into glutathione within the liver. Glutathione is needed by the liver to metabolize alcohol, hepatotoxins, and toxic substances. Milk Thistle has been observed to raise liver glutathione levels in the liver preventing its depletion. Hyperestrogenism, as well as Gilbert's syndrome will often respond to methionine and Milk Thistle therapy. Supplementing bile itself, or bile salts will also, of course, act as lipotropic agents. Using liver products, such protomorphogens or consuming organic liver as a food will also provide choline, methionine, sulfur, B Vitamins, fat soluble vitamins and many other substances. Protomorphogens are best for extremely debilitated, weakened, or elderly individuals.

Iodine, Nutritents, and Breast Health
Iodine also plays a role in not only thyroid, but many endocrine functions in the human body. Iodine helps maintain normal breast tissue architecture and function. Iodine may also have important antioxidant functions in breast tissue and other tissues that concentrate iodine via the sodium iodide symporter. Studies suggest that using 3.0- to 6.0-mg of Iodine may effectively treat fibrocystic breast disease.[1,2] Iodine may also protect against known carcinogens, including N-methyl-n-nitrosourea-induced mammary

carcinogenesis.[3] Molecular iodine treatment activates a caspase-independent and mitochondria-mediated apoptotic pathways in the breasts and helps to treat a variety of breast pathologies from fibrocystic breasts to cancer.

Folic acid also appears important to maintain health breast tissue.[4] Vitamin A in the form of Retinoic acid appears to be an important co-regulator of many hormone at the level of the nucleus of reproductive and endocrine organ cells. Retinoids act as agents of chemoprevention and differentiation in breast diseases. Retinoid mediate activity at nuclear receptors, retinoic acid receptors, and retinoid X receptors, and are modulated by cellular retinol binding proteins. Breast disease, including fibrocystic breast disease may be mitigated with retinoic acid supplementation.[5]

CALENDULA OFFICINALIS
POT MARIGOLD
Family: *Compositate (Asteraceae)*

These sunny flowered marigolds will blossom continually throughout the spring, summer, and fall, and then cheerfully reseed themselves when faced with the harshness of winter. This Mediterranean native has acclimatized itself to diverse climes becoming a valuable medicine of ancient healing, European folk medicine, early American pioneer medicine, and modern herbalism.

The orange and yellow flowers are gathered in the early stages of flowering to be tinctured or soaked in vegetable oil to create salves and topical medicines. Dry flowers may be used in teas or also used to prepare oils. The fresh plant including succulent stems and leaves may be juiced to use fresh or preserved with alcohol to prepare succi.

Calendula is commonly used as a wound healing medicine for external skin afflictions, and internal mucous membranes infections and inflammations. The herb is known to be antimicrobial to bacterial, viral, and fungal microbes. The herb is credited with anti-inflammatory, astringent, hemostatic, and vulnerary actions. *Calendula* may be infused and used as an astringent wash for suppurative, bleeding, or weeping skin conditions. Or infusions and successes may be taken internally for infection of the digestive tract, inflammatory conditions of the stomach, bowel, or bladder, and for bleeding and irritation of internal digestive and urinary passages. *Calendula* oils and salves may applied to abrasions, lacerations, dermatitis, diaper rash, dry cracking skin, chapped lips and chaffed or wind-burnt skin, and many other conditions. *Calendula* may also be used as a douche for vaginitis, and to irrigate the ears in cases of otitis externa and interna.

In addition to these topical usages for which *Calendula* is so well known, this herb may also have hormonal, lymphatic, and alterative actions. Where there are chronic infections of the sinuses, throat, tonsils, or ears with accompanying lymphadenopthy, consider Calendula teas, succi, and gargles. Where there are skin infections and lymphadenopthy, vaginitis and inguinal lymphadeopthy, or any chronic infection or inflammation associated with lymph node enlargement or tenderness, Calendula may be a gentle and effective tonic.

Calendula has not had extensive molecular or physiologic research, but appear to promote angiogenesis and support microvascular tissue. *Calendula* may support breast health via promotion of the glycosamino-glycan hyaluronic acid, and increase microvasculature in a manner that supports circulation.[6] *Calendula* has been shown to activate lymphocytes and increase cytotoxicity against breast cancer cell lines.[7]

Calendula Constituents:
Carotenoids and other *Flavinoids* – having an anti-inflammatory effect
Triterpenoid Saponins
Phytosterols
Resins – believed responsible for the astringent activity, as Calendula is not high in tannins
Bitters
Essential Oils
Mucilage

GALIUM APAREINE
CLEAVERS
Family: *Rubiaceae*

This low growing herbaceous herb possesses minute hooked hairs and burs that cause it to cling to passing fur and fabric. Effective medicines may be made from the fresh young plant by tincturing or juicing. Fresh juices may be combined with alcohol to create succuses (~1:5, low alcohol of 25%), or preserved in glycerol. (~40%) *Galium* is a gentle, nourishing eliminative herb that can be used to improve lymphatic flow. *Galium* is a diuretic and depurative capable of improving renal function and thereby enhancing lymphatic circulation. *Galium* is also high is organic salts and alkali minerals and is thought to improve electrolyte and solute balance in the tissues. *Galium* may have anti-inflammatory and tonifying effects specifically on the urinary and lymphatic systems. *Galium* is also credited with anti-inflammatory effects on the bladder and ureters, and was recommended for painful conditions of the urinary tract. Lymphadenopathy accompanying chronic infections and inflammations will often respond to *Galium*. Lymphatic stagnation, resulting in edema and urinary tract infections, may also be improved by *Galium*. Scudder, a well-known early American physician, reported *Galium* to be indicated where there were nodular growths or deposits in the tissues. *Galium* was considered an alterative agent specifically called for in scrofulous disorders.

Galium has sometimes been mentioned in folkloric literature for lymphatic congestion and lymphatic tumors of the throat, and was recommended both internally and topically for such purposes. One recent study suggested activity against head and neck cancer cell lines[8], and another showed activity against laryngeal cancers.[9] *Galium* is shown to be highly inhibitory to cancer initiation, whether due to benzenes or cigarette smoke, and is therefore credited with preventative, as well as therapeutic activity.[10] An Algerian species of *Galium, Galium mollugo,* is noted to reduce inflammatory responses in fibroblasts, which may help deter fibroblast proliferation and inflammation in various fibrotic diseases.[11] *Galium* species have strong antioxidant activity and have been shown to have anti-haemolytic effects[12], and to help with the re-epithelialization of wounds and burns.[13]

Galium Constituents
- Iridoid glycosides: *monotropein, acubin*. Credited with lymphatic effects
- Phenolic acids
- Flavinoids: *quercitin, isorutin, hesperidin, luteolin*
- Mineral salts and nutrients.
- Small quantity of anthroquinone glycosides including *galiosin*. Galiosin is found in associatiion with a reddish pigment, like it's Rubiaciae family relative Madder.
- Coumarins: *asperuloside, umbelliferone, scopoletin*
- Organic acids including *citric acid, gallitannic acid, and rubichloric acids.*
- Tannins

IRIS VERSICOLOR
WILD IRIS, BLUE FLAG
Family: *Iridaceae*

Iris was used and written about extensively by the early American "eclectic" physicians, a group of MDs practicing in the late 1800s and early 1990s who used herbal medicines extensively. *Iris versicolor* is a small wild *Iris* found in marshy damp areas of the United States and goes by the common name Blue Flag as its presence should "flag" you to be aware of the marshy area. *Iris* contains iridin, volatile oils, resins, and alkaloids, but has not yet had its turn in the research arena and little molecular, cellular, or clinical research has been conducted on the plant. None the less, the plant has a long history of medicinal use, some of the particulars being to move all sorts of bodily fluids: saliva, lymph, bile, and digestive secretions. For all manner of sluggish metabolic functions, including the thyroid, *Iris* was used to clear congested tissues, move sluggish bowels, decongest the lymph, and reduce enlarged spleen, liver, and thyroid glands. For all of these important functions, the eclectic physicians classified *Iris* as an alterative, sailagogue (promotes salivation), cholagogue (promotes bile flow), and lymphogogue (promote gradual decongestion of lymphatic channels and tissues).

Traditional uses for the thyroid include topical use directly on goitrous thyroid glands to stimulate thyroid function and reduce enlargement, while taking the medicine internally simultaneously. One respected eclectic author and practitioner, HW Felter said that *Iris* "impresses the thyroid function", here meaning the opposite of suppresses, or supports and promotes thyroid function. The bulk of the early 1900s era literature purports that *Iris* mainly decongests and detoxifies tissues, including the breast and the thyroid, so that normal functioning can be restored. Iris is most indicated for hypo-rather than hyperfunctioning glands.

The freshly dug resinous bulbs are tinctured or dried and used in small doses to support fluid circulation. In large amounts, Iris preparations can be nauseating, irritating, and emetic. Specific indications include using *Iris* to stimulate bile flow, pancreatic, gastric and salivary secretions. H.W. Felter has reported Iris as being specific for soft pliable lymphatic enlargements, and rough, oily skin with sebaceous disorders. As a digestive alterative, Iris is thought specific for engorgement of the liver, spleen, and thyroid with a sensation of fullness, aching and pain. Where the skin is unhealthy, jaundice, or otherwise discolored, where tissues are full and boggy, and where there are deficient secretions in any and all of the body's glands, Iris may be helpful. The eclectic physicians espoused Iris for lymphatic disorders resulting in "bad blood" and recommended it for the various cachexias – lymphatic, scrophular, and syphillitic.

Iris Constituents
- Triterpenoids – *iriversical, isoiridogermanl*
- Oleoresins – *iridin*, an isoflavone, a type of flavonoid. It is the 7-glycoside of irigenin and can be isolated from several species of irises
- Steroidal resin
- Organic acids – *isophthalic, salicylic*
- Volatile Oil

PHYTOLACCA AMERICANA
(Synonymous with PHYTOLACCA DECANDRA)
POKEROOT, POKE

Even though Phytolacca is well known to have toxicity, this southern beauty has been used as a food and a medicine. The leaves of Phytolacca are sometimes eaten as a spring green, but must be boiled in fresh water several times to remove the potentially toxic alkaloids. The therapeutic use of Phytolacca requires some skill, so it is best left to a trained herbalist until the plant is well understood. The alkaloid phytolaccine is toxic in high doses, but occurs only in small amounts in the root and is considered safe in moderation, in small doses, and short-term. The tempting purple berries should be avoided as they are quite high in Phytolaccine and outright toxic, although they do produce a lovely red dye. The word Pokeroot is thought to have come from "puccoon" meaning a red dye. The Latin Genus Phytolacca is derived from the root words *phyto-* meaning plant, and *lacca*, meaning milk. The root can become very large and when chopped and processed will exude a milky fluid. When processing Phytolacca root, it is best to wear gloves, as prolonged contact with the milky juice can be irritating to the skin.

Small doses of 10 to 40 drops of tincture diluted in water or other botanicals can be taken several times a day for sore throats, and lymphatic swelling. Phytolacca oil is also applied topically to enlarged lymph nodes in the neck accompanying infections. For fibrocystic breast, Phytolacca oil may be combined with several drops each or Chamomile, Rosemary, and Thuja essential oils. Several tsp may be rubbed into the breasts and covered with heat.

Phytolacca has been used as a stimulating alterative herb, particularly for the lymphatic system.[14,15] *Phytolacca* appears to enhance resistance to viruses in particular. Like Echinacea, Pokeroot appears to enhance white blood cell efficiency. *Phytolacca* has been shown to inhibit the herpes virus in microbiology experiments[16]. The early American eclectic physicians and herbalists' used *Phytolacca* in small dosages internally for breast ailments, cancer and lymphatic engorgement.[17,18] Poultices of the fresh root were applied topically for breast, lymph, and skin cancers. This therapy is NOT recommended often since fresh Pokeroot used topically is rather caustic, and strong enough to ulcerate the skin and promote destruction of tissue. This was done purposely by some practitioners a century or more ago in an effort to promote expulsion of diseased tissues prior to the development of modern surgical skills. Oils made from the fresh roots, are much safer as the caustic substances are sufficiently diluted.

When used for infections, *Phytolacca* excels in treating the throat and tonsils since the tonsils are organs of the lymphatic system. Breast infections, such as those due to milk engorgement in a nursing mother, or breast cysts will often respond to the administration of *Phytolacca* tincture. Swollen lymph nodes are another indication for Pokeroot. *Phytolacca* oil may be applied topically and covered with heat, while *Phytolacca* tincture may be taken in small dosages internally. Lymph node tenderness or enlargement can be a sign of a serious problem, and when unexplained or persistent, require professional attention.

Phytolacca is used in traditional anticancer, warming, anti-phlegm clearing formulas in China.[19]
Highly diluted and homeopathic forms of *Phytolacca* have also been deter breast cancer cell lines, although the full strength mother tincture had the greatest cytotoxic effect.[20] Activity against human breast

adenocarcinoma has been demonstrated.[21] *Phytolacca* contains a ribosomal inactivating protein (RIP) with antiviral effects. It is not able to enter cells on its own, in isolation, but with other herbs, or perhaps even the broader constituents of the *Phytolacca,* it may. This protein is reported to act as a hormonotoxin, due to its ability to bind GnRH receptors that may be over expressed on breast cancer cells.[22]

Possible Toxicities and Side Affects
Phytolacca can be nauseating and irritating to throat and digestive tissues. When taken internally it should be diluted with water or with other herbal preparations. Large dosages of *Phytolacca* can grossly alter white blood cell activity, raising the WBC count, and mimicking leukemia. Do not consume *Phytolacca* berries as they are particularly high in the phytolaccine alkaloid. Use root preparations in small cautious dosages only. Limit the usage of Pokeroot to a short duration. Long-term use or overdose can cause a type of toxicity that comes on slowly and is slow to subside.

Phytolacca Constituents
Antimicrobial alkaloid, *Phytolaccine*
Anti viral protein substance, a substance known as pokeweed mitogen[23]
Triterpenoid saponins
Vitamin K in significant quantities

OTHER LYMPHOGOGUE BOTANICALS (LYMPH-MOVERS) INCLUDE:

Baptisia tinctoria **(Wild Indigo)** a stimulating potentially caustic plant used for chronic infections and suppuration. Contains immune polysaccharides and is specific for chronic tonsillitis, dampness of tissues, congested unhealthy tissues with purplish discoloration and swelling, tendency to ulceration and discharge. Foul breath, infectious secretion, chronicity to complaints with tissue breakdown.

Ceanothus americanus **(Red Root, New Jersey Tea)** the Eclectic physicians recommended *Ceanothus* for swollen tissues with a damp boggy character and for catarrh and excessive secretions. *Ceanothus* is reported to improve congestion in the spleen and to be specific for splenomegaly and malaria. *Ceanothus* is used during the Civil War for malarial and splenic enlargement.

Echinacea angustifolia, purpurea **(Purple Cone Flower)**
Echinacea is specific indicated for decay and when tissues become stagnant, foul smelling, discolored, congested and purulent.

*Urtica urens, dioica (***Nettles)** – Nourishing tonic acting as a renal depurant, mineral source, lymphatic stimulant, anti-inflammatory. Old herbals have reported Nettles to be useful in tuberculosis, lung infections, lymphatic stagnation, and scrophular diseases. Due to its high mineral content, Nettles are also useful for anemia, rickets, and malnutrition.

Viola tricolor, arvensis **and** *vulgaris* **sub-species (Violets, Johnny Jump-ups)** – used in pediatric infections and cradles cap. Useful for excema and tubercular skin conditions, especially when used topically.

---

[1] **Altern Med Rev.** 2008 Jun;13(2):116-27. *Iodine: deficiency and therapeutic considerations.* Patrick L1.
[2] **Can J Surg.** 1993 Oct;36(5):453-60. *Iodine replacement in fibrocystic disease of the breast.* Ghent WR1, Eskin BA, Low DA, Hill LP.
[3] **J Biol Chem.** 2006 Jul 14;281(28):19762-71. *Molecular iodine induces caspase-independent apoptosis in human breast carcinoma cells involving the mitochondria-mediated pathway.* Shrivastava A1, Tiwari M, Sinha RA, et al.
[4] **Int J Vitam Nutr Res.** 1998;68(1):59-62.*A high-affinity folate binding protein in fluid of benign cysts of human liver and mammary gland.* Holm J1, Hansen SI, Høier-Madsen M.
[5] **Eur J Endocrinol.** 1997 Oct;137(4):410-4. *Retinoic acid receptors alpha, beta and gamma, and cellular retinol binding protein-I expression in breast fibrocystic disease and cancer.* Pasquali D1, Bellastella A, Valente A, et al.

[6] **Phytomedicine.** 1996 May;3(1):11-8. *Induction of vascularisation by an aqueous extract of the flowers of Calendula officinalis L. the European marigold.* Patrick KF1, Kumar S, Edwardson PA, Hutchinson JJ.

[7] **BMC Cancer.** 2006 May 5;6:119.*A new extract of the plant Calendula officinalis produces a dual in vitro effect: cytotoxic anti-tumor activity and lymphocyte activation.* Jiménez-Medina E1, Garcia-Lora A, Paco L, Algarra I, Collado A, Garrido F.

[8] **Oncol Rep.** 2014 Sep;32(3):1296-302. *Galium verum aqueous extract strongly inhibits the motility of head and neck cancer cell lines and protects mucosal keratinocytes against toxic DNA damage.* Schmidt M1, Polednik C1, Roller J1, Hagen R1.

[9] Int J Oncol. 2014 Mar;44(3):745-60. Effect of *Galium verum aqueous extract on growth, motility and gene expression in drug-sensitive and -resistant laryngeal carcinoma cell lines.* Schmidt M1, Scholz CJ2, Gavril GL3, Otto C1, Polednik C1, Roller J1, Hagen R1.

[10] **Oncol Rep.** 2014 Sep;32(3):1296-302. *Galium verum aqueous extract strongly inhibits the motility of head and neck cancer cell lines and protects mucosal keratinocytes against toxic DNA damage.* Schmidt M1, Polednik C1, Roller J1, Hagen R1.

[11] **J Pharm Biomed Anal.** 2016 Jan 5;117:79-84. *Unusual compounds from Galium mollugo and their inhibitory activities against ROS generation in human fibroblasts.* Chaher N1, Krisa S2, Delaunay JC2, et al.

[12] **Arh Hig Rada Toksikol.** 2014 Dec;65(4):399-406. *Antihaemolytic activity of thirty herbal extracts in mouse red blood cells.* Khalili M, Ebrahimzadeh MA, Safdari Y.

[13] **Res Pharm Sci.** 2013 Jul;8(3):197-203.n*Antioxidant and burn healing potential of Galium odoratum extracts.*nnKahkeshani N1, Farahanikia B, Mahdaviani P, Abdolghaffari A, Hassanzadeh G, Abdollahi M, Khanavi M.

[14] Felter, H., The Eclectic Materia Medica, Phyarmacology, and Theraputics Cincinatti, OH 1922, pp 535-538.

[15] The British Herbal Pharmacopea, published by the British Herbal Medecine Association, Cowling, 1983

[16] Aron, G., and Irvin, J., *'Inhibition of herpes simplex virus multiplication by the pokeweed antiviral protein'*, Antimicro. Agents Chemother., 1980, 17, pp. 1,032-3.

[17] . Ellingwood, F. American Materia Medica, Theraputics, and Pharmacognosy Eclectic Medical Publications, Reprinted inPortland, OR. 1983

[18] Culbreth, D. A Manual of Materia Medica and Pharmacology, Eclectic Medical Publications, Reprinted in Portland, OR 1983

[19] **Chin J Integr Med.** 2012 Aug;18(8):599-604. *Anticancer effects of 5-fluorouracil combined with warming and relieving cold phlegm formula on human breast cancer.* Wang XL1, Ma F, Wu XZ.

[20] **Homeopathy.** 2013 Oct;102(4):274-82.. *Anti-proliferative effects of homeopathic medicines on human kidney, colon and breast cancer cells.* Arora S1, Aggarwal A, Singla P, Jyoti S, Tandon S.

[21] **Int J Oncol.** 2010 Feb;36(2):395-403. *Cytotoxic effects of ultra-diluted remedies on breast cancer cells.* Frenkel M1, Mishra BM, Sen S, Yang P, Pawlus A, Vence L, Leblanc A, Cohen L, Banerji P, Banerji P.

[22] **Endocrinology.** 2003 Apr;144(4):1456-63. *Cytotoxic activity of gonadotropin-releasing hormone (GnRH)-pokeweed antiviral protein conjugates in cell lines expressing GnRH receptors.* Yang WH1, Wieczorck M, Allen MC, Nett TM.

[23] Lewis, W., and Elvin-Lewis, M., Medical Botany, John Wiley and Sons, New York, NY, 1977, pp. 98-9

Autism Spectrum Disorders and the Search for Answers

©2014 updated 2015, David Winston, RH(AHG)

Autism spectrum disorders (ASD) are pervasive neurodevelopmental disorders that are characterized by delayed or abnormal ability to communicate and interact with others, as well as patterns of repetitive, restricted or stereotypical behavior. These problems occur early in childhood (before age 3) and are more frequent in boys than girls (4 boys have ASD to every girl who has it). The occurrence of this disorder has increased dramatically over the past 30 years. According to the CDC in the past decade alone, the incidence of ASD has increased 78%. In 2000 and 2002 it is estimated 1 in 150 children had the disorder, by 2006 the number had increased to 1 in 110 and current data suggests that 1 in 88 children have autism (CDC, 2012). While there is no doubt that greater awareness and early detection have had some influence on this, it is also clear that neither of these factors is a major component to the fast paced increase of ASD cases.

In the DSM-IV, ASD was divided into several types. These include autism, Asperger's syndrome, and pervasive developmental disorder not otherwise specified (PDD-NOS). Two other conditions are upon occasion included in this list, Rett's syndrome and childhood disintegrative disorder. Both are pervasive developmental disorders, but are thought to be unrelated to ASD. In the recently published DSM-V, the differentiated conditions, autism, Asperger's syndrome and PDD-NOS have been replaced by the umbrella term Autism Spectrum Disorders and will now be rated by severity (level 1, 2 or 3).

The new DSM-V criteria for ASD include the following, and a person must fit all 4 criteria:
A. Persistent deficit in social communication and social interaction across contexts, not accounted for by general developmental delays, and manifest by all 3 of the following:
   1. Deficits in social-emotional reciprocity: ranging from abnormal social approach and failure of normal back and forth conversation through reduced sharing of interests, emotions, and affect and response to total lack of initiation of social interaction.
   2. Deficits in nonverbal communicative behaviors used for social interaction; ranging from poorly integrated-verbal and nonverbal communication, through abnormalities in eye contact and body-language, or deficits in understanding and use of nonverbal communication, the total lack of facial expression or gestures.
   3. Deficits in developing and maintaining relationships, appropriate to developmental level (beyond those with caregivers); ranging from difficulties adjusting behavior to suite different social contexts through difficulties in sharing imaginative play and in making friends to an apparent absence of interest in people.
B. Restricted, repetitive patterns of behavior, interests, or activities as manifested by at least two of the following:
   1. Stereotyped or repetitive speech, motor movements, or use of objects (such as simple motor stereotypes, repetitive use of objects or idiosyncratic phrases).
   2. Excessive adherence to routines, ritualized patterns of verbal or nonverbal behavior, or excessive resistance to change (such as insistence on same route or food, repetitive questioning or extreme distress at small changes).
   3. Highly restricted, fixated interests that are abnormal in intensity or focus (such as strong attachment to or preoccupation with unusual objects, excessively circumscribed or perseverative interests).
   4. Hyper- or hypo-reactivity to sensory input or unusual interest in sensory aspects of environment (such as apparent indifference to pain/heat/cold, adverse response to specific sounds or textures, excessive smelling or touching of objects, fascination with lights or spinning objects).

C. Symptoms must be present in early childhood (but may not become fully manifest until social demands exceed limited capacities),

D. Symptoms together limit and impair everyday functioning.

The Causes of ASD
Currently there is no single known cause for ASD, but numerous risk factors and possible causes have been identified. Research suggests that ASD most likely results from a complex combination of causes including genetic, environmental, immunological and neurological factors. Genetics certainly can be involved, and at least 15 possible gene interactions have been identified as being involved with ASD (Cook, 2001). The siblings of people with ASD (or the children of parents with this condition) have a 15-30 times greater risk of developing this disorder. Whether this is due to innate genetic factors, a similar environment or a combination of both is not known. In ASD with concomitant tuberous sclerosis, Fragile X syndrome, neurofibromatosis or chromosomal abnormalities there is evidence of a strong genetic component (Ashwood, et al, 2006). Other risk factors include increased parental age (>35 for women and 40 for men), gestational diabetes or maternal obesity, the use of some prescription drugs during pregnancy, low birth weight, exposure to a number of environmental toxins, immune dysfunction, abnormal folate and methionine metabolism, excessive glutamate and decreased oxytocin production, impaired cellular and systemic detoxification with reduced endogenous antioxidant levels, increased neuro-inflammation, phenylketonuria, low vitamin B-12, D and folate levels, pre and postnatal viral infections (measles, rubella, varicella, CMV, herpes simplex, mumps), and mitochondrial dysfunction.

Poor parenting and vaccines, both of which were blamed as causes of ASD, have been shown not to be causative factors (Jain, et al, 2015; Uno, et al, 2015 & 2012). While vaccines are not the cause of ASD, the large number of anecdotal reports of behavior regression after vaccination is troubling and should be studied further. Additional discussion of some of these potential causes is warranted.

Immune dysfunction - over the past 20 years, research has revealed the incredible complexity and interconnectedness of immune and neurological function. Children (and adults) with ASD have been found to have abnormal Th-1 and Th-2 T lymphocyte ratios, decreased peripheral lymphocytes, inhibited T cell mitogen response, increased autoimmunity, and elevated monocytes and interferon-Υ. Immune imbalances such as these can modulate brain function, impair learning and emotional processing and cause inflammation with resultant damage to neurological tissue (Ashwood, et al, 2006). In a fascinating article in the journal, The Scientist, a father used worm therapy, which alters Th-1/Th-2 T-lymphocyte balance and has been used to treat autoimmune disease, with his autistic son. With a regular dose of porcine whipworm eggs (Trichuris suis), the boy's extreme behavior (smashing his head into a wall dozens of times per day, biting himself until he bled, gouging his eyes and face, screaming and kicking tantrums) disappeared and the father stated that he had his son back "or in many ways, it was like giving me a son that I didn't ever have" (Grant, 2011). A healthy Th-1/Th-2 T lymphocyte balance is also dependent on a healthy gut flora (Critchfield, et al, 2011). Many people with ASD have abnormally high levels of Clostridium and Desulfovibrio bacteria, some of which can produce neurotoxins. Research has also shown that the gut-microbiota-brain axis has significant control over immune and nervous system function (Petra, et al, 2015).

In addition, immune response to dietary proteins and peptides (casein, caseomorphins, gluten and gluteomorphins) can stimulate T-cells and cytokine production and induce peptide-specific T-cell response, all of which can cause autoimmune reactions, disrupt neuroimmune communications and promote inflammation (Vojdani, et al, 2004). Children with ASD often have impaired digestion with increased gut permeability and gluten or casein peptides can be easily absorbed. Numerous studies show that the levels of urinary peptides are much higher in people with ASD than in normal subjects (Nelson, et al, 2001). This has led to many parents of children with ASD to adopt a gluten-free, casein-free (GFCF) diet.
Research also shows that increased neuro-inflammation, as evidenced by elevated levels of phospholipase A-2 (PLA2) and inflammatory cytokines [including interleukins, interferon-γ, tumor necrosing factor-alpha (TNF-α), heatshock proteins (HSP70), caspase 7 and transforming growth factor] probably plays a significant role in autism. It is also postulated that testing for these markers and changes in their levels

could be an objective method of determining efficacy and safety of ASD treatments (El-Ansary & Al-Ayadhi, 2012). Certain herbs and supplements have been shown in laboratory research to inhibit PLA2, including Turmeric, Gotu Kola and Ginkgo (Ong, et al, 2015). High levels of PLA2 incrase arachidonic acid levels, inflammatory prostaglandins, leukotrienes and lysophospholipids, which are converted into platelet-activating factors.

Exposure to environmental toxins – laboratory, animal and human studies clearly indicate that the prenatal/fetal period is very susceptible to epigenomic dysregulation that can cause neuro-developmental deficits as well as many diseases (Perera & Herbstman, 2011). Many environmental chemicals, as well as pharmaceuticals and a lack of essential nutrients, have been shown in preliminary research to affect neurological development. Air pollution, especially polycyclic aromatic hydrocarbons (PAHs) such as benzo[a]pyrene can induce DNA damage, cause mutations, they are neurotoxic and act as endocrine disruptors. They are fat-soluble and can cross the placenta and fetal blood brain barrier (Perera & Herbtsman, 2011). Exposure to these chemicals is associated with developmental delays, reduced IQ, reduced birth weight, slow development and increased behavioral disorders. Bisphenol A (BPA) is commonly used in plastics and to line cans containing food. It is also fat soluble and recent epidemiological studies suggest that low dose prenatal exposure to this ubiquitous compound interferes with sexual dimorphism in brain structure and behavior, while negatively affecting social behavior and cognitive function. BPA is also linked to increased inflammation, it interfered with thyroid hormone, and in animal studies it increased hyperactive behavior and disrupted neocortical patterning (Nakamura, et al, 2007). In addition to these two compounds, prenatal exposure to pharmaceutical medications (Valproate, SSRIs, Misoprostol and possibly acetaminophen), phthalates, PCBs and organophosphate pesticides, have all been found to have negative effects on neurodevelopment and may possibly be a factor in the development of ASD. Studies have also found that exposure to environmental pollutants can cause mitochondrial dysfunction, which is significantly more common in children with ASD than in normal children (Napoli, et al, 2013; Rossginol & Bradstreet, 2005). Mitochondrial disorders can cause seizures, ataxia, and cardiac conduction problems and have been associated with developmental regression and growth retardation in children with ASD (Poling, et al, 2008).

Impaired cellular and systemic detoxification and endogenous antioxidant systems. - people with ASD have increased levels of oxidative stress and a reduced ability to eliminate metabolic wastes via methylation. They also have reduced levels of endogenous antioxidants such as sulfates, glutathione, superoxide dismutase and catalase (Ghanizadeh, et al, 2012). This means that environmental toxins (see above) and heavy metals are more difficult to eliminate, and the cellular antioxidant systems needed to mediate their effects are less active. Studies have repeatedly shown that children with ASD have higher levels of heavy metals including aluminum, arsenic, cadmium, mercury, antimony and lead (Blaurock-Busch, et al, 2012). In addition, some people with ASD have a dysfunctional folate-methionine metabolism, and elevated serum levels of homocysteine (Kaluzna-Czaplinska, et al, 2013). Methionine is needed to synthesize SAMe, which is essential for proper methylation and it is converted into S-adenosyl-homocysteine (SAH), which provides cysteine for glutathione production (Main, et al, 2010). In multiple human studies nutrients that enhanced methylation, sulphation and act as antioxidants have also shown the ability to improve some ASD behaviors. Recent research indicates that prenatal inflammation is a significant risk factor for development of ASD (Napoli, et al, 2013). Mothers who had elevated C-reactive protein (Top 20th percentile) had a 43% greater chance of having a child with autism (Brown, et al, 2013).

To further complicate this already challenging problem, many people with ASD have other disorders including epilepsy (11-39%), mental retardation (40-69%, more likely in females than males), learning disabilities (25-75%), chronic anxiety (7-84%), sensory processing disorder (42-88%), chronic gastrointestinal problems (67.6%), allergies (62.2%), sleep disturbances and depression (4-58%). Studies have also found significant overlap with people with high functioning ASD and ADHD (Rommelse, et al, 2010). Research clearly shows that ASD is a complex multi-system disorder and thinking of it as one condition with one cause or one treatment is a flawed concept. In order to adequately understand, prevent and treat this disorder we need to think beyond the brain and look at each person, subtypes of disorders and family. Prevention may have more to do with the environment and maternal health/nutrition or inflammation than genetics. Treatment of someone with level 1(high functioning) ASD, who has GI problems and allergies may differ significantly from another person who is also level 1 but has seizures, depression and sleep issues.

Orthodox Treatment and Management of Autism Spectrum Disorders

Standard treatments of this challenging condition aim to reduce the behavioral/emotional or intellectual deficits and increase the person's quality of life and independence. Early behavioral therapy, social skills therapy, specially tailored education, as well as speech and occupational therapy are often implemented. Three programs, Early Intensive Behavioral Intervention (EIBI), Applied Behavior Analysis (ABA) and Relationship Development Intervention (RDI) are well studied and can help improve communication skills, behavior, relationships and learning in children with ASD. The drawback to this type of therapy is that they are time and staff intensive, requiring each child to undergo as many as 30-40 hours per week of therapy for several years with highly trained therapists (Lofthouse, et al, 2012). Other programs have found that autistic children respond well to interactions with a human therapist and specially engineered teaching robots. Children with ASD are often fascinated with objects and technology and robots are easier to understand as they have no complicated facial expressions, body language or tonal changes in their voices (Woolston, 2011).

A number of SSRIs, antipsychotic, psychostimulants, and other pharmaceutical medications have been used to reduce ASD behaviors such as irritability, hyperactivity, aggression and repetitive actions. Only Risperidone and Aripiprazole (Abilify) are FDA-approved for treating ASD-associated irritability (in 5-16 year olds). Many other medications are used "off label". Some work best for children, other for adolescents or adults and all can have significant adverse effects. Research suggests that 47% of children and adults with ASD are taking these medications (Lofthouse, et al, 2012).

Some Commonly Used Pharmaceutical Medications for ASD Symptoms

Medication-type	Benefits	Adverse Effects	Used for Children	Adults
Clomipramine-Tricyclic antidepressant	Reduces repetitive behavior and stereotypies, may reduce aggressive behaviors and hyperactivity	Sleep disturbances, constipation, fatigue, depression, dystonia, seizures, behavioral problems		√
Fluxoxamine-SSRI	Reduces repetitive behaviors, maladaptive behaviors and aggression	Well tolerated in adults. In children, increased insomnia, aggression, ritual behavior, anorexia, anxiety and irritability		√
Fluoxetine (Prozac™)-SSRI	Reduces stereotypy, irritability, inappropriate speech and angry outbursts	Adverse effects more common in children and adolescents. Hypomania, anxiety, agitation		√
Sertraline-SSRI	Moderately reduced repetitive behaviors and aggression	Increased anxiety, agitation, skin picking, weight gain	√	√
Citalopram-SSRI	None-no better than placebo in large study	Increased impulsiveness, hyperactivity, stereotypy, diarrhea, insomnia and pruritus	√	
Haloperidol-antipsychotic	Reduced stereotypies and social withdrawal alleviated aggression, irritability	Increased sedation, dystonia, rare dyskinesias	√	
Risperidone-atypical antipsychotic	Reduces irritability, stereotypy, hyperactivity and non-compliance behavior	Increased appetite, weight gain, fatigue, anxiety, rhinitis, upper respiratory tract infection and dyskinesias	√	√
Methylphenidate-psychostimulant	Moderately reduces hyperactivity	Increased irritability. Is more effective for ADHD alone	√	√
Aripiprazole-atypical antipsychotic	Reduces irritability, hyperactivity and stereotypies	Increased weight gain, sleepiness, drooling and tremors	√	

CAM Treatments for ASD

Dietary Therapies
A significant number of people with ASD also have major GI problems, including chronic diarrhea, GERD, constipation, flatulence, and abdominal pain. Studies of autistic children reveal that they often have a distinct GI pathology with duodenitis, abnormal bowel flora, increased gut permeability and decreased small intestine enzymes (Geraghty, et al, 2010a). For this large sub-group of ASD patients the gluten-free, casein-free (GFCF) diet has been shown to not only alleviate many of their digestive issues, but also reduce ASD behaviors and improve social behaviors (Pennesi & Klein, 2012; Harris & Card, 2012). This may be explained by the effect of the gluten and casein peptides known as gluteomorphins and caseomorphins. These compounds have been shown to cross the blood-brain barrier, negatively effect neurotransmission and they may inhibit CNS maturation (Geraghty, et al, 2010b). The challenge of implementing the GFCF diet is two-fold. First sources of gluten and casein are ubiquitous in the western diet. Eliminating dairy and wheat is not adequate. Gluten is also found in rye, spelt, triticale and in some oats. Gluten and gluten-products are often added to processed foods and this is also true of casein. According to some sources, the GFCF diet must be adhered to strictly for at least 7-9 months, before results are evident and maximal improvement may take two years to achieve (Kidd, 2003). The second issue is that many children with ASD are picky eaters and resistant to dietary changes. Other foods which may act as excitotoxins include refined sugars, artificial additives (aspartame, artificial food colorings and preservatives) and foods which the person has an intolerance to. Food sensitivities are especially problematic with ASD, as increased gut permeability, abnormal gut flora and impaired eliminatory abilities are all co-factors for creating food intolerances. After wheat/gluten and dairy, the most common problem foods are soy, corn, eggs and citrus fruits.

Herbal Therapies
There is little research into the use of herbs for ASD. Ginkgo, in a case study (3 patients), helped to reduce ASD symptoms (Niederhofer, 2009). In a RCT Ginkgo given with Risperidone did not improve treatment outcomes (Hasanzadeh, et al, 2012). In a 12 week, prospective, open label study with 40 children. a Kampo formula, Yokukansan was shown to improve ASD symptoms. This formula contains Atractylodes lancea, Poria, Cnidium, Gambir spines, Japanese Angelica root, Bupleurum and Licorice and it reduced irritability, stereotypic behavior, hyperactivity and inappropriate speech (Miyoka, et al, 2012). The herbs in this formula enhance digestion, inhibit inflammation, reduce hyperactivity and help re-regulate immune and endocrine function. This may explain some of its benefits exhibited in the study.

Based on what we know about ASD and its probable underlying mechanisms there are several herbal approaches that, while untested, would seem to make sense and offer little in the way of risk (especially compared to pharmaceutical medications).

A Theoretical Protocol for Treating ASD Symptoms and Metabolic Abnormalities
People with ASD often have allergies and abnormalities in their immune and inflammatory response system (IRS). Studies have found elevated levels of inflammatory cytokines including tumor necrosis factor-α (TNF-α), interferon γ, heat shock proteins (HSP 70), transforming growth factor (TGF-β_2), caspase 7 and interleukins 1, 6, 8, 10, 12 and 1β (El-Ansary & Al-Ayadhi, 2012; Lee & Kong, 2012). If pro-inflammatory cytokines are chronically activated, it can not only cause systemic and neurological inflammation but GI symptoms as well.

There are several categories of herbs that can be effective for re-regulating a disordered immune/endocrine system. They include immune amphoterics, immuno-regulators, some adaptogens, and antioxidant/ antiinflammatory herbs. Immune amphoterics are "foods for the immune system". They strengthen and nourish immune function, allowing a disordered immune system to regain its normal regulatory capacity. Maitake, Cat's Claw or Astragalus are effective immune amphoterics. Other herbs such as Licorice, Reishi, Eleuthero, Asian and American Ginseng, Ashwagandha and Schisandra berry are both immune amphoterics and adaptogens.

Adaptogens help to re-regulate the immune, nervous and endocrine systems while enhancing an organism's ability to tolerate and deal with acute and chronic stress. The term immuno-regulator is one I coined to describe antiinflammatory herbs which reduce pro-inflammatory cytokine levels and help to moderate an abnormal Th-1 and Th-2 T lymphocyte balance. Herbs in this category include Baikal Scullcap, Sarsaparilla, Gotu Kola, Unprocessed Rehmannia, Dan Shen/Salvia miltiorrhiza, Madder root, Turmeric, Boswellia and Bupleurum.

Studies have shown that people with ASD also have decreased ability to excrete metabolic wastes (⇓methylation) and ineffective endogenous antioxidant systems which allows increased damage and inflammation from these wastes. Antioxidant/antiinflammatory herbs can help to reduce oxidative stress and the resultant inflammation. Herbs in this category include Amla fruit, Turmeric, Blueberry/Bilberry, Green tea, Rosemary, Hibiscus, Rose hips, Lycium fruit, Beets, Hawthorn, Grape Seed extract, Pine bark extract, and Triphala.

In addition, several herbs and supplements have been shown to enhance hepatic glutathione levels allowing for more effective excretion of wastes by the liver ((Phase II detoxification). Herbs that increase hepatic glutathione levels include Turmeric, Schisandra, Milk Thistle and Picrorhiza. Nutritional supplements which can enhance hepatic glutathione levels include alpha lipoic acid, N-acetylcysteine and SAMe.

Herbs that can enhance systemic elimination are known as alteratives. These herbs gently promote kidney, liver, lymph, skin and bowel function. Many mild alterative herbs could be useful as a part of an ASD protocol including Cleavers, Dandelion root, Yellow Dock root, Sarsaparilla, Oregon Grape Root, Burdock root, Violet leaf and Red Clover.

Botanicals that help reduce anxiety, hyperactivity, insomnia and irritability are also indicated. Nervines are calming herbs that help to reduce irritability, agitation and hyperactivity. Useful herbs might include Linden flower, Scullcap, Chamomile, Passion Flower and Blue Vervain. Anxiolytics relieve anxiety and Bacopa, Motherwort, Blue Vervain and Chinese Polygala are good choices. Nootropics enhance cerebral circulation, improving memory, focus and concentration. Effective nootropics include Bacopa, Ginkgo, Gotu Kola, Rosemary, Eclipta and White Peony. In an animal model of autism, Bacopa significantly improved behavioral abnormalities, decreased oxidative stress markers and helped to restore normal histoarchitecture of the cerebellum (Sandhya, et al, 2012).Many of the herbs mentioned as nervines, anxiolytics or nootropics also are effective for treating insomnia, seizures and depression, which are common co-morbidities in ASD.

A significant number of people with autism also have digestive issues which are clearly linked to increased agitation, irritability, hyperactivity and anxiety. Carminatives and GI antispasmodics (along with probiotics-see under Supplements) would be a useful addition to their protocols. Effective carminatives include Ginger, Chamomile, Fennel seed and Angelica. Gastrointestinal antispasmodics/analgesics include Xiang Fu/Cyperus, Wild Yam, Hops, Mu Xiang/Saussurea root and Catnip.

Nutritional Therapies
A number of nutritional supplements have been studied for treating ASD symptoms. The number of studies and the quality of them makes it difficult to accurately access the true benefits of many of these nutrients. With the scarcity of significant adverse effects in supplement studies and the lack of effective pharmaceuticals with their propensity for side effects, the benefit to risk ratio is in favor of supplement use.

B-6 and magnesium - in several clinical trials high dose B-6 (600-1,125 mg) combined with magnesium (400-500 mg per day), as well as magnesium alone have shown the ability to improve alertness and reduce outbursts, self-mutilation and stereotyped behaviors (Mousain-Bosc, et al, 2006; Martineau, et al, 1985). Other studies have found either negligible or no benefits. Some research suggests that people with ASD have elevated serum B-6 levels. This may indicate an inability to convert pyridoxal to pyridoxal-5-phosphate (P-5-P), the active metabolite of B-6.

Folic acid – in children with early onset low-functioning autism and Rett's Syndrome, folate receptor (FR) autoimmunity has been found to be a common problem. This inhibits folate binding to the choroid epithelial cells and produces cerebral folate deficiency (Ramaekers, et al, 2012). Oral supplementation of folinic acid improved cerebral folic acid levels and reduced ASD behaviors (Ramaekers, et al, 2007). The use of pre-natal folic acid supplements has also been found to significantly reduce the risk of having children with ASD (Surén, et al, 2012).

B-12 (methylcobalamin) - both children and adults with ASD have impaired metabolic detoxification pathways (transmethylation and transsulfuration) and reduced cellular antioxidant activity (glutathione, methionine, SAMe, homocysteine and cysteine). Some researchers believe this may be a contributing factor to developing ASD and its clinical manifestations. Several studies have looked at supplementing methylcobalamin, which is needed for production of SAMe used for methyltransferase reactions. Folate is also essential to these processes, and in two studies supplementing methylcobalamin (75 mcg/kg 2 x per week) and folinic acid (400 mcg BID) improved these metabolic imbalances and may have also improved speech and cognitive function (James, et al, 2009 & 2004).

Essential Fatty Acids – many studies of children with ASD have found that a large percentage have low levels of Omega-3 fatty acids. These compounds are essential for normal brain development and healthy neurological functioning. Evidence suggests maternal Omega 3 levels during pregnancy and early ingestion while an infant are protective against developing ASD. It is unclear if taking it later has benefits for people with ASD. Early small studies of EPA/DHA suggested they might offer modest benefits for ASD but the results were not conclusive (Lofthouse, et al, 2013). More recent RCT trials found no benefits from 6 months of Omega 3 fatty acid consumption in children with ASD (Mankad, et al, 2015; Voight, et al, 2014). In a double blind, placebo-controlled randomized trial, teenagers with ASD were given arachidonic acid (ARA) and docosahexaenoic acid (DHA). ARA is proinflammatory and usually thought to be harmful, but it is essential for signal transduction needed for neuronal maturation. In this study the fatty acids improved plasma antioxidant levels, social responsiveness and social interactions (Yui, et al, 2012).

Probiotics – a large number of people (67.7%) with ASD have GI dysfunction (constipation, diarrhea, IBS, GERD, dyspepsia, flatulence, etc.), which has been linked to increased irritability, tantrums, aggressive behavior and sleep disturbances (Critchfield, et al, 2011). Children with ASD also have abnormalities of the gut flora. Studies have found 10-fold increases in Clostridium spp., some of which produce neurotoxins. A small study of ASD patients with chronic diarrhea found that vancomycin (8 weeks) significantly improved behavior and communication skills (Sandler, et al, 2000). Probiotics offer a healthier and more sustainable method of promoting a healthy GI microbiome. In addition many people with ASD also have increased gut permeability and GI-based immune dysfunction. Probiotics have been shown to have antiinflammatory, anxiolytic and immune regulatory effects and may offer significant benefits for improving not only GI problems associated with ASD, but behavioral problems as well.

Vitamin/mineral combinations – nutrient deficiencies are common in ASD. While some may be due to picky eating habits, others may be due to impaired digestive function, reduced methylation and gut dysbiosis. In a RCT 141 children and adults with ASD were given a vitamin/mineral supplement containing a broad range of nutrients. Not only did nutritional and metabolic status improve (including methylation, sulfation, glutathione levels and reduced oxidative stress), there were also reductions in hyperactivity and tantrums (Adams, et al, 2011).

Vitamin D – is essential for normal brain development and people with ASD have been found to have lower than normal levels of this antiinflammatory nutrient. In a case report a 32-month-old child with autism and a vitamin D deficiency was given supplemental vitamin D. His core ASD symptoms significantly improved with supplementation (Jia, et al, 2015). Further research is needed to determine whether this single case has any significance for the greater ASD population.

Flavonoids – a proprietary formula containing luteolin, quercetin and rutin was given to 50 children with ASD in an open-label trial over 26 weeks. There was improvement in communication, adaptive functioning and daily living skills as well as reduced aberrant behavior (Taliou, et al, 2013).

L-carnitine – was given to 30 children with ASD. The dose was 50 mg L-carnitine/kg bodyweight per day for three months. In this RCT, significant improvements in cognitive skills and other measures of autism severity were observed (Geier, et al, 2011). The researchers looked at using this amino acid because it has been shown to enhance mitochondrial function, fatty acid metabolism and it acts as a cellular antioxidant.

Melatonin – has been found to help alleviate sleep problems in children with autism and fragile X syndrome. In several RCTs, 1-10 mg of melatonin per day reduced sleep latency and prolonged sleep duration (Malow, et al, 2012; Wright, et al, 2011; Wirojanan, et al, 2009).

L-carnosine – is a dipeptide made up of two amino acids, beta-alanine and histidine. It is abundant in brain tissue and muscles. It has antioxidant and neuroprotective activity and has been shown in laboratory studies to protect against shortening of the telomeres. In a small RCT, autistic children were given 800 mg per day of carnosine. The study found that it improved behavior, communication and socialization (Chez, et al, 2002),

TCM and Autism

In Traditional Chinese Medicine (TCM), the person being treated and the unique patterns of their condition are more important than the disease they have. Five people could be diagnosed with Rheumatoid Arthritis (or ASD) and they would receive five different protocols depending on their constitution, symptoms and unique differential diagnosis (tongue and pulse diagnosis). It is difficult to do RCT with this type of individualized prescribing, but clinical reports suggest that various TCM modalities (herbs, massage, acupuncture, moxabustion, cupping and therapeutic exercises) can have some benefits for ASD patients. In one published account of TCM treatment for autism, the condition was divided into two types (Zhang, 2010). Type I ASD displays physical and emotional retardation (head lag, inability to roll over at 6 months of age, inability to sit up by 9-12 months, inability to stand, lack of recognizable speech), as well as stereotypical behaviors, poor sleep and digestive problems. This is believed to be caused by a severe depletion of pre-natal jing (depleted kidney qi and jing). The treatment was changed according to the season and relies on kidney and spleen qi tonics (Red Ginseng, Pantocrin, Processed Rehmannia, Atractylodes, Placenta, Dang Gui, etc.) as well as herbs that calm the shen and relieve phlegm stagnation in the heart orifice (Calamus, Zizyphus seed, Chinese Polygala, Musk). In addition, acupressure, massage, music therapy and moxabustion were recommended. The symptoms of Type II ASD are described as apathy, poor communication skills and repetitive behaviors. This is believed to be caused by a congenital blockage of the heart and is treated with herbs to move and build blood (Cinnamon, Dan Shen, Ginger), clear phlegm (Calamus, musk) and tonify the kidney essence (Red Ginseng, Psoralea, Pantocrin, Codonopsis). According to this report 2 months of treatment in a 2-year-old improved his ability to speak and walk.

Acupuncture – in a RCT of acupuncture versus sham Acupuncture, children with ASD responded significantly better to the actual therapy. Hand-eye coordination, language comprehension, cognitive function and self-care all improved during the 8 weeks of therapy (Wong & Sun, 2010).

Other Therapies for ASD

Animal assisted therapy – people with autism often find interacting with animals easier than with people. Anecdotal reports suggested that equine-assisted therapy may be of benefit for children with ASD. A six-month long study of children with ASD aged 3-12 found that therapeutic horseback riding reduced the severity of autism symptoms as determined by the Childhood Autism Rating Scale (CARS) (Kern, et al, 2011).

Hydrotherapy – a specific form of hydrotherapy, the Halliwick method, has been shown to improve muscle strength, attention, motor performance and social interactions in children with ASD (Mortimer, et al, 2014). In some cases there was also a decrease in anxiety and hyperactive behavior.

Music therapy – has been found to improve language skills (verbal and body language), compliant behavior, social engagement and eye contact in children with ASD (Akins, et al, 2010).

Exercise – has been found in preliminary studies to reduce self-stimulatory behavior and it improved academic performance in autistic children (Lofthouse, et al, 2013).

Massage – in several small studies daily massage has been found to modestly improve attention span, decrease stereotypic behaviors and enhance sleep in autistic children (Akins, et al, 2010).

Neurofeedback (NF) – is a technique which enhances self-regulation of the brain by providing real-time video/audio information about EEG function. In several studies NF improved attention span, sensory/cognitive awareness, communication skills and social interactions in people with ASD (Lofthouse, et al, 2013).

Art therapy – there are case studies and clinical observations that claim art therapy can improve behavior, attention and motor performance in autistic children. There is little objective research to confirm these anecdotal reports.

Drama therapy – has been found to improve social deficient (facial recognition, social awareness and social cognition) in young people aged 8-17 years old with ASD (Corbett, et al, 2014).

Ineffective Therapies for ASD
Many pharmaceutical medications used to treat ASD symptoms have been found to have a higher risk to benefit ratio for children (and adults) and so are not effective as a treatment. This includes Ritalin, Citalopram and Fluoxamine (in children). Porcine Secretin has also failed to show benefits (Krishnaswami, et al, 2011). Chelation therapy has not been shown to be effective and there are safety concerns with this practice (Akins, et al, 2010). In addition, EEG biofeedback (Kouijzer, et al, 2012) and hyperbaric oxygen therapy (Sampanthavivat, et al, 2012) have not proven to be useful treatments.

References available in the downloadable version of this book, for purchase at
www.botanicalmedicine.org

Making Love – An Herbal/Nutritional Guide to Sexual Health

©2005/ Revised 2015 David Winston, RH(AHG)

Sexual activity is a normal and healthy part of most adult human lives. Unfortunately, we come from a culture that is seriously confused and conflicted about sexuality. Our media (television, movies, magazines) is awash in covert and overt sexual images, while at the same time many religions, our government, and "moral leaders" have an almost puritanical view of sexuality. A healthy view of human sexuality lies somewhere between these two extremes. As Alfred Kinsey showed in his groundbreaking books, human sexuality is diverse and what is considered normal is a subjective decision based on culture, religion, and class. Without spending too much time on such a broad topic, I believe there are a few basic practices that promote healthy and fulfilling sexual relations:

- Sexual activity is most appropriate between consulting adults who are mature enough to deal with the potential psychological, social and physical consequences of this act.
- While some people like or prefer casual sex, sex between committed partners allows for an intimacy that is unlikely to occur with a stranger. Promiscuous sex, precocious sex, and sexual activity under the influence of alcohol or drugs are more like to lead to unhealthy consequences (STD's, unwanted pregnancy, date-rape)
- As long as both partners are truly consenting and no one is hurt physically or emotionally, nothing is abnormal or deviant.

Real intimacy requires trust, respect, commitment, empathy, and love. Sexual problems are opportunities for open dialogue, growth in relationships, and personal healing. Healthy sexuality can be much more than the physical act, it is an opportunity for deep emotional connectedness, emotional healing, and it can be viewed as a spiritual practice. For more on this I recommend reading Margo Anand's book, The Art of Sexual Ecstasy.

Women's Sexual Health

Vaginal Dryness

Vaginal dryness can be occasional or chronic. Occasional vaginal dryness can be caused by lack of stimulation or foreplay, fluctuations in hormonal cycles, candidiasis, or lack of essential fatty acids and dehydration. Chronic vaginal dryness is usually associated with menopause, but can also be caused by Sjögren's Syndrome. In addition to herbs, adequate intake of vitamin E (mixed tocopherols with tocotrienols-200 iu per day), Omega 3 fatty acids (fish oils-2-4 g per day) and water, as well as topical applications of natural progesterone creams can help restore normal vaginal secretions.

Dang Gui root (Angelica sinensis) – increases circulation to the uterus and pelvis and also lubricates the bowel and vagina. It is a blood, cardiac and liver tonic and it benefits anemia, dysmenorrhea, amenorrhea, PMS, and menopausal symptoms. In animal research it enhanced cornification of vaginal tissue (Circosta, et al, 2006), which supports a healthy vaginal mucoas.
Tincture (1:5): 1.5-3 mL TID
Tea: 1-2 tsp. dried herb, 8-10 oz. water, decoct 10 minutes, steep 40 minutes, take 4 oz. TID

Fresh Oat (Avena sativa) – is a nervous system trophorestorative and yin tonic that, used with other herbs, helps relieve vaginal dryness.
Tincture (1:2): 4-5 mL TID

Licorice rhizome (Glycyrrhiza uralensis, G. glabra) – is a yin tonic that contains isoflavones which act as phytoestrogens. The combination helps relieve dryness and also has a mild estrogen-like effect which promotes vaginal mucous membrane elasticity and health.
Tincture (1:5): 1-2 mL TID
Tea: 1/2 tsp. herb, 8-10 oz. water, decoct 15 minutes, steep 1/2 hour. Take 4 oz. BID.

Shatavari root (Asparagus racemosus) – is a major Rasayana in Ayurvedic medicine. It acts as a yin tonic to the mucous membranes (lung, throat, GI tract, bladder, and vagina). Long-term use, along with other yin tonics, can help to reestablish normal vaginal secretions.

Tincture (1:5): 1.5-2.5 mL TID
Tea: 1-2 tsp. dried herb, 8-10 oz. water, decoct 15 minutes, steep 45 minutes, take 4-6 oz. BID/TID

White Kwao Krua root (Pueraria mirifica) – is a Southeast Asian plant used in traditional Thai medicine as a rejuvenative tonic for aging men and women. It is rich in isoflavones and has been the subject of numerous human and animal studies, which have found it relieves a number of menopausal symptoms (osteoporosis, hot flashes and night sweats), especially vaginal dryness (Manonai, et al, 2007). Interestingly, other isoflavone-rich supplements such as soy, Black Cohosh or Red Clover have not been found to alleviate vaginal dryness.
Capsules: 50 mg per day

White Pond Lily rhizome (Nymphaea odorata) – has both demulcent and astringent effects. It tonifies the urinary tract, bowel, and mucous membranes. I use it clinically for vaginal dryness (with other yin tonics), uterine or bladder prolapse, leucorrhea (as a douche), and for a boggy, atonic uterus.
Tincture (1:2): 1-2 mL TID
Tea: 1 tsp. cut/sifted dried rhizome, 8 oz. water, steep 40 minutes, take 4 oz. TID/QID

Painful Intercourse
Painful intercourse can be caused by lack of lubrication (see above), sexual trauma, vulvodynia, vaginismus, uterine fibroids, STD's, cervicitis, and uterine prolapse. Men with larger penises may also hit the cervix during sexual intercourse in some positions. The woman on top position allows a women to control the depth of penile penetration, avoiding painful deep thrusts.

Pain due to vulvodynia – I believe vulvodynia has an autoimmune component and in fact it is very similar etiologically to interstitial cystitis (in women) and chronic nonbacterial prostatitis (in men). I use a combination of urinary analgesics (Hydrangea, Kava, Gravel root, Yucca root), antiinflammatories (Eryngo, St. John's wort, Marshmallow, Couch Grass, or Saw Palmetto), and immune amphoterics (Maitake, Reishi, American Ginseng) to treat all 3 conditions.

Pain due to vaginismus – a number of anxiolytic and antispasmodic herbs can help treat vaginismus including:

Motherwort herb (Leonurus cardiaca)	Black Cohosh root (Actaea racemosa)
Kava root (Piper methysticum)	Butterbur rhizome (Petasites spp.)–PA free only
Black Haw bark (Viburnum prunifolium)	Cyperus tuber (Cyperus rotundus)
Pulsatilla herb (Anemone patens)	Cramp bark (Viburnum opulus)

Increasing magnesium intake can be a useful therapy for vaginal spasms and Lady's Mantle essence seems to help decrease some of the emotional trauma caused by sexual abuse or rape.

Pain Due to Uterine Prolapse
Mild to moderate uterine prolapse can be treated by the use of physical manipulation, exercise, and herbs. Severe cases may require surgery. Uterine adjusting is a technique utilized in Naprapathy or the old naturopathic "bloodless surgery" practices. Rosita Arvigo has popularized a combination of Mayan uterine massage and naprapathic adjustment, which can help with uterine prolapse. Pelvic floor exercises (aka Kegal exercises) can tonify the uterine ligaments, strengthen bladder control and enhance the intensity of women's orgasms. Herbs that help strengthen the uterus include:

Raspberry leaf (Rubus villosa)	Lady's Mantle herb (Alchemilla vulgaris)
Partridge berry herb (Mitchella repens)	Rose hips (Rosa laevigata)
White Pond Lily rhizome (Nymphaea odorata)	Agrimony (Agrimonia spp.)

A Chinese formula containing equal parts Zhi Shi (immature orange fruit) and Motherwort seed taken for 30 days was 83.87% effective in relieving uterine prolapse in a study of 924 patients (Chen & Chen, 2001).

A classic TCM formula for uterine prolapse as well as bladder or rectal prolapse is Bu Zhong Yi Qi Tang (decoction for strengthening the middle jiao and benefiting vital qi). This formula combines Astragalus, Codonopsis, Dang Gui, Atractylodes, Orange peel, Processed Licorice, Chinese Black Cohosh/Sheng Ma, Bupleurum, Jujube dates, and fresh Ginger root. It is usually taken as a decoction.

Anorgasmia

Anorgasmia is an inability to achieve orgasm in women (and men as well). In women, it is most often caused by inadequate clitoral stimulation, relationship issues, medication (SSRIs, anticonvulsants, hydrochlorothiazide and antipsychotic drugs), fear, depression, or anxiety. An excellent book on enhancing women's sexual pleasure is Sheri Winston's Women's Anatomy of Arousal.

Celery seed (Apium graveolens) – has a long history of use as a urinary remedy. It enhances uric acid excretion (gout, gouty arthritis), is an antibacterial diuretic, and it stimulates libido in some women. It should be taken with other herbs to prevent urinary irritation.
Tincture (1:5): 1-2 mL TID
Tea: ¼ - ½ tsp. fresh ground seeds, 8 oz. hot water, steep covered for 20 minutes, take up to 4 oz. 3x/day

Ginkgo standardized extract (Ginkgo biloba) – has been shown to relieve anorgasmia in both men and women caused by antidepressant medication. While it had slight benefit for men, it was more effective for anorgasmia in women (Cohen & Bartlik, 1998). In another RCT, a Ginkgo extract significantly improved sexual desire in post-menopausal women (Pelodani, et al, 2014).
Capsule-standardized extract: 120 mg. BID

Grief Relief – is a formula I have used for over 12 years containing Mimosa bark, Hawthorn berries and flowers, and Rose petals. It is a phenomenal remedy for grief, sadness, post-traumatic stress disorder, and depression. It is also a mood elevator and makes people feel happier. It can be useful for anorgasmia caused by grief or PTSD.
Dosage: 2-4 mL TID

Lack of Libido

Lack of libido can be caused by depression, unhappy relationships, medications (SSRIs, hydrochlorothiazide), fear of pregnancy, low testosterone levels, and sexual trauma. Herbs can be of use, but a thorough medical exam and counseling (psychiatric or marital) may be necessary.

Asian Ginseng root (Panax Ginseng) – has long been used in TCM as a qi tonic and to enhance male reproductive functioning. In a human trial of menopausal women with lack of libido Ginseng was found to significantly enhance sexual arousal (Oh, et al, 2010).
Tincture (1:5): 2-3 mL TID
Capsule/Tablet-900 mg TID

Celery seed (Apium graveolens) – see Anorgasmia.

Chaste Tree berries (Vitex agnus-castus) – is appropriate for decreased libido due to hormonal imbalances, as it helps to re-regulate FSH & LH produced by the pituitary. It can be especially useful for women who have lack of libido after stopping contraceptive pills, or after pregnancy or menopause.
Tincture (1:5): 3-5 mL BID
Tea: 1-2 tsp. dried berries, 8 oz. water, steep covered 1 hour, take 1-2 cups/day

Damiana herb (Turnera diffusa) – has a long folk history of being an aphrodisiac and nerve tonic. Whether it directly stimulates libido in women is unclear, but it is a mild antidepressant that seems to be useful for low-grade depression with loss of libido as a prominent symptom. It also acts as a nervine and antidepressant for stagnant depression.
Tincture (1:5): 2-3 mL TID

Tea: 1 tsp. dried herb, 8 oz hot water, steep 20 minutes (covered), take 4 oz TID/QID

Dang Gui root (Angelica sinensis) –increases circulation to the uterus and pelvis and also lubricates the bowel and vagina. It is a blood, cardiac, and liver tonic and it benefits anemia, dysmenorrhea, amenorrhea, PMS, and menopausal symptoms. Enhanced circulation can increase sexual pleasure and desire for some women.
Tincture (1:5): 1.5-3 mL TID
Tea: 1-2 tsp. dried herb, 8-10 oz. water, decoct 10 minutes, steep 40 minutes, take 4 oz. TID

Fresh Oat (Avena sativa) – is a superb nervous system trophorestorative that helps restore emotional balance and relieves anxiety. It was used by the Eclectics for sexual neurasthenia, a lack of sexual energy causing impotence and lack of libido.
Tincture (1:2): 4-5 mL TID
Glycerite (1:2): 5-7.5 mL 4-5x/day

Maca root (Lepedium meyenii) – this herb is widely promoted as a male and female sexual tonic. Studies for both men and women show that in large doses (3 g/day) it does seem to have some benefits. In a RCT women with SSRI-induced sexual dysfunction who took the higher doses of Maca (a dose of 1.5 g per day showed no effect) had improved libido (Dording, et al, 2008). A second study found Maca worked better in post-menopausal women than pre-menopausal women for relieving SSRI-induced sexual dysfunction (Dording, et al, 2015).
Tincture (1:4 or 1:5): 3-5 mL (60-100 gtt.) TID
Capsules/tablets: 3 g per day

Muira Puama root or bark (Ptychopetalum olacoides) – in a human trial (Waynberg & Brewer, 2000), a product with Muira Puama and Ginkgo was given to 202 women who had a low sex drive. After one month of treatment sixty-four percent noted increased libido, intensity of orgasm, and an increased sexual satisfaction.
Tincture (1:5): 1-2 mL TID
Tea: 1 tsp. cut/sifted herb, 10 oz water, decoct 20-30 minutes, steep 1/2 hour, take 4 oz BID

Tribulus/Gokshura herb/seed (Tribulus terrestris) – has been widely promoted as an anabolic agent and male sexual tonic. In animal and human studies it has failed to increase testosterone levels or enhance strength. In a human clinical trial, Tribulus extract improved desire and arousal in women with female sexual dysfunction (Gama, et al, 2014). Interestingly, it reduced testosterone levels but increased DHEA, which is believed to be more significant for enhancing sexual desire in women.
Tea: 2 tsp. dried herb, 8 oz. water, steep 30 minutes, take 4 oz. TID
Capsules: 100-250 mg TID

Supplements for Lack of Libido

A supplement containing arginine plus Ginseng, Ginkgo, Damiana, vitamins, and minerals has been shown in several double-blind placebo controlled studies to enhance sexual desire, frequency of sexual activity, and reduced vaginal dryness in peri- and post-menopausal women (Ito, et al, 2006). A second proprietary formula containing L-arginine, Pycnogenol®, L-citrulline and a Rose hip extract also improve sexual functioning in healthy women aged 37-45 years old (Bottari, et al, 2013).

Sexual Anxiety

Sexual anxiety is usually rooted in fear. Fear of not being loved, fear of STD's or pregnancy, previous sexual trauma, fear of inadequacy, lack of self-esteem, etc. Herbs can help relieve the anxiety, but better communication (if possible) and therapy are more likely to deal with the root issues.

Blue Vervain herb (Verbena hastata) – is used in combination with Motherwort for sexual, PMS, or menopausal anxiety. It also relieves petit mal seizures associated with menses and can be of benefit for vaginismus.
Tincture (1:2.5): 1-2 mL TID
Tea: 1 tsp. dried herb, 8 oz. water, steep, covered, 45 minutes, take 4 oz. TID

Fresh Oat (Avena sativa) – see Lack of Libido.

Motherwort herb (Leonurus cardiaca) – is an excellent anxiolytic agent and nervine that reduces the effects of stress, irritability, PMS anxiety, menopausal agitation, and insomnia.
Tincture (1:2): 2-4 mL TID
Tea: 1 tsp. dried bark, 8 oz. water, steep 20-30 minutes, take 4 oz. up to 4x/day

Passion Flower leaves/vine (Passiflora incarnata) - is a nervine especially indicated for circular thinking, constant worry, and anxiety. It can be used with Fresh Oat, Motherwort, or other anxiolytics.
Tincture (1:2): 2.5-3 mL TID
Tea: 1 tsp. dried herb, 8 oz. water, steep 1 hour, take 2-3 cups/day

Pulsatilla herb (Anemone patens) - is a powerful herb used in very small doses for anxiety and irritability. The specific indications are for people who cry easily or get a deep sense of sadness with little or no provocation or known reason.
Tincture (1:2): 1-3 gtt TID

Female Sexual Tonics
In Chinese medicine, herbs that tonify the blood (xue) are used to strengthen and nourish the female reproductive system. Blood tonics include processed Rehmannia, He Shou Wu, Nettle Leaf, and White Peony. Herbs that have a more direct effect on the female reproductive system include:

Ashwagandha root (Withania somnifera) – is a calming adaptogen, anxiolytic and nutritive tonic (it is a rich source of iron). It is mostly thought of as a male reproductive tonic but has also been used as a sexual tonic for women as well. In a RCT, women given a concentrated Withania extract had improved libido, vaginal lubrication, ability to achieve orgasm and sexual satisfaction than those taking a placebo (Dongre, et al, 2015).
Tincture (1:5): 2-3 mL TID
Tea: 1/2 tsp. dried, powdered root, 8 oz. water, decoct 10 minutes, steep 30 minutes, take 4 oz. 3x/day

Helonias root (Chamaelirium luteum) – is a threatened species, so only cultivated roots should be used. It is the most effective herb for correcting minor hormonal imbalances that cause infertility. It acts as a trophorestorative to the female reproductive system and helps correct menstrual abnormalities.
Tincture (1:5): 1-1.5 mL TID

Rose petals (Rosa gallica) – are given as a symbol of love. Rose petals have a long history of use as an antidepressant and nervine. Roses improve mood, heal broken hearts, and enhance concentration and focus.
Tincture (1:5): 10-20 gtt TID
Tea: 1/2 tsp. Rose petals with other herbs, steep covered 10-15 minutes, take 4 oz. BID.

Shatavari root (Asparagus racemosus) – is the most prominent tonic herb for women in Ayurvedic medicine. It helps promote vaginal lubrication, fertility, and normalizes hormone levels.
Tincture (1:5): 1.5-2.5 mL TID
Tea: 1-2 tsp. dried herb, 8-10 oz. water, decoct 15 minutes, steep 45 minutes, take 4-6 oz. BID/TID

Men's Sexual Health

Impotence/Erectile Dysfunction (ED)
Impotence, or as it's now more frequently referred to, Erectile Dysfunction, is a problem that few men would want to admit to. Fortunately, with all the publicity surrounding Viagra®, Cialis® and Levitra® ED has come out of the bedroom and is being discussed more openly.

This is important for the estimated 15-30 million men who suffer with this condition and their partners. Impotence is the inability to achieve or maintain an erection and it is often subdivided into 2 broad categories, physiological or psychological. 10-20% of ED is psychological; the other 80-90% has physiological causes. A simple diagnostic test can often determine which form it is by seeing if a man has normal erections during sleep. With physiological impotence, no or partial erections will occur during sleep. The reverse is true of psychological impotence. Once it has been determined which type of ED a man has, it is important to find the underlying cause. Common causes of physiological impotence include:

- Atherosclerosis
- Heart disease
- Hypertension
- Diabetes
- Obesity
- Thyroid or Pituitary dysfunction
- Medications (antidepressants, tranquilizers, cimetidine, hypertensive medications, and antihistamines)
- Recreational drug use (steroids, alcohol, marijuana, tobacco, cocaine, heroin)
- Penile deformities including Peyronie's disease
- Kidney disease
- Multiple Sclerosis and other neuro-degenerative diseases
- Bladder and prostate cancer surgery
- Lack of testosterone
- Stage III or IV BPH and prostate resection surgery (TURP)

Causes of psychological impotence include:

- Performance anxiety (fear of failure)
- Depression
- Guilt
- Sexual abuse
- Chronic stress
- Chronic anxiety
- Unhappy relationships

For psychological impotence, family therapy and psychotherapy may be of significant benefit. The orthodox treatments for physiological ED include the oral "impotence medications" sildenafil (viagra®), tadalafil (cialis®), and vardenafil (levitra®), injectable drugs such as caverject®, oral testosterone (for men with low testosterone levels), urethral suppositories (alprostadil), vacuum pumps, and inflatable implants which require a surgical procedure.

All of these approaches have benefits (the ability to achieve erection), but they all have drawbacks as well. Since the oral medications are now the most widely used, I will only discuss the problems with these drugs. Men who take nitroglycerin or nitrates should not take these medications, and men taking alpha-blockers cannot take Levitra. These medications work by enhancing the effects of nitric oxide (NO) which relaxes smooth muscle tissue in the penis and thus increases penile blood flow. Side effects associated with these medications include headaches, flushing, dyspepsia, nasal congestion, and back and muscle pain. All of these drugs can cause priapism (an erection that lasts more than three hours). While uncommon, it is a serious adverse reaction that, left untreated, can cause severe damage to the penis.

In a study published in JAMA, 110 obese men with ED were put on diets. A loss of 10% of body mass was associated with improved sexual function in 1/3 of the men (Esposito, et al, 2004).

Alternatives for ED

There are a significant number of herbal medicines that offer benefits to men suffering from ED. None have the immediate effects of orthodox therapies. The only herb which seems to offer relatively quick stimulus is **Yohimbe bark** (Pausinystalia yohimbe) which works well for some men. Yohimbe or yohimbine hydrochloride acts as a vasodilator to increase peripheral blood flow and it is a pre-synaptic alpha$_2$-adrenergic blocking agent.

The exact mechanism of how Yohimbe works is unclear, but it does increase norepinephrine release as well as affecting dopamine and serotonin levels. The effects I describe here sound quite "drug-like" and the drawbacks to Yohimbe are also significant. It should not be used if taking antidepressants or antihypertensive agents, and its use should be avoided by men who have angina or other heart disease, hypertension, kidney or liver disease, anxiety, or BPH. It can also cause headaches, sweating, anxiety, abdominal pain, nausea, tachycardia, hypertension, and insomnia (Kearney, et al, 2010). The dosage for Yohimbe: tincture (1:5): 15 gtt BID, Yohimbine hydrochloride tablets – 5.4-6 mg TID

Other herbs for Erectile Dysfunction
Asian Ginseng root (Panax ginseng) – is a very useful adaptogen with broad reaching effects on the nervous system, endocrine system, and immune system. It also has a reputation as an "aphrodisiac" for men. For many years I believed that it was only useful for exhausted, depleted men with little or no sexual desire, but discounted its broader use for impotence.
Human studies suggest the popular wisdom about Ginseng may be true after all. In a double-blind crossover study published in the *Journal of Urology*, over 60% of the participants using Panax reported improved erections (Hong, et al, 2002). A review of six human trials found that Asian Ginseng is effective for ED (Jang, et al, 2008).
Tincture (1:5): 2-3 mL TID
Capsule/Tablet-900 mg TID

Damiana herb *(Turnera diffusa)* – has a long folk history of being an aphrodisiac and until recently I would have told you it is not. Animal studies found that, at least in rats, it does stimulate sexual behavior (Estrada-Reyes, et al, 2009; Arletti, et al, 1999). It is also a mild antidepressant that seems to be especially useful for low-grade depression with loss of libido as a prominent symptom.
Tincture (1:5): 2-3 mL TID
Tea: 1 tsp. dried herb, 8 oz hot water, steep 20 minutes (covered), take 4 oz TID/QID

Ginkgo standardized extract *(Ginkgo biloba)* – is primarily thought of as a cerebral tonic, but studies indicate it also has benefits for impotence caused by antidepressant medications. In a trial (Cohen and Bartlik, 1998) with 63 men and women with antidepressant induced sexual dysfunction, 84% of the participants found Ginkgo effective for relieving this troubling side-effect.
Standardized capsule: 120 mg BID

Maca root *(Lepidium meyerii)* – internet companies promoting "herbal viagra" has touted this small radish-like tuber for its reputed male sexual enhancement properties. Also frequently mentioned is the long history of this plants use for infertility and impotence. The actual evidence for this is less clear. There is little to no mention of Maca as anything but a food for people living in the high Andes until the late 20th century. It became popular in Peru and surrounding countries but a long history of medicinal use is lacking. Many early animal and human studies on this herb show little or no effect for improving sexual functioning. Recent studies using Maca extracts have shown some benefit. In a 2008 human trial (Dording, et al, 2008) a high-dose of Maca (3 g per day) helped to alleviate SSRI-induced impotence. A lower dose (1.5g per day) was not effective. A second human trial found that 2400 mg of a Maca extract produced a small but significant improvement in sexual performance and feelings of well-being (Zenico, et al, 2009). In a pilot trial, trained male cyclists taking Maca had increased sexual desire but also improved cycling time trials (Stone, et al, 2009). Some research suggests that Maca's high level of absorbable nutrients and antioxidants may explain its activity rather than any direct effect on the male (or female) reproductive systems.
Tincture (1:4): 5-9 mL TID
Capsules – Standardized Extract: 2400-3000 mg per day

Morinda/Ba Ji Tian root *(Morinda officinalis)* – is another Chinese herb used to tonify the kidney yang. It is commonly used with Epimedium, Red Ginseng, or Rou Cong Rong for impotence, urinary frequency, premature ejaculation, and low back pain. In an animal study, an isolated constituent of Morinda (Bajijiasu) given orally enhanced sexual activity, testosterone levels and sperm quality (Wu, et al, 2015).
Tincture (1:5): 2-4 mL TID
Tea: 1-2 tsp. dried root, 10 oz water, decoct 15 minutes, steep 45 minutes, take 4 oz TID

Muira Puama root or bark (Ptychopetalum olacoides) – also known as potency wood, is commonly used in Brazil as an aphrodisiac and nerve tonic. It is official in the Brazilian pharmacopoeia and it is used for impotence, loss of libido, and to enhance pelvic circulation. Its effects are somewhat similar to Yohimbe, but much milder and with much less potential of drug interactions or adverse reactions. In several small studies Muira Puama enhanced erectile function and improved libido (Rowland, 2003). In animal studies it has been found to have antidepressant, neuroprotective and nootropic effects.
Tincture (1:5): 1-2 mL TID
Tea: 1 tsp. cut/sifted herb, 10 oz water, decoct 20-30 minutes, steep 1/2 hour, take 4 oz BID

Nutmeg seed (Myristica fragrans) – has a long history of use in Ayurvedic, Chinese and Unani-Tibb (Graeco-Arabic) medicine. It is used as a carminative, sleep aid and to treat diarrhea. In the Unani-Tibb system it is also used to stimulate male sexual functioning and libido. Although there are no human studies confirming this traditional use, an animal study found that it did significantly increase sexual activity (Tajuddin, et al, 2005).
Tincture (1:10): .25-.5 mL (5-10 gtt.) TID

Red Kwao Krua (Butea superba) – is a Thai medicinal plant with a reputation as a male aphrodisiac. Animal studies suggest it does enhance male sexual activity and in a human trial, 82.4% of patients with ED showed significant improvement in their ability to achieve and maintain an erection (Cherdshewasart & Nimsakul, 2003). In rat studies large doses of this herb (150-200 mg/kg BW per day) increased blood levels of alkaline phosphatase and AST, decreased neutrophils, increased eosinophils and lowered serum testosterone levels. This suggests that large doses in humans may have possible risks.
Capsules: 250 mg herb powder BID

Rhodiola root (Rhodiola rosea) – is a superb adaptogen, antioxidant, cardiotonic, and nootropic. It has also been shown to enhance erectile function in men. In an open study, 35 men with erectile dysfunction took Rhodiola for 3 months (150-200 mg per day). Twenty-six of the thirty-five men had improved sexual functioning and normalization of prostatic fluid (Brown, et al, 2002).
Tincture (1:5): 4-6 mL TID

Suo Yang herb (Cynomorium songaricum) – this Chinese herb is used to tonify the kidney yang and treat erectile dysfunction, spermatorrhea, and premature ejaculation. It is most often combined with a related herb, Rou Cong Rong (Cistanche salsa). There are no human studies to confirm traditional uses of Suo Yang, but in an animal study a water extract of this herb increased testicular weight and development (Abdel-Magied, et al, 2001).
Tincture (1:5): 2-3 mL TID
Tea: 1-2 tsp. dried herb, 8 oz water, decoct 15 minutes, steep 45 minutes, take 4 oz TID

Tongkat Ali root *(Eurycoma longifolia)* – also known as Pasak Bumi, is native to Malaysia and Indonesia where it is used as an aphrodisiac, antimalarial, antibacterial and antiulcer medicine. This herb has become popular in the west due to some very aggressive internet marketing and videos by several well-known herb/supplement promoters. There are more than a half dozen animal studies (unfortunately all by the same research team, Ang, et al) suggesting the herb increases sexual desire and performance in rats. There are only two human trials with this herb. The first did not look at the aphrodisiac effects, but rather its ability to build muscle. In this small study, men who took Tongkat Ali had increased muscle strength and size along with reduced body fat (Hamzah, et al, 2003). In the second study, men with late-onset hypogonadism took two 100 mg capsules of a standardized Tongkat Ali product. There was a significant increase in testosterone production in most of the men (Tambi, et al, 2012). This study had several flaws, among them there was no control group.. Reports from people using this herb for ED are mixed, with some claiming great benefit and others none. Several factors may be affecting people's response including dosage, product quality, and the placebo effect.
Capsules - Standardized extract:
    20:1 – 1000 mg capsule, 1-2 capsules BID
    100:1 – 500 mg capsules, 1-2 capsules per day
    200:1 – 300 mg capsule, 1 per day

Velvet Bean/Cowhage (Macuna pruriens) – is a traditional medicine used in the Ayurvedic and Unani-Tibb traditions. It has a long history of use as a nerve tonic, sexual stimulant and is a rich source of L-dopa (it has been found to be effective in treating Parkinson's disease). Research suggests the herb works via the HPA axis enhancing testosterone, LH, dopamine, adrenaline and nonadrenalin levels, while inhibiting FSH and prolactin (Shukla et al, 2009). There are no human studies on the use of this herb for ED. It has been shown in a human trial to alleviate stress and improve semen quality in infertile men (Shukla, et al, 2007). An animal study showed that in rats it produced a significant and sustained increase in sexual activity.
Standardized extract: 200 mg capsule once per day
Powdered seed: ¼-1/2 tsp. once or twice per day in ghee, water, milk or honey

Xian Mao rhizome *(Curculigo orchioides)* – is considered one of the most effective remedies in TCM for impotence. Due to its slight toxicity it is not recommended for long-term use. It is always combined with other herbs, including Epimedium, Suo Yang, and Morinda, often in an alcohol base. While human studies are lacking, several animal studies have shown increased sexual activity in test animals given Curculigo (Thakur, et al, 2012; Thakur, et al, 2009; Chauhan, et al, 2007).
Tincture (1:5): .5-1 mL BID

Yin Yang Huo leaf *(Epimedium spp.)* – is used in TCM to tonify the kidney yang and enhance libido. Sold in the U.S. as Horny Goat Weed, this herb has a long history of use for impotence, premature ejaculation, spermatorrhea, infertility (including low sperm count) and "loss of libido". In animal studies it has been shown to increase testosterone production and improve erectile function (Makarova, et al, 2007; Chiu, et al, 2006) while lowering cholesterol and elevated blood sugar levels. Epimedium is best used in formulas and long-term use as a simple may damage the kidney yin.
Tincture (1:5): 1.5-2.5 mL BID/TID
Tea: 1 tsp. herb, 8 oz hot water, steep 40 minutes, take 4 oz BID

There are several popular as well as many lesser-known herbs that are used throughout the world for stimulating male sexual behavior. Many of these herbs have never been studied or have shown benefits in rat studies, but human studies are lacking. Some of these herbs include Tribulus terrestris seed or root, Trichopus zeylanica, Cnidium monnieri, Aframomum melegueta, Ferula harmonis, Montanoa tomentosa, Fadogia agrestis, Boar Hog root (Ligusticum canadense or Angelica venenosa), Chione venosa (Bois Bande) and Elosema krassianum.

Supplements for Erectile Dysfunction
Several nutritional supplements including carnitine (it has also been shown to have benefit for Peyronie's disease and male infertility) and arginine (see below) have been shown to be effective for treating mild to moderate ED in human clinical trials.

<u>Arginine</u> – this amino acid has been shown to promote erectile function when combined with Pycnogenol® (Ledda, et al, 2010; Stanislavov, et al, 2003) or with Yohimbe (Lebret, et al, 2002). A combination of Arginine aspartate (8 g.) and adenosine monophosphate (200 mg.) taken 1-2 hours before sexual activity was effective in relieving mild to moderate erectile dysfunction (Neuzillet, et al, 2013).

<u>L-carnitine</u> – has been shown to enhance penile blood flow in diabetics, men who have had radical prostate surgery and for those with ED. It enhances erectile function when used by itself (Cavallini, et al, 2004) and increases the benefits of viagra® or testosterone when used concurrently (Cavallini, et al, 2004; Cavallini, et al, 2005). A combination of propionyl-L-carnitine, L-arginine and niacin improved penile rigidity (Granfrilli, et al, 2011).

<u>Zinc</u> – this essential mineral is known to be important for normal sperm production and motility. Animal research suggests it also is important for enhancing libido (Dissanayake, et al, 2009).

Exercise for erectile dysfunction – pelvic floor exercises are often recommended for women with poor bladder control and uterine prolapse. They are also useful for men. In a RCT, men with ED were taught how to do these simple exercises and did them for 3 months. In that time 40% regained normal erectile function, 35.5% had improved function and 24.5% failed to respond to treatment (Dorey, et al, 2005).

Premature Ejaculation

Premature ejaculation is usually not so much a medical issue as a quality of life issue. Ejaculating, which often ends sexual intercourse, is a normal response to sexual stimuli. The problem is difficult to accurately quantify because what is premature for one couple may be satisfactory for another. The causes for this problem include an excessively sensitive glans penis, inexperience, a quick habitual response learned while masturbating when young (get it over before anyone catches you), and a lack of knowledge about healthy sexual practices. In our society we titillate our youth with images of nearly naked men and women, give them little or no knowledge of how to be a good and considerate lover, and tell them that abstinence is appropriate behavior. What a confusing, conflicting set of ideas we teach our young, hormonally challenged boys and girls. From a TCM perspective, premature ejaculation is caused by deficient kidney yin and yang and/or a leaky jing gate. A substantial number of mildly astringent herbs are used to treat this condition, but in clinical practice herbs alone are not effective.

Western urologists and sex therapists often recommend desensitizing creams to delay ejaculation. This mirrors the common men's trick of thinking about something else during sex (rebuilding a carburetor, counting to 100) to delay orgasm.

While both techniques may work, both distance a man, physically and/or emotionally, from his partner and what for many men is one of the most life affirming, intimate acts in their lives. In Eastern traditions (India, China), the art of being a good lover is a recognized body of knowledge. In Margo Anand's classic book, The Art of Sexual Ecstasy, she teaches westerners this important information. I highly recommend this book because it is accessible to the average American, eliminating much of the arcane and stylized language of the ancient Kama Sutra and Oriental pillow books. Individuals or couples can learn to enhance lovemaking and intimacy and some men can actually learn to have orgasms without ejaculating. Pelvic floor exercises can also help enhance ejaculatory control.

Herbs to Help with Premature Ejaculation

Cornus/Shan Zu Yu fruit (Cornus officinalis) – tonifies the Chinese kidney and liver, and it astringes the jing. It benefits deficient kidney yang conditions (use with Epimedium, Rou Cong Rong, or Morinda) such as impotence, low back pain, urinary frequency, premature ejaculation, plus it helps prevent excessive sweating, bedwetting, urinary dribbling, and uterine bleeding.
Tincture (1:5) 2 mL TID
Tea: 1 tsp. dried fruit, 8 oz. water, decoct 5 minutes, steep 45 minutes, take 4 oz. BID/TID

Eucommia/Du Zhong bark (Eucommia ulmoides) - is a Chinese kidney and liver tonic. It is most often used for chronic low back pain especially after sex, during pregnancy, or after menses. It is also of benefit for hypertension, weak knees, to heal bone fractures, and for deficient kidney yang symptoms such as nocturia, urinary frequency, impotence, and premature ejaculation.
Tea: 2 tsp. dried bark, 16 oz. water, decoct slowly until reduced by half, take 4 oz. BID

Psoralea seed /Bu Gu Zhi/(Psoralea corylifolia) – also tonifies the kidney yang and helps astringe a leaky jing gate. It is also used for impotence, urinary frequency, nocturia, premature ejaculation, as well as low back pain (especially if worse after sex), chronic pelvic pain syndrome (CPPS), and diarrhea. It is contraindicated in patients with yin deficiency. It can be stir-fried in salt water to reduce its astringency or you can add moistening herbs such as Couch Grass, Suo Yang, or Rou Cong Rong.
Tincture (1:5): 1-2 mL TID
Tea: 1 tsp. dried seed, 10 oz. water, decoct 10-15 minutes, steep 1/2 hour. Take 4 oz. BID

Schisandra berry/Wu Wei Zi (Schisandra chinensis) – is a mildly stimulating adaptogen which enhances HPA axis function and benefits asthma with wheezing, neurasthenia, and adrenal exhaustion. It is used in TCM to astringe a leaky jing gate, symptoms of this include premature ejaculation, spermatorrhea, a heavy non-specific vaginal discharge, and urinary frequency in either sex.
Tincture (1:5): 2-4 mL TID
Tea: 1 tsp. dried berries, 8 oz. water, decoct 5-10 minutes, steep 1/2 hour, take 4 oz. 3-4 times per day

Painful Ejaculation
Painful ejaculation can be caused by epididymitis, STD's, testicular spasms, scarring of the vas deferens, or spermatic chord, or Peyronie's Disease. Each of these conditions needs to be dealt with in a specific way. There are a number of herbs that act as urinary analgesics that help relieve painful ejaculation:

Black Cohosh root (Actaea racemosa) – is an antispasmodic, analgesic, and antiinflammatory agent. It is especially useful for testicular pain, testicular spasms, and the pain caused by orchitis or epididymitis.
Tincture (1:2): .5 – 1.5 mL TID

Cleavers herb (Galium aparine) – relieves pain and inflammation of the spermatic chord and vas deferens. I use it for men who have scarring and inflammation caused by long-term untreated chlamydia infections.
Tincture (1:2): 2-4 mL TID

Hydrangea root bark (Hydrangea arborescens) – is probably the best of the urinary anodynes. It relieves pain in the bladder, kidneys, prostate, urethra, and seminal vesicles. It is indicated for pain in the lower back and for pain that originates in the groin and wraps around the thighs.
Tincture (1:5): 2-3 mL TID

Kava root (Piper methysticum) – was originally introduced into western herbal medicine as a urinary analgesic. The Eclectics used it for urinary or pelvic pain caused by urinary infections, epididymitis, orchitis, renal colic, or testicular or vaginal spasms.
Tincture (1:5): 2-4 mL TID/QID

Performance Anxiety
Performance anxiety is best dealt with by good communication and compassion between sexual partners. Unfortunately for some couples neither communication nor compassion are evident. Once the fear of failure is eliminated, herbs and exercises can help to relieve anxiety and any underlying problems.

Bacopa herb (Bacopa monnieri) – is an Ayurvedic herb used for anxiety, irritability, mental fog and nervous exhaustion. It can be combined with Passion Flower or Fresh Oat for sexual anxiety.
Tincture (1:5 or 1:2): 1.5-2.5 mL TID/QID
Tea: 1 tsp. dried herb, 8 oz. water, steep 45 minutes, take 4 oz. TID

Fresh Oat (Avena sativa) – is a superb nervous system trophorestorative that helps restore emotional balance and relieves anxiety. It was used by the Eclectics for sexual neurasthenia, a lack of sexual energy causing impotence and lack of libido.
Tincture (1:2): 4-5 mL TID
Glycerite (1:2): 5-7.5 mL 4-5x/day

Passion Flower leaves/vine (Passiflora incarnata) – is a nervine especially indicated for circular thinking, constant worry, and anxiety. It can be used with Fresh Oat, Motherwort, or other anxiolytics.
Tincture (1:2): 2.5-3 mL TID
Tea: 1 tsp. dried herb, 8 oz. hot water, steep for 40-50 minutes, take 2-3 cups/day

Pulsatilla herb (Anemone patens) – is a powerful herb used in very small doses for anxiety, irritability, and "grumpy old man" syndrome (use it with Saw Palmetto and Fresh Oat for this). For anxiety attacks I use small doses of this herb with Bacopa, Chinese Polygala, Fresh Oat and Motherwort.
Tincture (1:2): 1-3 gtt TID

Male Sexual Tonics
The following herbs enhance libido, increase sperm count and sperm motility, and help nourish the male reproductive system.

Ashwagandha root (Withania somnifera) – is a Rasayana (rejuvinative herb) and adaptogen frequently used in Ayurvedic medicine. It is used as a sexual tonic for men and over time increases testosterone levels and libido as well as overall energy. In a human study it improved semen quality in infertile men (Ambiye, et al, 2013; Ahmad, et al, 2010).
Tincture (1:5): 1.5-2.5 mL TID
Tea: 1 tsp. dried root, 8 oz water, decoct 15 minutes, steep 1/2 hour, take 4 oz TID

Asian Ginseng root (Panax ginseng) – is a very useful adaptogen with broad reaching effects on the nervous system, endocrine system, and immune system. It also has a reputation as an "aphrodisiac" for men. For many years I believed that it was only useful for exhausted, depleted men with little or no sexual desire, but discounted its broader use for impotence. Recent studies suggest the popular wisdom about Ginseng may be true after all. In a double-blind crossover study published in the *Journal of Urology*, over 60% of the participants using Panax reported improved erections (Hong, et al, 2002). In a second RCT 66% of men reported improved erectile function (de Andrade, et al, 2007).
Tincture (1:5): 2-3 mL TID
Capsule/Tablet-900 mg TID

Cordyceps fungus (Cordyceps sinensis, C. militaris) – is one of the great adaptogenic tonic remedies in Chinese medicine. It is an immune, endocrine, kidney, and nervous system restorative. As such it enhances HPA axis function and supports healthy sexual function. It has been shown in animal studies to stimulate sperm production and motility (Chang, et al, 2008; Huang, et al, 2004) as well as enhancing energy and libido.
Tincture (1:5): 1-2 mL TID
Capsules: 2 capsules BID

Fresh Oat (Avena sativa) – is a phenomenal nervine and nervous system tropho-restorative. It is a wonderful nourishing tonic remedy for fatigue, chronic stress, anxiety, and neurasthenia. The Eclectic physicians who introduced this remedy also recommended it for sexual neurasthenia from excess sexual activity, nervousness, or lack of libido. It was often combined with celery seed and very small amounts of the toxic stimulant Nux Vomica.
Tincture (1:2): 4-6 mL TID
Glycerite (1:2): 5-7.5 mL 4-5x/day

He Shou Wu root (Polygonum multiflorum) – is a blood or xue tonic in Chinese medicine. It is primarily used for dizziness, premature graying of the hair, lower back and kidney pain, and anemia. It also enhances sperm count and motility, plus it increases hormonal secretions by the adrenals and thyroid.
Tincture (1:5): 1.5-2.5 mL TID
Tea: 1-2 tsp. dried root, 12 oz. water, decoct 20 minutes, steep 40 minutes, take 4 oz. 3x/day

Maca root (Lepidium meyenii) – has been touted as a sexual tonic for men and women, but until recently only rat studies have indicated possible efficacy. Several human trials have added to the previously scanty evidence showing large doses of Maca enhanced male libido and increased the volume of seminal fluids as well as sperm count and sperm motility (Lentz, et al, 2006).
Tincture (1:5): 3-5 mL TID Capsules: 3 g per day

Morinda/Ba Ji Tian root (Morinda officinalis) – is used in TCM as a kidney yang tonic. It is often combined with Epimedium and Curculigo root (in wine) as a male reproductive tonic for impotence, infertility, premature ejaculation, and low back pain after sex. It has mild adaptogenic activity.
Tincture (1:5): 40-60 gtt TID
Tea: 1 tsp. dried root, 10 oz. water, decoct 15 minutes, steep 45 minutes, take 4 oz. 3x/day

Rou Cong Rong herb (Cistanche salsa) – and the following herb, Suo Yang, are related to the American plant Broomrape (Conopholis americana). It is possible the American plant shares some similar activity to the 2 Asian plants. Cistanche tonifies the kidney yang, jing, and blood. It is used for impotence, lack of libido, low sperm count, and low back pain. It is mild acting and needs to be combined with other stronger herbs.
Tea: 1-2 tsp. dried herb, 8-10 oz. water, decoct 15 minutes, steep 40 minutes. Take 4 oz. TID

Suo Yang herb (Cynomorium songaricum) – is stronger than Rou Cong Rong, but less tonifying to the blood and jing. It is used with Morinda, Epimedium, and Red Ginseng for deficient kidney yang with lack of libido, erectile dysfunction, and male infertility. In an animal studies a water extract of Cynomorium prevented decreased testicular function caused by reduced daylight (Lee, et al, 2013).
Tea: 1-2 tsp. dried herb, 8-10 oz. water, decoct 15 minutes, steep 40 minutes. Take 4 oz. TID

Yin Yang Huo (Epimedium spp.) – is used in TCM to tonify the kidney yang and enhance libido. Sold in the U.S. as Horny Goat Weed, this herb has a long history of use for impotence, premature ejaculation, spermatorrhea, infertility (including low sperm count) and loss of libido. In studies it has been shown to increase testosterone production while lowering cholesterol and elevated blood sugar levels. Animal studies show it can relax the corpus cavernosum, enhancing potential erections (Chiu, et al, 2006). Epimedium is best used in formulas and excessive or long-term use can damage the kidney yin.
Tincture (1:5): 1.5-2.5 mL BID/TID
Tea: 1 tsp. herb, 8 oz hot water, steep 40 minutes, take 4 oz BID

Nutritional Supplements for Enhancing Male Reproductive Function
Several essential nutrients are associated with healthy reproductive functioning and male fertility, including Omega 3 fatty acids (fish oils), zinc, vitamin E (mixed tocopherols with tocotrienols), vitamin C, selenium, and Co-Q-10.

References available in the downloadable version of this book, for purchase at
www.botanicalmedicine.org

Herbs and Nutrition For Cardiovascular Health and Disease
David Winston, RH (AHG) ©2010, revised 2012

Cardiovascular diseases (CVD) are the leading cause of death in the U.S. and developed countries. The CDC reports that in 2007 there were 616,067 deaths caused by heart problems and that many, if not most, were preventable. According to the WHO, the major CVDs are myocardial infarction/MI (heart attack), hypertension, stroke (cerebrovascular disease), congestive heart failure and rheumatic heart disease. The majority of these diseases (rheumatic heart disease is the exception) are caused by obesity, insulin resistance, lack of exercise, diabetes, nutritional deficiencies, hypertension, smoking, and chronic stress. Certain risk factors (age, being male, family history, ethnic group) are beyond our control. Many other risk factors, as seen below, can be favorably altered to reduce CVD risk.

The following chart lists major risk factors for CVD.

RISK FACTOR	CAN CAUSE OR EXACERBATE
Obesity (especially abdominal obesity), Insulin resistance, Type 2 Diabetes *(these are closely related)*	Hypertension Elevated cortisol levels Increased inflammation Atherosclerosis Low HDL cholesterol High LDL cholesterol High triglycerides Elevated Hemoglobin A1c (HbA1c) Elevated C-reactive protein (CRP) Elevated Homocysteine levels *(these are related)*
Sedentary lifestyle	Obesity
Smoking	Erectile dysfunction Impaired circulation Decreased vitamin C levels Buerger's Disease
Chronic Stress	Elevated cortisol levels Decreased sleep Hypertension Increased inflammation
Negative emotions (chronic anxiety, rage, fear, anger)	Increased cortisol and adrenaline levels Impaired sleep Hypertension Decreased digestion/absorption Decreased libido
Low HDL cholesterol, High LDL cholesterol, High triglycerides, Elevated Hemoglobin A1c, Elevated CRP *(these are related)*	Atherosclerosis Increased blood viscosity Elevated blood sugar levels (insulin resistance/diabetes) Increased inflammation

Elevated Homocysteine levels

Risk Factor	Can Cause or Exacerbate
Nutritional Deficiencies	
Omega 3 fatty acids	Increased inflammation, blood viscosity and risk of atherogenesis
Magnesium	Increased risk of muscle spasm and arrythmia
Vitamin D	Increased risk of inflammation and atherogenesis
Vitamin C	Increased risk of inflammation and atherogenesis, unstable plaque
B-12	Increased risk of inflammation and atherogenesis
Recreational Drug Use [Cocaine, amphetamines, methadone, ephedrine, MDMA)	Increased risk of stroke, cardiomyopathy, MI, hypertension, cardiotoxicity
Alcohol (in excess of 1-2 drinks per day)	Hypertension, increased triglycerides, liver disease
Pharmaceuticals	
Doxorubicin, 5-Flourouracil, Adriamycin	Cardiotoxic – can cause heart damage
Cisplatin, Cyclophosphamide	Cardiotoxic – can cause heart damage
Novantrone (antileukemic), antihistamines	Cardiotoxic – can cause heart damage
Anti-retroviral drugs, NSAIDs (Vioxx)	Cardiotoxic – can cause heart damage
Tricyclic antidepressants	Cardiotoxic – can cause heart damage
Vinorebine and other fluoropyrimidine drugs	Cardiotoxic – can cause heart damage
Other diseases	
Kidney disease	Congestive heart failure
Thalassemia major (iron excess)	Increased risk of MI or stroke
Environmental pollutants	
Smog/air pollution (aldehydes)	Increased risk of MI
Lead	Increased CV mortality, hypertension
Mercury	Endothelial dysfunction, hypertension
Cadmium	Hypertension, kidney damage
Diet	
High intake of trans fats	Increased atherosclerosis
Excess iron	Increased risk of MI

Prevention of CV disease is obviously the clinicians' primary goal, but even simple changes in diet (low glycemic load diet, sodium reduction, 1 glass of red wine per day, regular use of olive oil and increased soluble fiber), improved nutritional status (add fish oils, L-carnitine, magnesium, vitamins C and E, Co-Q-10), lifestyle changes (increased exercise, moderate weight loss, quitting smoking, stress reduction techniques) and the use of herbal CV tonics (Hawthorn, Tienqi Ginseng, Dan Shen, and antioxidant-rich herbs/foods) can reduce risk of disease and help to reverse many mild to moderate CV conditions.

A Short List of Major Cardiotonic Herbs

Arjuna (Terminalia arjuna)
Part Used: Bark
Active Constituents: Triterpenoids, Tannins
Taste: Bitter
Energy: Cool and Dry
Activity: Cardioprotective, lowers LDL cholesterol levels and triglycerides, elevates HDL cholesterol levels
Cardiovascular uses: Increases O_2 to the heart, strengthens contractions, and slows the heart rate (it is negatively chronotropic and positively inotropic).
It is used for stable angina pectoris (it is not effective for unstable angina), especially with ectopic beats (Bharani, et al, 2002), mild congestive heart failure, palpitations, and mild to moderate mitral valve prolapse with regurgitation (Dwivedi, et al, 2005). Use it with Hawthorn, Night Blooming Cerus, and Collinsonia for MVP.
Dosage: Fresh tincture (1:5) 2-4 ml TID
    Tea (Decoction) 1 tsp. dried, powdered, bark, 10 oz. water, decoct 15 minutes, steep 40 minutes take 4 oz. 3x/day
CI/Drug Interactions: Unstable angina, patients with recent myocardial infarctions. Dry constipation, pregnancy.

Astragalus (Astragalus membranaceous)
Part Used: Root
Active Constituents: Astragalosides, flavonoids
Taste: Sweet
Energy: Warm and Moist
Activity: Cardiovascular tonic, it mildly lowers blood pressure, dilates the coronary arteries and stimulates peripheral circulation. It can be used with Dan Shen, Dang Gui and Tienqi for angina and mild congestive heart failure.
There are a multitude of Chinese studies using this herb and isolated constituents for treating CV conditions. Animal studies show it improves impaired endothelial function (Deng and Yu, 2009) and can ameliorate abnormal cardiac function, especially diastolic function in heart failure (Su, et al, 2009). Other studies show it can protect the heart against Coxsackie B virus, a major cause of myocarditis and that if taken orally it prevented diabetic rats from developing cardiomyopathy by down-regulating angiotensin II type 2 (AT 2) receptors (Li, et al, 2004).
Dosage: Tincture (1:5, cook 4-6 hours) 2-4 ml TID
    Tea (Decoction) 2 tsp. dried root, 12 oz. water, decoct 20 minutes, reduce to 6 oz., steep 30 minutes, take 3 cups/day

Dan Shen (Salvia miltiorrhiza)
Part Used: Root
Active Constituents: Diterpene quinones, Salvenolic acids
Taste: Bitter
Energy: Cool and Dry
Activity: Cardioprotective, Analgesic, Peripheral vasodilator
Cardiovascular uses: It increases circulation to the heart and reduces blood viscosity. Dan Shen is used for angina pain, hypertension, and palpitations. It also lowers cholesterol and triglyceride levels.
Dosage: Tincture (1:4 or 1:5) 1.5-3 ml TID/QID
    Tea (Decoction) 1-2 tsp. dried root, 8 oz. water, decoct 10-15 minutes, steep 1 hour, take 2-3 cups/day
CI/Drug Interactions: Pregnancy or heavy blood flow. It can potentiate Warfarin and other anticoagulant medications, avoid concurrent use.

Dang Gui (Angelica sinensis)
Part Used: Root
Active Constituents: Z-Ligustilide, Ferulic acid
Taste: Pungent and Sweet
Energy: Warm and Moist
Activity: In TCM Dang Gui is used to nourish the blood and enhance circulation. It improves cardiac circulation and can be used with Dan Shen, Tienqi, Astragalus and Corydalis for angina pain. It can also be useful for intermittent claudication and Buerger's disease. In animal studies, Dang Gui prevented doxorubicin-induced cardiotoxicity (Xin, et al, 2007) and it inhibited atherogenesis (Zhui, et al, 2000).
Dosage: Tincture (1:4 or 1:5) 2-4 ml TID
    Tea (Decoction) 1-2 tsp. dried root, 8 oz. water, decoct 10-15 minutes, steep covered 45 minutes, take up to 3 cups/day
CI / Drug Interactions: Use carefully with blood thinning medication.

Hawthorn (Crataegus monogyna, C. oxycanthoides)
Taste: Sweet, Sour, Bland

Part Used: Fruit, Flowers and Leaf
Energy: Warm and Slightly Moist
Active Constituents: Flavonoids
Activity: Cardiotonic (trophorestorative), nervine, antiinflammatory, mild diuretic.
Cardio-vascular uses: Hawthorn is a "Food for the Heart". It can be used for nourishing, strengthening and repairing the heart.
Functional and organic heart conditions benefit from Hawthorn (angina, mild congestive heart failure, hypertension, mitral valve weakness). It is also a tonic for the veins, capillaries, and arteries and is useful for atherosclerosis and intermittent claudication.
Dosage: Tincture (1:4): 4-5 ml QID
       Tea (Infusion): 1-2 tsp. dried berries, 8 oz. hot water, steep for 1 hour, take 3 cups/day
       Solid extract: 1/4 teaspoon BID
CI / Drug Interactions: Crataegus may potentiate Beta blockers

⊗**Lily of the Valley** (Convalleria majalis)
Taste: Bitter
Part Used: Leaves and Flowers
Energy: Neutral, Moist, Toxic
Active Constituents: Cardiac Glycosides (convallatoxin, convallamarin), flavonoids.
Activity: Cardiac stimulant, diuretic.
Cardiovascular uses: Convalleria is used with Crataegus and Night Blooming Cereus for congestive heart failure (CHF), mitral insufficiency with dyspnea, cardiac edema, bradycardic forms of heart failure and cardiac arrhythmias with a rapid, feeble pulse.
Dosage: Tincture (1:5) 3-5 gtt BID/TID
CI / Drug Interactions: It will potentiate Digitalis glycosides (Digoxin, Lanoxin, Digitoxin).

Night Blooming Cereus (Selenicereus grandiflorus)
Taste: Bitter and Slightly Sweet
Part Used: Stem and Flower
Energy: Neutral and Moist
Active Constituents: Cactine, Flavonoid Glycosides (Cacticin, Grandiflorin, Rutin).
Activity: Cardiotonic, antidepressant, demulcent.
Cardio-vascular uses: Palpitations with shortness of breath, the patient is irritable, with tightness in the chest and a feeble, irregular pulse. It can be used (along with Hawthorn and Arjuna) for angina and "Tobacco Heart". For mitral and aortic regurgitation use it with Hawthorn, Collinsonia and Gotu Kola.
Dosage: Fresh tincture (1:2), 5-15 gtt TID
CI / Drug Interactions: Hypertension, may interact with prescription cardiac medications

Tienqi Ginseng (Panax notoginseng)
Taste: Sweet, Slightly Bitter
Part Used: Root
Energy: Warm and Dry
Active Constituents: Arasaponins, Ginsenosides, Notoginsenosides
Cardiovascular uses: Tienqi is used in TCM for angina pectoris and congestive heart failure. It increases oxygen flow to the coronary artery and heart while decreasing oxygen consumption by the heart. It is used with Dang Gui, Astragalus, and Salvia miltiorrhiza for fatty degeneration of the heart.
Dosage: Tincture (1:5), 1.5-2.5 ml QID
       Tea (Decoction) 1 tsp. dried, powdered, root, 12 oz.water,, decoct 15-20 minutes, steep 45 minutes to 1 hour , take 4 oz. 4x/day
CI/Drug Interactions: Anticoagulant medications, pregnancy.

HYPERTENSION

Hypertension, or high blood pressure (>140/90 mm/Hg) is a condition where the blood pressure in the arteries is elevated. This may be acute, caused by pain, anxiety or exertion, or a chronic condition. Chronic hypertension is a major risk factor for heart disease, peripheral vascular disease and stroke. Hypertension is usually classified as either primary (essential) hypertension or secondary hypertension. Approximately 90-95% of all hypertension is primary hypertension, which has no obvious medical cause. Secondary hypertension is caused by cardiac, kidney or endocrine/thyroid problems.

⊗ **Toxic: Should be used only with directions from a trained practitioner!**
Even through there is no identifiable cause of primary hypertension, many factors can influence this condition including genetics, stress (white coat hypertension), diet (excess salt and carbohydrates, low potassium and magnesium intake), insulin resistance, obesity, chronic insomnia or poor quality sleep, a sedentary lifestyle, vitamin D deficiency, excessive alcohol consumption, use of stimulants (ephedrine, cocaine, amphetamines), and some medications (NSAIDs, decongestants).

Herbs and Supplements for Hypertension

Chrysanthemum flower (Chrysanthemum morifolium)
Is used in China as a beverage tea and medicine. It mildly reduces blood pressure and a tea made of Chrysanthemum flower, Hibiscus flower, Linden flower, Olive leaf and Lemon Balm can be effective for relieving pre-hypertension and mild cases of high blood pressure.
Dosage: Tincture (1:5) 2-4 ml TID/QID
      Tea 1-2 tsp. dried flowers, 8 oz. hot water, steep covered for 20-40 minutes, take 1-3 cups/day

Coenzyme Q-10
Co-Q-10, or its more active form, ubliquinone, has been shown in human trials to lower blood pressure in patients with type II diabetes (Hodgson, et al, 2002).
Dosage: 60-100 mg BID

Dan Shen root (Salvia miltiorrhiza)
This herb has a long history of use in TCM for relieving blood stasis and blood heat (infection). It is used for gynecological, liver and cardiac problems. Much of the research on this herb for cardiovascular issues has used injectable isolated constituents, so it is not applicable to herbal usage. Even though clinical data on oral use is limited (Kang, et al, 2002), this herb can be useful as part of a protocol for hypertension as well as angina, palpitations, and to inhibit atherosclerosis.
Dosage: Tincture (1:4 or 1:5), 1.5-3 ml TID/QID
      Tea (decoction) 1-2 tsp. dried root, 8 oz. water, decoct 10-15 minutes, steep 1 hour, take 2-3 cups/day

Du Zhong bark (Eucommia ulmoides)
Is used in TCM to strengthen the bones, tendons and the Chinese liver and kidney. It is also used for hypertension. The decoction (the tincture is not effective for this) can be combined with Chrysanthemum flower, Gambir vine, Dan Shen and Huang Qin. Animal studies have also confirmed this herb's ability to lower blood pressure (Lang, et al, 2005).
Dosage: Tea (decoction) 2 tsp. dried bark, 16 oz. water, decoct 1 hour, take 2-3 cups/day

Gou Teng spines (Uncaria sinensis)
The hooks or "cat's claws" of this Asian species of Uncaria, are used in TCM to calm the spirit (sedative) and extinguish wind (antispasmodic). It is useful for treating liver fire rising symptoms such as headaches, hypertension with dizziness, red, painful eyes and anxiety (Wu, et al, 1980).
Dosage: Tincture (1:4 or 1:5) 1-2 ml TID
      Tea (decoction) 1-2 tsp. dried stems, 8 oz. water, decoct 5 minutes, steep ½ hour, take 4 oz. QID

Hibiscus flower (Hibiscus sabdariffa)
This lovely red flower is used to make a sour tasting tea that is rich in anti-inflammatory and antioxidant polyphenols. In a clinical trial, Hibiscus tea was more effective than Lisinopril for lowering blood pressure, decreasing sodium levels (without affecting potassium) and inhibiting angistensin-converting enzyme/ACL activity (Herrera-Arellano, et al, 2007).
Dosage: Tincture (1:2 or 1:5), 2-4 ml TID
      Tea 1-2 tsp. dried flowers, 8 oz. hot water, steep for 20 minutes, take 2-3 cups/day

Kudzu root (Pueraria lobata)
Is commonly used in TCM for clearing wind heat (spasms) and headaches. It can also be used for hypertension with a stiff neck, headache, tinnitus or dizziness. It has only a mild effect on blood pressure (combine it with stronger herbs) but is very effective for the secondary symptoms.
Dosage: Tincture (1:5), 3-5 ml TID/QID
       Tea (decoction) 1-2 tsp. dried root, 10 oz. water, decoct 10-15 minutes, steep 1 hour, take 2-3 cups/day

Linden flower (Tilia platyphyllos)
Has been used in Europe as a delicious beverage tea as well as a nervine, mild hypotensive agent and pectoral. The tea gently reduces blood pressure and, when combined with Hibiscus flowers, Lemon Balm, Chrysanthemum flower, Hawthorn, and Olive leaf, makes a pleasant tasting tea for mild to moderate hypertension.
Dosage: Tincture (1:5), 2-3 ml TID/QID
       Tea 2 tsp. dried flowers, 8 oz. hot water, steep covered for 30-40 minutes, take 2-3 cups/day

Mistletoe herb (Viscum album)
Is an effective medicine for hypertension. It may cause a slight elevation in blood pressure for a few days, but this is usually followed by a drop with sustained use. Do not use it with pharmaceutical medications for hypertension (beta blockers, ACE inhibitors, calcium channel blockers) as it seems to increase blood pressure without the reduction in blood pressure seen when used by itself.
Dosage: Tincture (1:5), 1-2 ml TID

Motherwort herb (Leonurus cardiaca)
Has a long history of use for anxiety, stress-induced hypertension (white coat hypertension) and hyperthyroid-induced palpitations. It works best when combined with other stronger hypotensive herbs.
Dosage: Tincture (1:2.5 or 1:5), 2.5-4 ml TID/QID
       Tea 1 tsp. dried herb, 8 oz. hot water, steep for 20-30 minutes, take 4 oz. up to 4x/day

Olive leaf (Olea europaea)
Has been used for centuries in Europe for treating high blood pressure and diabetes. Animal and human studies (Cherf, et al, 1996; Perrinjaquet-Onoceato, et al, 2005) confirm that the leaf does lower blood pressure. It has strong antioxidant activity and mild ACF (angiotensin converting enzyme) inhibiting effects.
Dosage: Tincture (1:5), 2-4 ml TID
       Tea 1-2 tsp. dried leaf, 8 oz. water, decoct 10 minutes, steep 40 minutes, take 4 oz. TID

Rauwolfia herb (Rauwolfia serpentina)
This herb has been used for millennia in India to treat epilepsy, insanity, high blood pressure and insomnia. In the 1950's reserpine, derived from this plant, was a popular medication for hypertension. Its use was discontinued due to side effects including depression and fears that it might case breast cancer (it does not). The whole herb is much less problematic than the isolated alkaloid and in small doses is a highly effective short-term treatment for moderate to severe hypertension. In an animal study, green tea was able to ameliorate oxidative liver damage caused by the isolated reserpine (Alibloushi, et al, 2009). It might be a good idea to take antioxidants such as Milk Thistle, Turmeric or Schisandra when taking Rauwolfia.
Dosage: Tincture (standardized to 1% total alkaloids) 2-12 gtt TID combined with other milder herbs

PREVENTION AND TREATMENT OF ATHEROSCLEROSIS (ARTERIOSCLEROTIC VASCULAR DISEASE – ASVD) AND CORONARY ARTERY DISEASE (CAD)

Atherosclerosis, or arteriosclerotic vascular disease/ASVD is a common degenerative condition associated with aging and the western diet /lifestyle. Over decades (evidence shows atherosclerosis often begins by the age of 14-15), the artery walls thicken due to buildup of oxidative LDL/VLDL cholesterol. These inflammatory proteins stimulate an immune response (macrophages) which provokes an autoimmune response. As this process progresses the artery walls form plaques that narrow the arteries, decreasing blood flow. Plaques can be stable or unstable. Unstable plaques can and often do rupture, causing arterial stenosis, blood clots, and ischaemic damage to the heart.

Herbs and Supplements for the Prevention and Treatment of Atherosclerosis (Arteriosclerotic Vascular Disease – ASVD) and Coronary Artery Disease (CAD)

Amla fruit (Emblica officinalis)
This Ayurvedic rasayana strengthens the veins, arteries and capillaries, reducing capillary fragility. It is of benefit for vasculitis, varicose veins, spider veins and inhibiting atherogenesis. Amla also enhances hemoglobin levels, prevents excessive bruising and helps lower LDL/VLDL cholesterol levels.
Dosage: Tincture (1:4 or 1:5), 3-5 ml TID/QID
  Tea: ½ to 1 tsp. dried powdered fruit, 8 oz. water, decoct 10 minutes, steep 1 hour, take 2-3 cups/day

Blueberry fruit (Vaccinium spp.)
Blueberry and Bilberry are powerful antioxidants and antiinflammatories. They help to stabilize capillaries, veins and arteries and inhibit atherogenesis.
Dosage: Solid extract: ¼ - ½ tsp. BID

Dang Gui root (Angelica sinensis)
Is used with Salvia miltiorrhiza for constrictive aoritis and impaired circulation. In animal studies, Dang Gui reduced triglyceride levels, mildly thinned the blood and inhibited atherogenesis (Zhul, et al, 2000).
Dosage: Tincture (1:4) 2-4 ml QID
  Tea - 2 tsp. dried root to 8 oz. of water, decoct 10-15 minutes steep (covered) 1 hour. 2-3 cups per day

Garlic bulb (Allium sativum)
Long-term use of Garlic can inhibit atherosclerosis, modestly lower cholesterol levels and prevent arteriosclerotic changes (Siegal, et al, 2004).
Dosage: Fresh Garlic: to tolerance
  Capsule: 2 BID

Ginkgo leaf (Ginkgo biloba)
Can be used for cerebral artherosclerosis with impaired memory, peripheral neuropathies and impotence due to atherosclerosis. In a human study of high risk cardiovascular patients, standardized Ginkgo reduced LDL cholesterol levels, inhibited Lp(a) while increasing cAMP/cGMP (vasodilating effects) and the antioxidant SOD (Rodriguez, et al, 2007).
Dosage: Standardized Extract: 120 mg BID

Green Tea (Camellia sinensis)
High does of green tea catechins (518 mg pd) helped to protect men against oxidative damage caused by smoking (1 pack per day). It improved endothelial dysfunction and inhibited atherogenic factors (Oyama, et al, 2010). Regular consumption of green tea (4-8 cups per day) has also been found to inhibit atherosclerosis.
Dosage: 2-4 cups per day

Hawthorn fruit/flower (Crataegus oxycanthoides, C. monogyna)
Reduces plaque formation in the arterial walls. It also strengthens arteries, capillaries and veins, reducing endothelial dysfunctions.
Dosage: Tincture 4-6 ml QID
  Tea 1-2 tsp. dried herbs, 8 oz. hot water, steep for 1 hour, take 3 cups per day
  Solid Extract ¼ to ½ tsp. BID

Hibiscus flower (Hibiscus sabdariffa)
In animal and human studies the flowers of Hibiscus have been found to have antioxidant, antihyperlipidemic and antiinflammatory effects. In a human trial (Mozaffari-Khosravi, et al, 2009), type II diabetics who took Hibiscus tea had increased HDL cholesterol and decreased total cholesterol, LDL cholesterol, triglycerides, and Apo-B-100 (Apolipoprotein B).
Dosage: Tincture (1:2 or 1:5) 2-4 ml TID

Tea 1-2 tsp. dried flowers, 8 oz. hot water, steep for 20 minutes, take 2-3 cups per day

Horsetail herb (Equisetum arvense)
Is a rich source of silicic acid, the organic form of silica. Silica is one of the most common minerals in our bodies and is necessary for strong bones as well as healthy skin, veins and arteries. Horsetail has been used in Europe for preventing and treating atherosclerosis. A Chinese animal study showed that Equisetum lowered both cholesterol levels and triglycerides (Xu, et al, 1993).
Dosage: Tincture (1:5) 1-2 ml TID
    Tea (Decoction): 1 tsp. dried herb, 8 oz. water, decoct 15 minutes, steep for 1 hour, take 4 oz. 3x/day
    Tablets: 1-2 BID

Huang Qin/Baikal Scullcap root (Scutellaria baicalensis)
Is used to treat and prevent atherosclerosis. It is anti-inflammatory, antioxidant and antithrombotic and inhibits oxidation of LDL cholesterol and arterial plaque formation.
Dosage: Tincture (1:5) 2-3 ml TID
    Tea (Decoction) 1-2 tsp. dried root, 8 oz. water, decoct 10-15 minutes, steep 1 hour, take 2-3 cups/day

Khella seed (Ammi visnaga)
Is used in Europe for impaired coronary and vascular circulation with angina. It is a powerful antispasmodic and it relieves venospasm.
Dosage: Tincture (1:5) .5-1.5 ml TID

L-Carnitine
The propionyl form of L-Carnitine has been shown to improve the symptoms of peripheral arterial disease (PAD) including intermittent claudication (Andreozzi, 2009).
Dosage: 500-1500 mg

Periwinkle leaf (Vinca minor)
Can be used for mild forms of cerebral atherosclerosis with impaired memory and concentration. (use it with Rosemary, Ginkgo and Bacopa).
Dosage: Tincture (1:2) 5-10 gtt TID.
    Tea: 1 tsp. dried leaf, 8 oz. hot water, steep 30 minutes, take 2 oz. TID

Resveratrol
This powerful stilbene is found in Japanese Knotweed, Grape skins and seeds, wine and many berries. Numerous studies (in vitro, animal and human) have shown that it is a strong antioxidant and anti-inflammatory agent. It inhibits atherogenesis by inhibiting hepatic triglyceride synthesis, reducing atherosclerotic plaque formation and preventing oxidation of LDL cholesterol. Other research shows that Resveratrol down-regulates pro-inflammatory cytokines, promotes NO (nitric oxide) release, and inhibits platelet aggregation (Rampraseth and Jones, 2010).
Dosage: 20-100 mg per day

Safflower blossoms (Carthamus tinctorius)
Is used in TCM for heart blood stagnation. It is used with Dang Gui, Tienqi, Dan Shen and Astragalus for treating and preventing atherosclerosis, and relieving angina pain and thromboangiitis obliterens (with dark red or purplish feet).
Dosage: Tincture (1:5): 1.5-2 ml QID
    Tea: 2 tsp. dried flowers, 8 oz. water, steep covered 30-40 minutes, take 4 oz. 4x/day

Triphala powder (Terminalia chebula/T. belerica/Phyllanthus emblica)
Is one of the great Ayurvedic rasayanas. It is a powerful antioxidant and anti-inflammatory and can help prevent or treat atherosclerosis, improve eye health and bowel function.
Dosage: Powder: 1-2 tsp. in warm water before bedtime
    Capsules: 1-2 capsules BID

HYPERCHOLESTEROLEMIA

Elevated total cholesterol levels have been widely promoted as an important and controllable (using statins and diet) risk factor for CVD. In reality, the total cholesterol number (>200) is relatively meaningless. Just because someone has a total cholesterol of 240 is no reason to be alarmed or take potentially dangerous statins. The more important numbers are the total HDL cholesterol (>50 for men and >60 for women are good numbers) and total LDL cholesterol (<130). The HDL/LDL ratio is also important (0-3.6 is normal) and comprehensive cholesterol panels measure VLDL-3 (which should be <10) and LDL-R (which should be <100), both of which are risk factors. In addition, elevated levels of C-Reactive Protein (0-4.9 normal), hemoglobin A1c (4.8 – 5.9 normal), triglycerides (0-149 normal), cortisol levels (3.1-22.4 ug/dL) and serum glucose (65-99 ug/dL) are significant risk factors.

Many people with elevated cholesterol are given statin drugs, which are effective for lowering LDL and total cholesterol. Unfortunately, these medications can have serious side effects including brain fog, muscle weakness and pain, as well as liver damage. If someone is using statin drugs (or Red Yeast rice) they should take Co-Q-10 (200-400 mg per day) to help prevent statin-induced rhabdomyolosis and muscle pain. A number of herbs and supplements have been shown to help reduce LDL cholesterol, elevate HDL cholesterol and lower triglycerides and other pro-inflammatory markers.

Herbs and Supplements for Hypercholesterolemia

Artichoke leaf (Cynara scolymus)
Is traditionally used as a cholagogue, antiemetic and bitter tonic. Several clinical trials show that it also modestly lowers cholesterol levels (Wilder, et al, 2004).
Dosage: Tincture (1:2 or 1:4 or 1:5): 1.5-3 ml TID
Tea: 1 tsp. dried herb, 8 oz. hot water, steep for 15-20 minutes, take up to 3 cups per day

Fish Oils
Omega 3 fatty acids, especially fish oils, have been found to lower LDL and triglycerid levels as well as improve HDL levels. Fish oils with plant sterols had a synergistic effect better than either supplement by itself (Micallef and Garg, 2008).
Dose: 4-6 g per day

Gum Guggul gum resin (Commiphora mukul)
There are both positive and negative studies on the use of Gum Guggul for lowering cholesterol. One study (Singh, et al, 1994) found that 50 mg of a standardized Guggul product (Guggulipid) reduced total cholesterol 11.7%, LDL cholesterol 12.5%, and triglycerides 12%. A study published in 2003 in JAMA found no cholesterol lowering activity at all. A third study (Nohr, et al, 2009) found Guggul lowered total cholesterol but did not alter LDL levels or triglycerides.
Dosage: Tincture (1:4 or 1:5): 1-2 ml TID
Capsules: 1-2 capsules BID

Niacin
Is also known as B3 or nicotinic acid. It is an essential nutrient and part of the B-complex family of vitamins. Niacin is especially interesting because it not only lowers VLDL cholesterol levels and triglycerides; it increases protective HDL cholesterol levels. In human trials, Niacin also decreased lipoprotein-associated phospholipase A2 and C-reactive protein levels, both of which are pro-inflammatory, suggesting an atheroprotective effect (Kuvin, et al, 2006). There are several issues with Niacin. One is flushing that can occur in sensitive people. Secondly, it has been linked to liver damage in higher doses and can exacerbate gout and diabetes.
Dosage: 2000 mg a day of extended release Niacin. Do not use with pregnant women.

Plant Sterols/Stanols

Regular intake of plant sterols and/or stanols in fortified foods (yogurt, mayonnaise, butter-like spreads or salad dressings) or as supplements lowers LDL cholesterol levels in people with elevated levels (Abumweis, et al, 2008).
Dosage: 2 g daily

Polyphenols
Are antioxidant and anti-inflammatory and are found in abundance in many plants. Several studies show that plants rich in polyphenols can reduce cholesterol levels. Insoluble carob fiber, rich in polyphenols (4g BID) reduced total cholesterol (17.8%), LDL cholesterol (22.5%), and triglycerides (16.3%) (Ruiz-Roso, et al, 2010). Various human studies utilizing apple polyphenols (Nagasako-Akazome, et al, 2007), tomato polyphenols (Shen, et al, 2007), cocoa powder (Baba, et al, 2007), grape polyphenols (Zern, et al, 2005), dark chocolate (Mursu, et al, 2004), and kiwi fruit (Duttaroy, et al, 2004) were able to reduce total and LDL cholesterol levels. Fresh tomato juice (also rich in lycopene) also lowered triglycerides (as did kiwi fruit) and raised HDL cholesterol.
Cocoa powder inhibited LDL oxidation, decreased ApoB and also increased HDL cholesterol (as did dark chocolate). Other polyphenol-rich foods and herbs (turmeric, beets, green tea, coffee, rosemary, blueberries, and amla fruit) and supplements (pine bark, grape seed extract) are likely to also have benefits for improving blood lipid profiles, as well as reducing cardiovascular risk factors.

Red Yeast Rice
Is a natural source of statins. In human studies it was comparable to pharmaceutical statins for reducing LDL cholesterol levels (Halbert, et al, 2010) and was better tolerated by people who cannot take statins due to statin-associated myalgia (SAM).
In another study (Zhao, et al, 2008), Red Yeast Rice also reduced post-prandial triglyceridemia. Many red yeast rice products are contaminated with a possible mycotoxin, citrinin. Be sure to use products that are tested and guaranteed to be citrinin free.
Dosage: 600 mg BID (when I recommend this I often use lower doses – 600 mg every other day, and in most cases it is still effective)

Soluble fiber
Various soluble fibers including Oats (Avena sativa) (Robitaille, et al, 2005), Psyllium seed (Plantago psyllium) (Wei, et al, 2009), Chia seed (Salvia hispanica), Fenugreek seed (Trigonella foenum-graecum), Barley (Hordeum vulgare), Guar gum (Yamopsis tetragonoloba), flax seed (Linum usitatissimum) (Bloeden, et al, 2008), carrots (Daucus carota), beans (Bazzano, et al, 2009), lentils, chickpeas, and prune juice have been found to mildly reduce total cholesterol and LDL cholesterol levels.

Walnuts (Juglans regia)
In a human trial, 21 men and women with elevated cholesterol levels were placed on either a Mediterranean diet or one in which walnuts replaced 32% of their monosaturated fats for 4 weeks. People on the walnut diet had significantly reduced total and LDL cholesterol levels and improved endothelium-dependent vasodilation (Ros, et al, 2004). A similar study using almonds also found that they reduced cholesterol levels as well as improving glycemic control (Li, et al, 2010). Other nuts such as pistachios, pecans, filberts, and Brazil nuts probably have similar effects.

Yerba Mate leaf (Ilex paraguariensis)
Is used daily as a beverage throughout South America and has become more popular in the U.S. as well. In a human trial, people with normal cholesterol, abnormal blood lipids, and those with elevated cholesterol and taking statins were given Mate. All groups had improved lipid parameters including reduced LDL levels, elevated HDL levels and lowered Apolipoprotein B (deMorais, et al, 2009)
Dose: Tea: 2-3 cups per day

References available in the downloadable version of this book, for purchase at www.botanicalmedicine.org

Botanicals for Aromatase Excess Syndrome
– Reducing Estrogen Dominance in Men and Women for Optimizing Reproductive Health and Reducing Disease Risk

Presented by:

Donald R. Yance Jr., MH, CN, RH (AHG), SFO
Clinical Master Herbalist and Certified Nutritionist
Founder, Mederi Centre for Natural Healing
Founder and Formulator, Natura Health Products

THE ECLECTIC TRIPHASIC MEDICAL SYSTEM (ETMS)

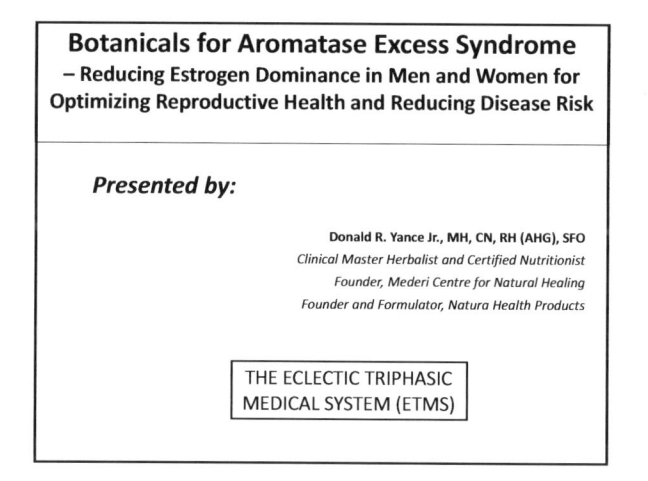

The Aromatase Enzyme

- Breaks the bonds on testosterone and creates estrogen.
- In postmenopausal women (and men), most estrogen is biosynthesized from cholesterol.
- This process takes place in various tissues, including normal breast tissue, and breast tumor tissue. Aromatase catalyzes the conversion of testosterone to estradiol in many tissues including the adrenal glands, ovaries, placenta, testicles, adipose (fat) tissue, and brain.
- There is also evidence that aromatase is involved in the production of DHT, which is well known for its negative effects on the prostate and male pattern baldness.

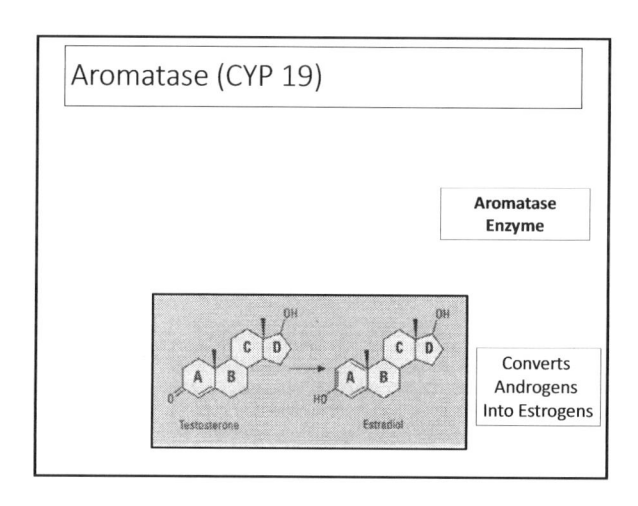

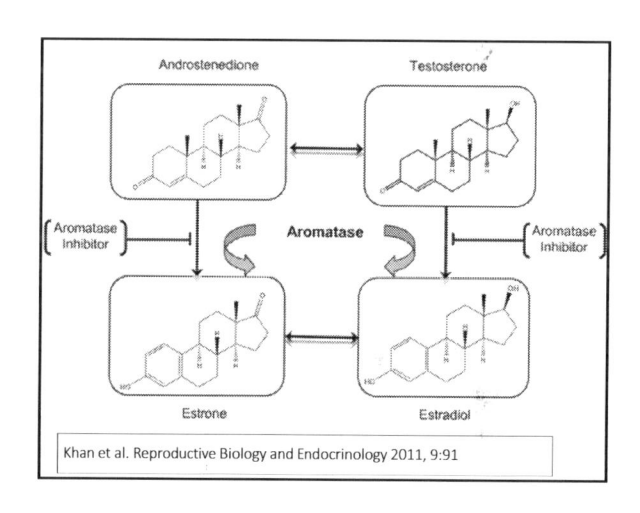

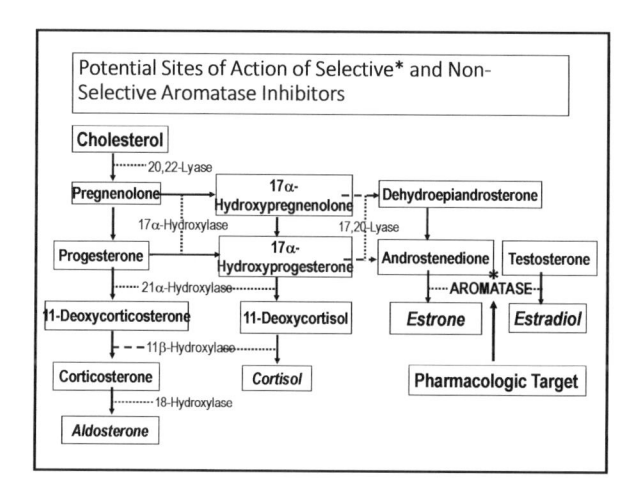

Aromatase (CYP 19)

Aromatase Enzyme

Converts Androgens Into Estrogens

Khan et al. Reproductive Biology and Endocrinology 2011, 9:91

Potential Sites of Action of Selective* and Non-Selective Aromatase Inhibitors

Cholesterol → (20,22-Lyase) → Pregnenolone → (17α-Hydroxylase) → 17α-Hydroxypregnenolone → (17,20-Lyase) → Dehydroepiandrosterone

Pregnenolone → Progesterone → (17α-Hydroxylase) → 17α-Hydroxyprogesterone → Androstenedione → Testosterone

Progesterone → (21α-Hydroxylase) → 11-Deoxycorticosterone

17α-Hydroxyprogesterone → 11-Deoxycortisol

AROMATASE → Estrone, Estradiol

11-Deoxycorticosterone → (11β-Hydroxylase) → Corticosterone → (18-Hydroxylase) → Aldosterone

11-Deoxycortisol → Cortisol

Pharmacologic Target

Diseases/conditions associated with over-active aromatase & excess estrogen

Female	Male
• **Breast and other HR+ cancers**	• Hypogonadism
• Benign tumors (breast, uterine fibroids)	• Gynecomastia
• Endometriosis	• Andropause
• Loss of muscle mass and gain of body fat	• Prostate problems
• Dense breasts	• Prostate Cancer
• Trauma	• Loss of muscle mass and gain of body fat
• Long-term Stress	• Trauma
	• Long-term Stress

Estradiol

- Is the most potent estrogen produced in the body.
- In post-menopausal women and in men, it is synthesized from testosterone or estrone via aromatase or 17β-hydroxysteroid dehydrogenase, respectively.
- In breast and other ER+ cancers, is a distinct aromatase promoter, leading to a marked increase in aromatase expression in tumors and adipose (breast) tissue adjacent to a tumor, and a consequential local overproduction of estrogen that promotes growth and progression of cancer.
- **Aromatase inhibitors (AIs) are now the treatment of choice for postmenopausal estrogen receptor-positive breast cancer.**

Anticancer Agents Med Chem. 2008 Aug; 8(6): 646–682.

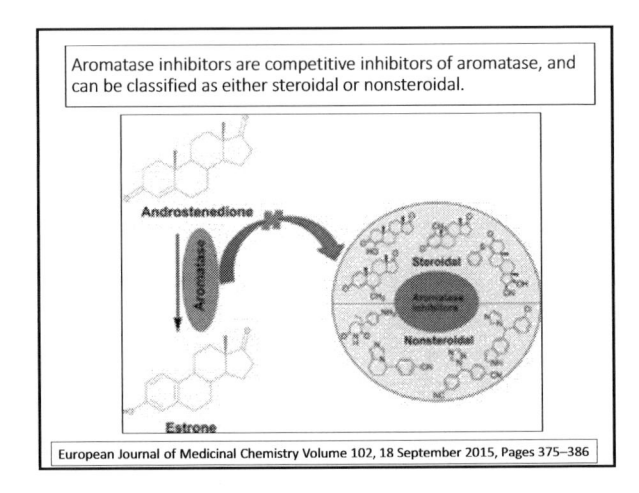

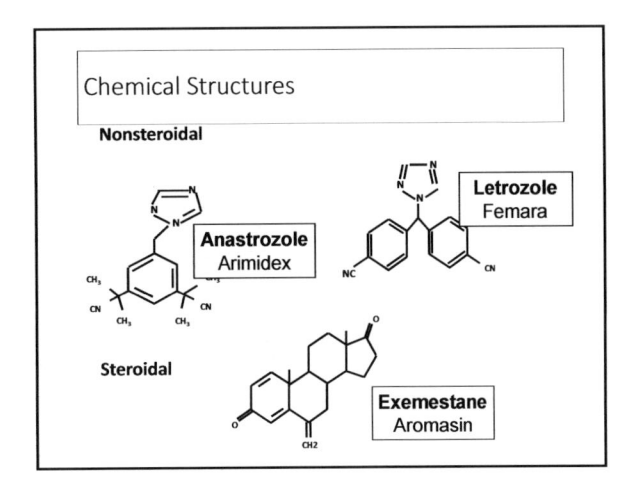

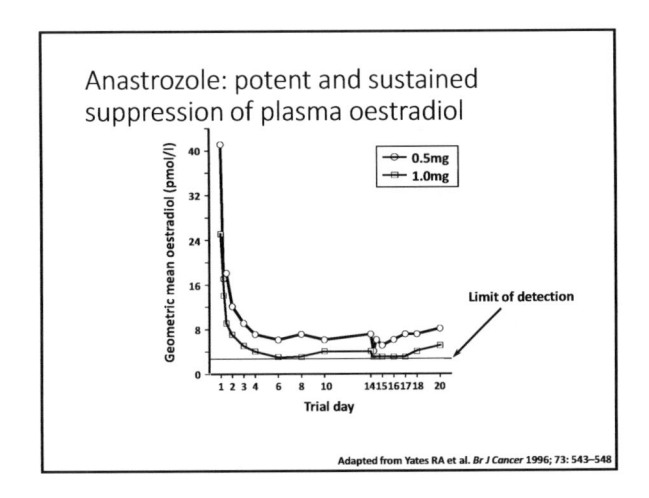

Aromatase inhibitors are competitive inhibitors of aromatase, and can be classified as either steroidal or nonsteroidal.

European Journal of Medicinal Chemistry Volume 102, 18 September 2015, Pages 375–386

Chemical Structures

Nonsteroidal
- Anastrozole — Arimidex
- Letrozole — Femara

Steroidal
- Exemestane — Aromasin

Anastrozole: potent and sustained suppression of plasma oestradiol

Adapted from Yates RA et al. *Br J Cancer* 1996; 73: 543–548

Clinical Pharmacology

	Anastrozole	Letrozole	Exemestane
Daily clinical dose	1 mg od	2.5 mg od	25 mg od
Monthly dose	30 mg	75 mg	750 mg
Time to steady state plasma levels	7 days	14-42 days	4 days
Half-life	48–50 hours	2–4 days	24 hours
Time to maximal E_2 suppression	3–4 days	2–3 days	7 days
Intratumoral activity	Yes	Yes	No data

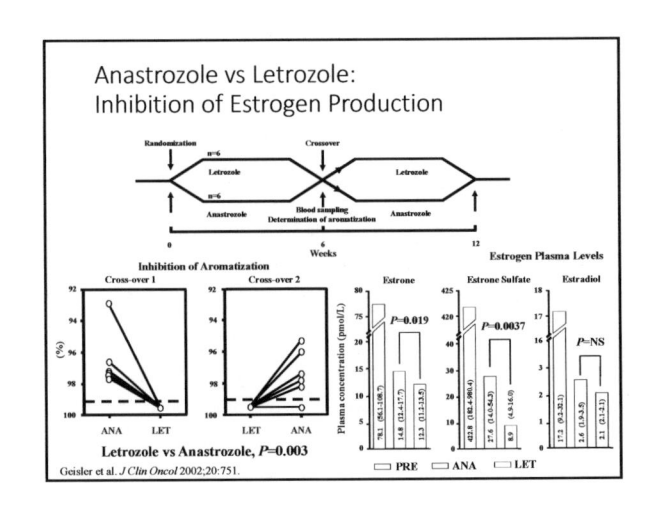

Anastrozole vs Letrozole: Inhibition of Estrogen Production

Letrozole vs Anastrozole, $P=0.003$

Geisler et al. *J Clin Oncol* 2002;20:751.

Phase II Trial of Exemestane and Tamoxifen : Peer-Reviewed Tumor Response and Time to Tumor Progression

	EXE (n=56) n	EXE %	TAM (n=56) n	TAM %
Complete response	5	8.9	1	1.8
Partial response	20	35.7	7	12.5
Objective response rate (95% confidence interval)	25	44.6 (38.2-51)	8	14.3 (9.7-18.9)
Clinical benefit (CR + PR + NC ≥6 months)	31	55.3	22	39.3
Median TTP*, months		8.9		5.2

*Based on 63 patients

Letrozole vs Anastrozole: Time Events

	ITT Population Letrozole (n=356)	ITT Population Anastrozole (n=357)	P value
Median TTP (mo) 90% CI	5.7 5.1-6.0	5.7 4.6-6.1	0.920
Median TTF (mo) 90% CI	5.6 4.4-5.8	5.6 4.0-6.0	0.761
Median OS (mo) 90% CI	22.0 19.6-24.6	20.3 18.0-23.1	0.624

Letrozole vs Anastrozole: Response Rate

Letrozole 19.1% (CR 6.7%, PR 12.4%), n=356
Anastrozole 12.3% (CR 3.6%, PR 8.7%), n=357
P=0.013

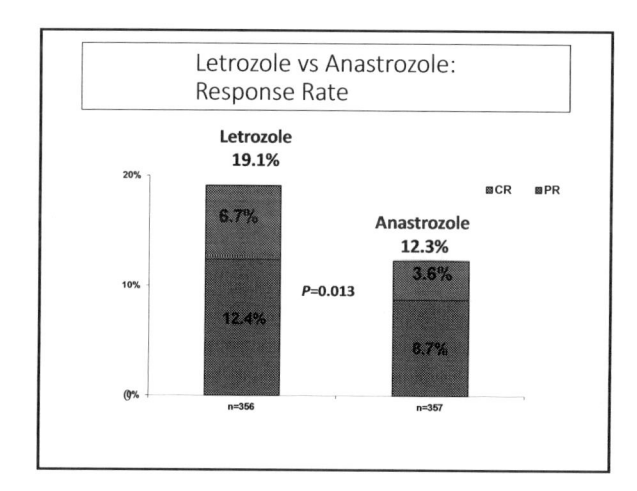

Serum E2 levels as a biomarker for Aromatase Inhibition

- Circulating estrogen levels have been shown to correlate with the expression of classically estrogen responsive genes in ER+ breast tumors, suggesting that E2 (estradiol) measurements may prove to be a valuable marker for endocrine sensitivity and for refining individualized treatment regimes.
- Nine prospective case-control studies conducted between 1990 and 2000 accrued evidence for this relationship between plasma estrogens and risk.

J Clin Oncol. 2014 May 10;32(14):1396-400; Brest Cancer Res Treat 138:157-165, 2013; Breast Cancer Res Treat. 2014 Jan;143(1):69-80.

Aromatase and Breast Cancer

- Targeting aromatase has proven beneficial in treating breast cancer since aromatase inhibitors are the most effective endocrine treatment of breast cancer to date.
- However, aromatase inhibitors cause major side effects such as bone loss, joint pain, weight gain, and abnormal lipid metabolism.

Cancer Lett. 2008 Jul 7.

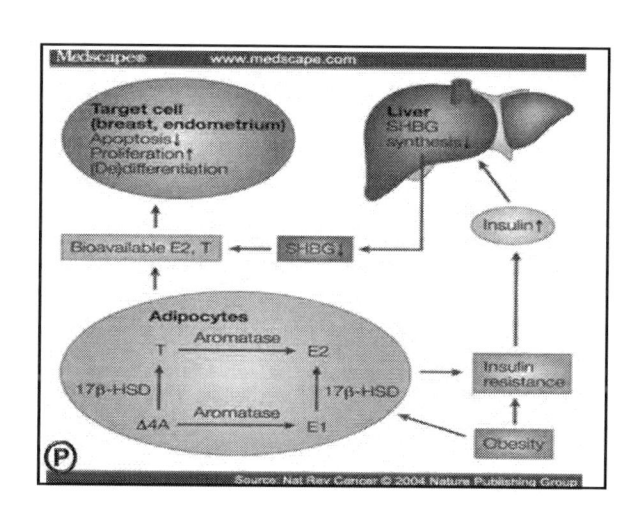

AI Resistance

- Even with the improved efficacy of AIs or other endocrine therapies, postmenopausal breast cancer patients eventually develop resistance to AIs causing relapse of the disease.
- Generally, resistance involves tumor regrowth after 12–18 months of treatment and stable disease.
- Several mechanisms are thought to be involved in resistance to synthetic AIs including circumventing normal cellular pathways, enhancing sensitivity to existing estrogens, and/or redistributing estrogen receptors to extra-nuclear sites.

Carol A Lange and Douglas Yee, Killing the second messenger, Endocr Relat Cancer. 2011 August; 18(4): C19–C24; Thangavel C, Dean JL, Ertel A, Knudsen KE, Aldaz CM, Witkiewicz AK, Clarke R, Knudsen ES. Therapeutically activating RB, Endocr Relat Cancer. 2011 Apr 28;18(3):333-45.

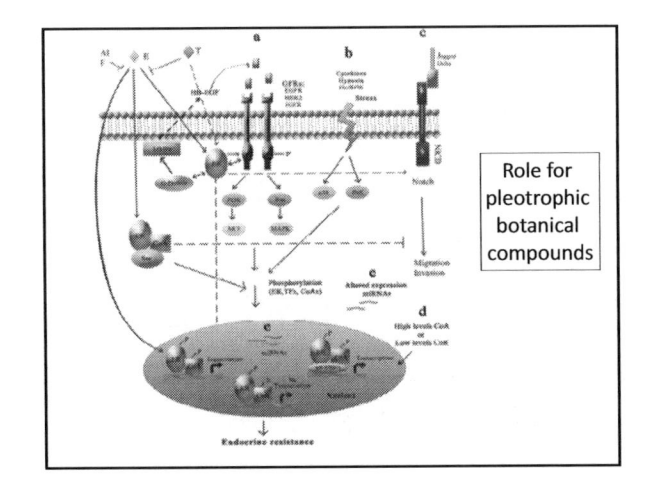

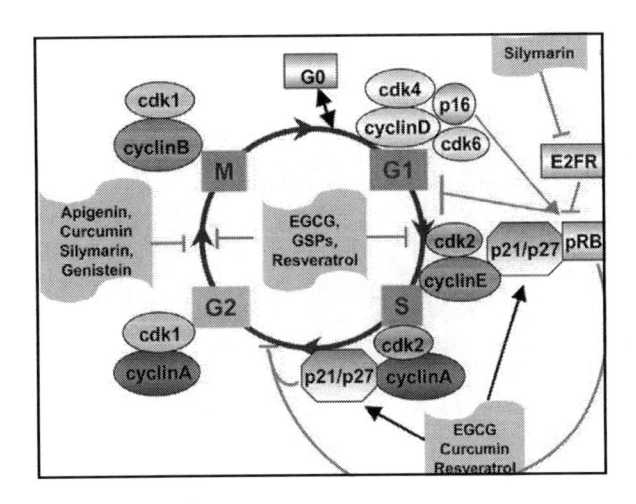

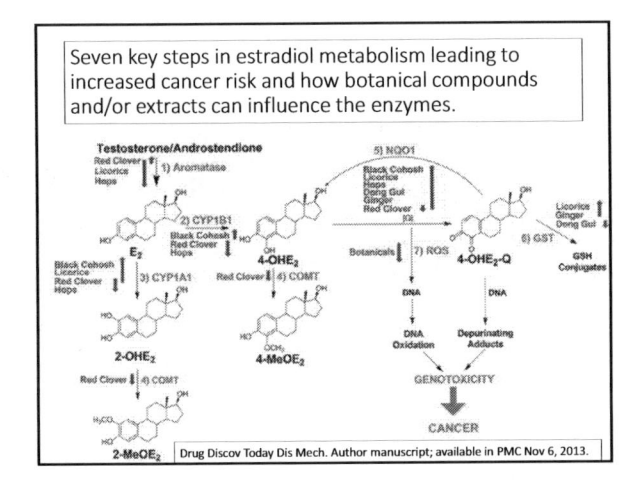

Role for pleotrophic botanical compounds

Seven key steps in estradiol metabolism leading to increased cancer risk and how botanical compounds and/or extracts can influence the enzymes.

Drug Discov Today Dis Mech. Author manuscript; available in PMC Nov 6, 2013.

Letrozole Synergistic with Curcumin in the Inhibition of Xenografted Endometrial Carcinoma Growth

- Letrozole enhanced the expression of Bax and cytochrome c release and suppressed the expression of estrogen receptor in tumor cells.
- Treatment with curcumin inhibited the expression of Bcl-2 in tumor cells at the mRNA and protein levels.
- Tumor cell apoptosis was observed in mice treated with either letrozole or curcumin; however, combination of letrozole and curcumin further enhanced the inhibitory rate in tumor growth.

Liang YJ, Hao Q, Wu YZ, Wang QL, Wang JD, Hu YL., Int J Gynecol Cancer. 2009 Oct;19(7):1248-52. doi: 10.1111/IGC.0b013e3181b33d76.

Major Hormones Involved in Age-Related Decline

- Testosterone
- Dehydroepiandrosterone (DHEA)
- Estrogens and Progesterone
- Growth hormone (GH)
- Thyroid stimulating hormone (TSH)
- Insulin, and IGF1 & II
- Melatonin
- Vitamin D (a hormone-vitamin)

Blood testing

- Serum Estradiol
- Estrone Sulfate
- Testosterone
  - total, free, and DHT
- DHEA Sulfate
- SHBG

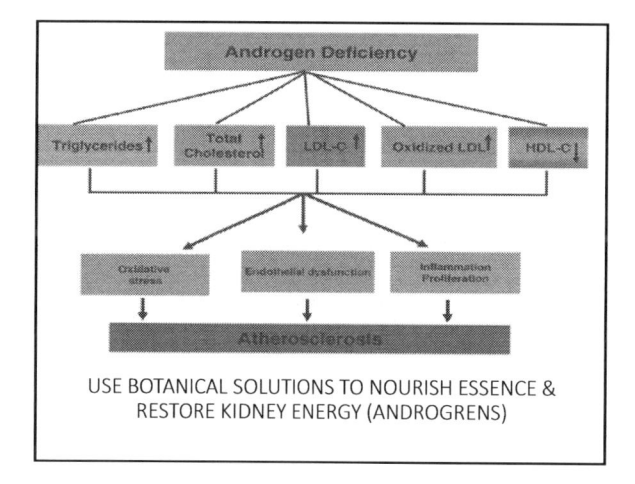

USE BOTANICAL SOLUTIONS TO NOURISH ESSENCE & RESTORE KIDNEY ENERGY (ANDROGRENS)

Testosterone (TES)

- Low serum TES, in elderly men, is a strong risk factor to CVD, a lack of QoL, and shortened lifespan. J Med Invest. 2003 Aug; 50(3-4): 162-9, Int Braz J Urol. 2008; 34: 302-12, International Journal of Cardiology, doi:10.1016/j.ijcard.2009.10.033
- Serum Estradiol is an Independent Predictor of Progression of Carotid Artery Intima-Media Thickness in Middle-Aged Men, J Clin Endocrinol Metab. 2006 Aug 29 and stroke in elderly men. Neurology. 2007 Feb 20;68(8):563-8.

Testosterone (continued)

- TES has protective effect against all CV-related diseases including: hypertension, diabetes, obesity, cardiomyopathy. CHF, J Endocrinol. 2003 Sep; 178(3): 373-80, J Med Invest. 2003 Aug; 50(3-4): 162-9.
- Low serum sex hormone-binding globulin (SHBG), is independently associated with abdominal obesity and insulin resistance in elderly men and women. Metabolism. 2007 Oct;56(10):1356-62.
- Lower total TES is associated with insulin resistance independently of measures of central obesity. Eur J Endocrinol. 2009 Oct;161(4):591-8. Epub 2009 Aug 6.

Testosterone (continued)

- Low serum TES levels are a risk factor for diabetes, metabolic syndrome, inflammation and dyslipidemia. Int J Impot Res. 2009 Jul-Aug;21(4):261-4. Epub 2009 Jun 18.
- Extremes of endogenous TES are associated with increased risk of incidence of coronary events in older women.
- An optimal range of TES may exist for cardiovascular health in women, with increased risk of CHD events at low levels of TES overall and at high levels of the bioavailable fraction of TES. J Clin Endocrinol Metab. 2009 Nov 24
- A high level of E(2)/T ratio has shown to be strongly associated with cardiovascular risk factors in postmenopausal women with CHD. Cardiology. 2012 May 5;121(4):249-254.

Prevalence of Abdominal Aortic Aneurysm (AAA) in Older Men

- AAA is associated with mortality in older adults, and increasing aortic diameter predicts incidence of cardiovascular events.
- Lower free TES and higher LH levels are independently associated with AAA in older men. Impaired gonadal function may be involved in arterial dilatation as well as occlusive vascular disease in older men. J Clin Endocrinol Metab. 2010 Jan 8.

Testosterone and Insulin Resistance in Men

- Relationship Between Testosterone Levels, Insulin Sensitivity, and Mitochondrial dysfunction.
- Hypogonadism can cause insulin resistance via dysregulation of fatty acid metabolism and low TES levels may represent an additional environmental factor contributing to decreased expression of genes involved in oxidative metabolism.

Diabetes Care July 2005 vol. 28, Clin Endocrinol. 2005;63(3):239-250, Eur J Endocrinol. 2006 Jun;154(6):899-906

Aromatase and 5-aReductase co-contribute to androgen deficiency, prostate diseases and other male health issues

17-Hydroxyprogesterone → DHEA → Androstenedione →[Aromatase]→ Estraone

↑↓

Testosterone → Estradiol

[5-a Reductase] ↓

DHT

Androgen Independence in Prostate Cancer (PC) Risk and Progression

- Two male reproductive hormonal changes that contribute to increased PC risk with age, and promote existing PC growth, are:
  - **Dihydrotestosterone** (DHT) - promotes prostate-cell proliferation and suppresses apoptosis, blocking the programmed cell-death process; plays a role in the development of both normal and malignant PC
  - **Estrogens** via conversion through aromatase

Increase in Aromatase Leads to Higher Levels of Estradiol

- High levels of estradiol can suppress the expression of GLUT-4, leading to insulin insensitivity.
- Morbidly obese infertile man, treated with an AI (anastrozole) showed a normalization of the pituitary-testis axis, spermatogenesis and fertility; as well as a significant reduction in body fat.

Obesity in men: the hypogonadal-estrogen receptor relationship and its effect on glucose homeostasis. Cohen PG Med Hypotheses. 2008; 70(2):358-60; Roth MY, Amory JK, Page ST. Treatment of male infertility secondary to morbid obesity. Nat Clin Pract Endocrinol Metab. 2008;4:415–419.

Aromatase and Prostate Cancer

- Paradoxically, the incidence of prostate disease increases with age when serum androgen levels are in decline and emerging evidence suggests that estrogens may also be important in the normal prostate, as well as in the etiology of prostate disease.
- Aromatase expression and activity has been reported in prostate tumor tissues and cells, implying that androgen aromatization to estrogens may play a role in prostate carcinogenesis or tumor progression.
- Accumulating evidence indicates that prostate cancer stem cells lack the androgen receptor and are, indeed, resistant to androgen deprivation therapy.
- In contrast, these cells express classical (α and/or β) estrogen receptors, which represent a new target in prostate cancer treatment.

Minerva Endocrinol. 2006 Mar;31(1):1-12; J Cell Biochem. 2007 Nov 1;102(4):899-911; Oncotarget. 2015 Oct 24. doi: 10.18632/oncotarget.6220.

Model of Androgen Action in Target Cells

Oncotarget. 2015 Oct 24. doi: 10.18632/oncotarget.6220.

Function of AR and ERs in Prostate cancer (PC) epithelial cells and prostate Stem cells (SCs)
The role of estradiol/ER axis in PC and prostate CSCs is undeniable

Oncotarget. 2015 Oct 24. doi: 10.18632/oncotarget.6220.

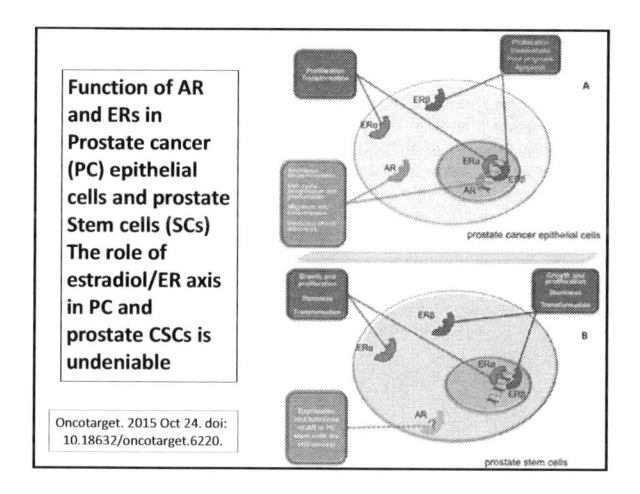

Convergence of Hormones, Inflammation, Blood stagnation, and Energy-Related Factors: Pathways of Cancer Etiology

- Inflammatory processes; hormones such as estrogen, androgen, and insulin; and energy-related factors together contribute to cancer.
- Critical genes involved, such as PTEN, and p53, are tumor suppressor genes and are often mutated.
- These and other genes are vulnerable to inactivation by reactive oxygen species, especially chemically reactive lipid mediators of inflammation and redox stress.

Cancer Prev Res (Phila). 2009 November; 2(11): 922–930..

Association of aromatase and the relationship between obesity and decreased sperm concentration.

- Obesity in men is associated with low sperm count.
- Men with high aromatase exhibit increased E(2) with increased weight.
- A decrease in testosterone: E(2) ratio with increasing BMI is more pronounced in men with high versus low aromatase.

Hum Reprod. 2010 Sep 29.

Testosterone (TES)

- Never use hormone replacement therapy

  Instead

- Use Natural compounds to reduce aromatase, thus preventing conversion to ER
- Use natural alternatives to assist in the natural production of testosterone
  - Plant extracts
  - Life style

Hormone Replacement Therapy

Testosterone Therapy Linked With Adverse CVD Events

- The use of testosterone therapy in men is associated with an increased risk of death, MI, or ischemic stroke.
- According to a study published in the November 6, 2013 issue of the Journal of the American Medical Association, the use of testosterone therapy was associated with a 29% increased risk of death, MI, or ischemic stroke (p=0.02), and this risk was unchanged after adjustment for the presence of coronary artery disease.
- Why?

JAMA 2013; 310:1829-1835; JAMA 2013; 310:1805-1806.

Paradoxical Effects of Androgens in Prostate Cancer (PC)

- Testosterone levels decrease with age and elderly men are usually androgen deficient; yet PC increases with age, also low free testosterone levels in serum are associated with aggressive PC.
- Patients with newly diagnosed, untreated PC yielded significantly higher cortisol levels compared to those without PC.
- Many herbs, such as Epimedium, Pygium, Serenoa (Saw palmetto), Urtica (Nettles root) and Panax ginseng, known as "male tonic" herbs, have demonstrated inhibitory effects on PC.

Mechanism of Action: 5-alpha Reductase Inhibitor

- 5-alpha reductase inhibitor converts testosterone to DHT
- DHT causes an increase in cell proliferation of the prostate, thus enlarging the gland
- Less conversion to DHT means less blood DHT and a decrease in cell proliferation
- Other drugs: Finasteride and Dutasteride

Aromatase inhibitors (AIs) in Male Reproductive Health

- Estrogen excess in turn has been associated with premature closure of the epiphyses, gynecomastia and low gonadotropin and testosterone levels.
- Lowering estrogen levels in men has emerged, consequently, as a potential treatment for a number of disorders including pubertas praecox, the andropause and gynecomastia.

Nat Clin Pract Endocrinol Metab 2007, 3:414-421.; Reprod Biol Endocrinol. 2011 Jun 21;9:93.

Aromatase inhibitors (AIs) in Male Reproductive Health (Continued...)

- AIs have been used in the treatment of idiopathic short stature, and constitutional delay of puberty in boys to increase adult height.
- AIs have been used in the management of gynecomastia, oligospermia and male hypogonadism related to obesity and aging.
- AIs have shown to improve testosterone levels in adult men.

Indian J Endocrinol Metab. 2013 Oct; 17(Suppl1): S259–S261; Reprod Biol Endocrinol. 2011 Jun 21;9:93.

Aromatase Inhibitors in Men: Effects and Therapeutic Options

- AIs are an attractive alternative for traditional testosterone substitution in elderly men.
- Natural compounds that down-regulate aromatase together with herbs that restore Kidney 'yang' Essence are an effective solution to managing this common age-related event in men (and woman).

Reprod Biol Endocrinol. 2011; 9: 93. Online 2011 Jun 21. doi: 10.1186/1477-7827-9-93

Aromatase Inhibitors and ER+ Cancer

- **Aromatase inhibitors** (AIs) have proven to be more effective than Tamoxifen in treating ER+ breast cancer.
- However, AIs cause major side effects such as bone loss, joint pain, weight gain, and abnormal lipid metabolism.
- BMI affects AI dosage and response. Low BMI = poor response.
- Combining an AI with Metformin, an **insulin sensitizer**, is more effective than an AI alone at inhibiting breast cancer recurrence.
- Also, combining an AI with a **mTOR**, **COX-2**, and/or **HDAC** inhibitor can be much more effective than AI alone. ← Herbs

Cancer Chemother Pharmacol. 2012 Sep 28., Cancer Lett. 2008 Jul 7. WWW.SCIENCEDAILY.COM /RELEASES/2011/12/111207201747.HTM, ENDOCRINE-RELATED CANCER (2006) 13 863–873, ANN ONCOL. 2009 MAR 2, CANCER RES. 2011 MAR 1;71(5):1893-903. EPUB 2011 JAN 18, J Clin Oncol 28:3411-3415. © 2010 by American Society of Clinical Oncology, The Breast 21 (2012) 40e45

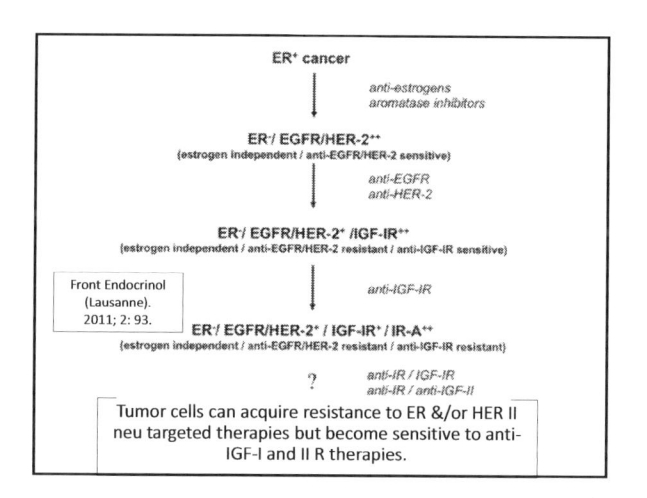

ER⁺ cancer

ER⁺ cancer
↓ anti-estrogens / aromatase inhibitors
ER⁻/ EGFR/HER-2⁺⁺
(estrogen independent / anti-EGFR/HER-2 sensitive)
↓ anti-EGFR / anti-HER-2
ER⁻/ EGFR/HER-2⁺ /IGF-IR⁺⁺
(estrogen independent / anti-EGFR/HER-2 resistant / anti-IGF-IR sensitive)
↓ anti-IGF-IR
ER⁻/ EGFR/HER-2⁺ / IGF-IR⁺ / IR-A⁺⁺
(estrogen independent / anti-EGFR/HER-2 resistant / anti-IGF-IR resistant)
↓ ? anti-IR / IGF-IR / anti-IGF-II

Front Endocrinol (Lausanne). 2011; 2: 93.

Tumor cells can acquire resistance to ER &/or HER II neu targeted therapies but become sensitive to anti-IGF-I and II R therapies.

Risks versus Benefits in the Clinical Application of Aromatase Inhibitors

- Aromatase inhibitors have non-specific toxic side effects including (but not limited to): **arthralgia** (joint discomfort), asthenia, headache, nausea, peripheral edema, fatigue, vomiting and dyspepsia.
- In addition, certain endocrinological side effects in postmenopausal women are notable, namely hot flushes and vaginal dryness.
- Long-term risk: Osteoporosis, heart disease

Ann Oncol (2013) doi: 10.1093/annonc/mdt037;
Endocrine-Related Cancer (1999) 6 325-332

Arthralgia incidence among large adjuvant trials, comparing ATAC [3], ITA [49], IES [5], BIG 1-98 [4], MA-17 [50], MAP.3 [51].

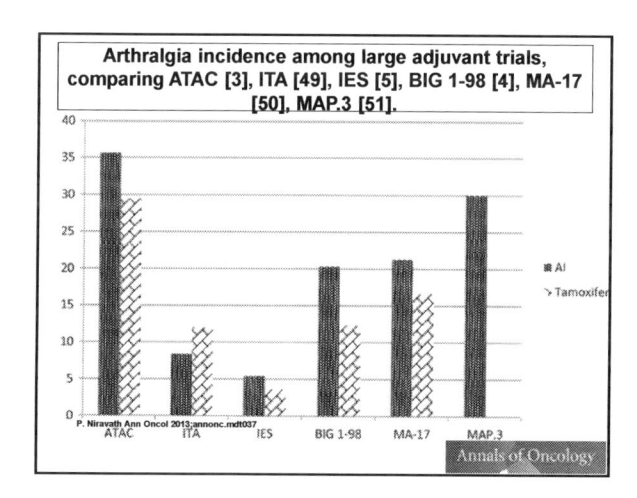

(bar chart: AI vs Tamoxifen across ATAC, ITA, IES, BIG 1-98, MA-17, MAP.3)

P. Niravath Ann Oncol 2013;annonc.mdt037

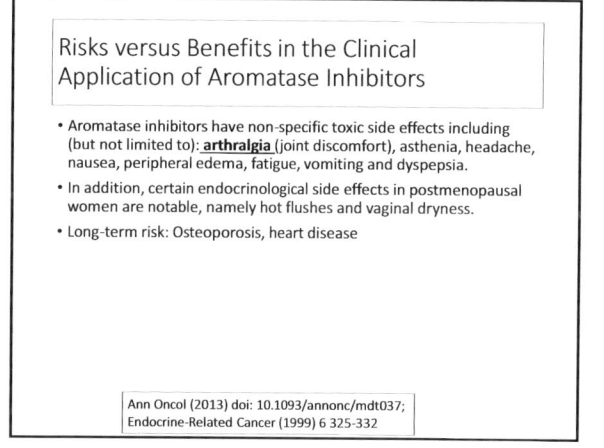

Compliance with AI therapy over time

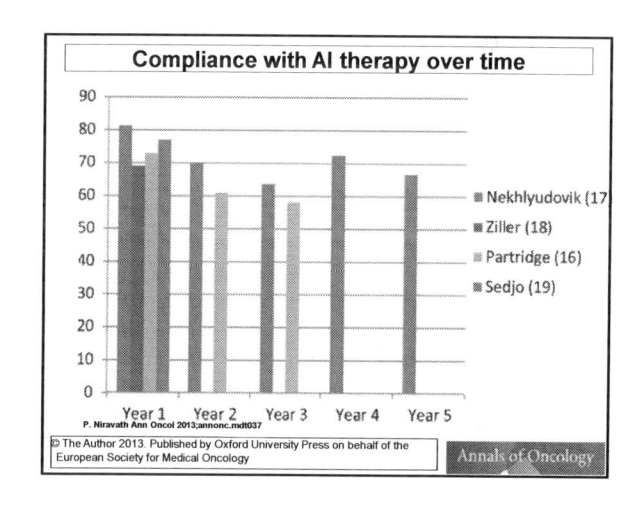

(bar chart comparing Nekhlyudovik (17), Ziller (18), Partridge (16), Sedjo (19) across Year 1–Year 5)

P. Niravath Ann Oncol 2013;annonc.mdt037
© The Author 2013. Published by Oxford University Press on behalf of the European Society for Medical Oncology

Decreased Recurrence with Arthralgia while on Anastrazole or Tamoxifen

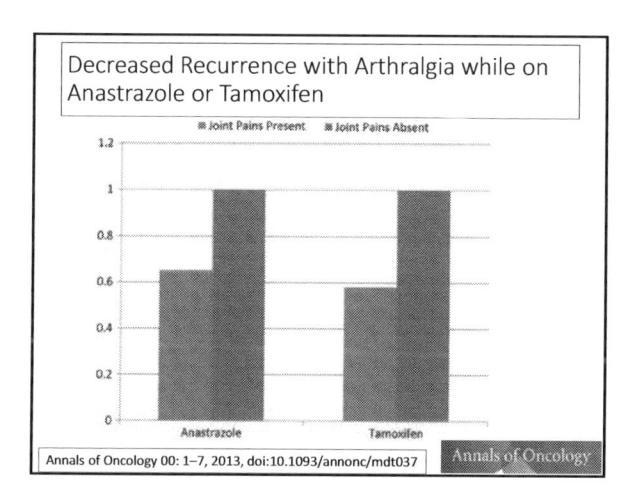

(bar chart: Joint Pains Present vs Joint Pains Absent for Anastrazole and Tamoxifen)

Annals of Oncology 00: 1–7, 2013, doi:10.1093/annonc/mdt037

Natural Aromatase Inhibitors/Modulators

- Lignans and flavonoids are naturally-occurring diphenolic compounds found in high concentrations in whole grains, legumes, fruits, and vegetables.
  - **Chrysin**, Grape seed OPC, EGCG, RES, ellagic acid, luteolin, kaempferol, Ursolic acid and apigenin
- Medicinal and common mushrooms
- Isoflavones biochanin A, genistein, and coumestrol
- The lignan agent enterolactone (flax seeds)
- Coptis (Berberine), also ↓ EGFR, HER II, COX-2
- Insulin and Leptin-trophic compounds also reduce ER, via aromatase pathways

Herbal Compounds that Inhibit Aromatase & Suppress Cancer

Herbal Compound	Source & Reference
Chrysin	*Passiflora spp.*, Bee propolis Persson I. J. Steroid Biochem. Mol. Biol. 2000;74:357; Reprod Nutr Dev. 2005 Nov-Dec;45(6):709-20.
Ursolic acid	*Salvia off.* (Sage) European Journal of Medicinal Chemistry Volume 43, Issue 9 2008 1865 – 1877
Berberine	*Hydrastis canadensis* (Goldenseal), *Coptis*, *Berberis aquifolium* (Oregon grape) etc.
Resveratrol & grape polyphenols	*Vitis L. sp* Breast Cancer Res. Treat. 2001;67:133; Ann. N. Y. Acad. Sci. 2002;963:239; Cancer Res. 2003;63:8516;
White button mushrooms	*Agaricus bisporous* Cancer Res 2006; 66(24): 12026-34
Apigenin	Major compound in Chamomile/celery J Steroid Biochem Mol Biol. 2006 Sep 9
Isoliquiritigenin	Licorice (*Glycyrrhiza glabra* & other species) Int J can 2009, 124:1028-1036. Exp Biol Med. 2007

Herbal Compounds that Inhibit Aromatase & Suppress Cancer

Herbal Compound	Source & Reference
Ginkgo Standardized extract	*Ginkgo biloba* Phytother Res. 2013 Dec;27(12):1756-62.
Damiana extract	*Turnera diffusa* J Ethnopharmacol. 2008 Dec 8;120(3):387-93.
Hesperetin	Citrus flavonoid J Nutr Biochem. 2012 Oct;23(10):1230-7.
Biochanin A	Isoflavone in red clover (*Trifolium pratense*) Br J Nutr. 2007 Aug 29;:1-8.
Ellagic acid	Pomegranates (*Punica granatum*), also strawberries, walnuts, raspberries Breast Cancer Research & Treatment. 71(3):203-17, 2002 Feb.

Chrysin
from Passiflora spp. & Bee Propolis

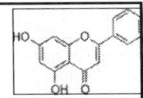

- Shows structural similarity to androgens
- Flavone-based aromatase inhibitors are of growing interest, and chrysin in particular provides a (natural) lead structure.
- Chrysin administered (1 mg/kg) to 2-year-old male rats for a period of 30 days lead to increased sperm count, greater fertilization potential, and greater litter size.
- Potent broad-spectrum anti-cancer effects

Nat Prod Commun. 2011 Jan;6(1):31-4; J Med Food. 2002 Spring;5(1):43-8; Kasala ER, Bodduluru LN, Barua CC. **Chrysin and its emerging antineoplastic effects.** Cancer Gene Ther. 2016 Jan;23(1):43.

Chrysin

- Significantly inhibits cancer and cancer related angiogenesis by decreasing the expression of:
  - Aromatase
  - HIF-1α (Hypoxia)
  - PG_2, COX-2, NF-kB
  - Histone deacetylase,
  - VEGF, IL-6 Inhibits Bcl-2, activates Bax
- Increases the expression of AMPK, p38, Bax, NK cells, p21/27, and Notch 1

The Journal of Steroid Biochemistry and Molecular Biology Vol. 107, Issues 1-2, Oct 2007, Pages 127-129; International Journal of Molecular Sciences, vol. 11, no. 5, pp. 2188–2199, 2010; J Nutr. 2006 Jun;136(6):1517-21, Toxicol Lett. 2012 Nov 27; J Agric Food Chem. 2012 Nov 28;60(47):11748-58; FEBS Lett. 2005 Jan 31;579(3):705-11; Biochem Biophys Res Commun. 2012 May 31; Int J Oncol. 2011 Feb;38(2):473-83; AANA J. 2008 Apr;76(2):113-7. Cancer. 2012 Sep 18; Anticancer Agents Med Chem. 2014;14(6):901-9.

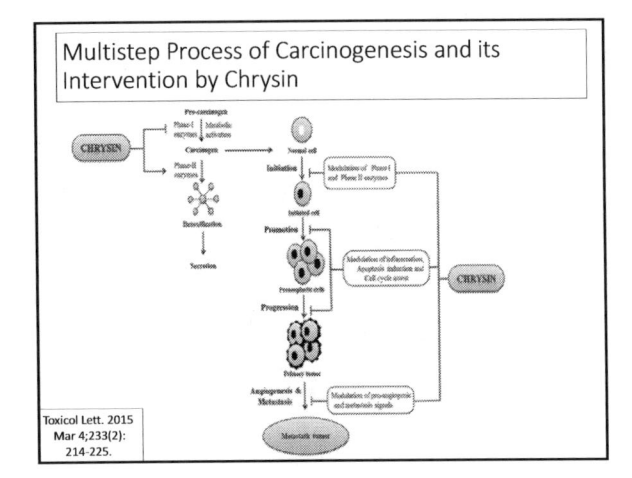

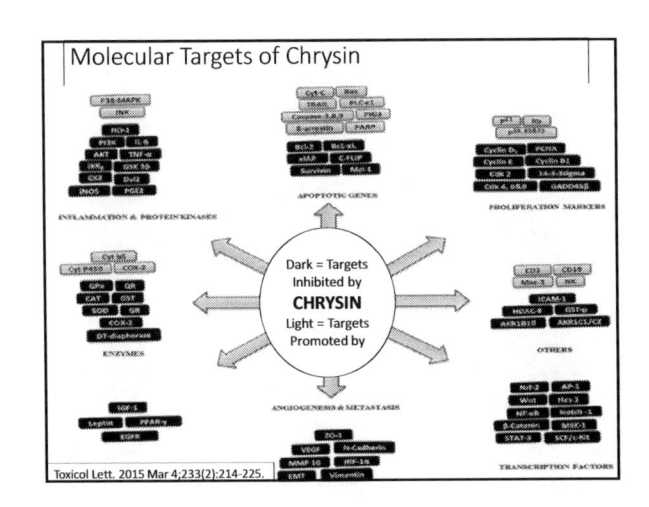

Multistep Process of Carcinogenesis and its Intervention by Chrysin

Toxicol Lett. 2015 Mar 4;233(2): 214-225.

Molecular Targets of Chrysin

Dark = Targets Inhibited by **CHRYSIN** Light = Targets Promoted by

Toxicol Lett. 2015 Mar 4;233(2):214-225.

Structures of Ursolic Acid and Its Isomer Oleanolic acid (pentacyclic triterpene), Apigenin (flavone) and Androstenedione (steroid), the Substrate of Aromatase.

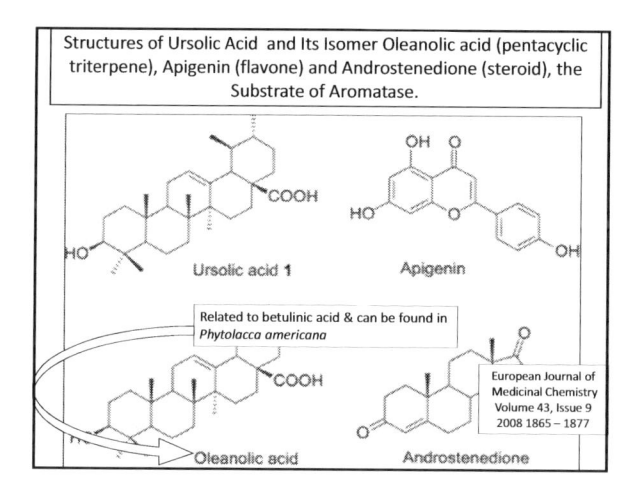

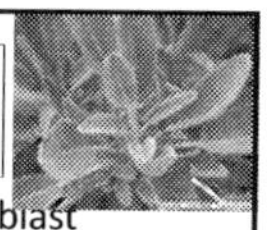

Ursolic acid 1
Apigenin
Related to betulinic acid & can be found in *Phytolacca americana*
Oleanolic acid
Androstenedione

European Journal of Medicinal Chemistry Volume 43, Issue 9 2008 1865–1877

Ursolic acid
Sage (*salvia off.*) powdered extract 75%

- Anabolic activity in the bone: Stimulating osteoblast differentiation *and inducing new bone* formation *in vivo* (Pharmacological Res, Vol 58, Iss 5-6, Nov.-Dec. 2008, Pages 290-296)
- Suppresses migration and invasion of human breast cancer via inhibition of: mTOR, MMP-9, u-PA, caspase-3 and PARP expression, NF-kB, LOX-5, and aromatase
- Activates (1) human dendritic cells via TLR2 and/or TLR4 and induces the production of IFN-gamma by CD4+ naïve T cells; (2) AMPK
- **100 mg/kg oral showed significant anticancer activity**

Mol Nutr Food Res. 2010 Mar 29, Zhongguo Zhong Yao Za Zhi. 2006 Jan;31(2):141-4; Eur J Pharmacol. 2010 Jun 28; 2011 Jul;46(7):2652-61. Epub 2011 Apr 3; Biochem Biophys Res Commun. 2012 Mar 23;419(4):741-7. Epub 2012 Feb 24

Potential of **ursolic acid** as a chemopreventive and anticancer compound

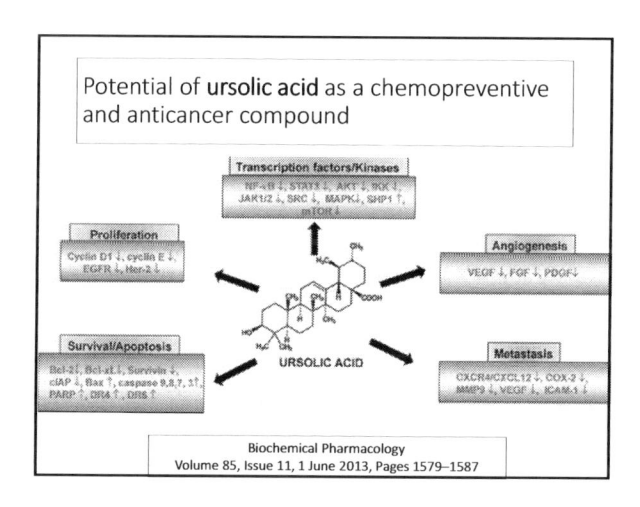

Transcription factors/Kinases: NF-κB ↓, STAT1 ↓, AKT ↓, SKt ↓, JAK1/2 ↓, SRC ↓, MAPK ↓, SHP1 ↑, mTOR ↓

Proliferation: Cyclin D1 ↓, cyclin E ↓, EGFR ↓, Her-2 ↓

Angiogenesis: VEGF ↓, FGF ↓, PDGF ↓

Survival/Apoptosis: Bcl-2 ↓, Bcl-xL ↓, Survivin ↓, cIAP ↓, Bax ↑, caspase 9,8,7, 3↑, PARP ↑, DR4 ↑, DR5 ↑

Metastasis: CXCR4/CXCL12 ↓, COX-2 ↓, MMP9 ↓, VEGF ↓, ICAM-1 ↓

URSOLIC ACID

Biochemical Pharmacology Volume 85, Issue 11, 1 June 2013, Pages 1579–1587

Evaluation of Ursolic acid on Aromatase inhibition

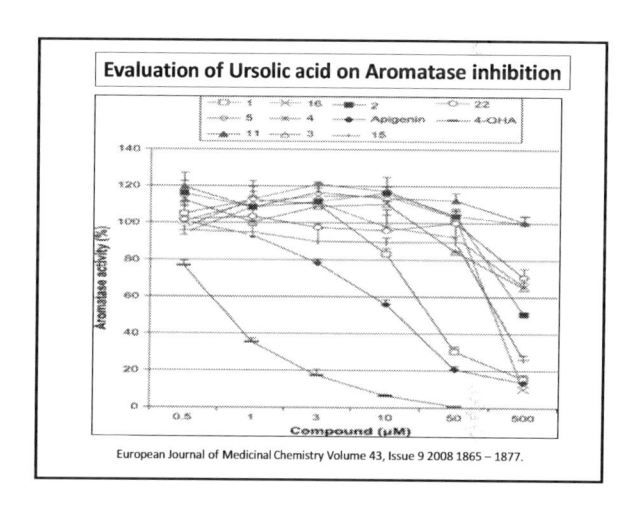

European Journal of Medicinal Chemistry Volume 43, Issue 9 2008 1865–1877.

Green tea (*Camellia sinensis*) extract

- Epigallocatechin gallate (EGCG) has been tested using an *in vivo* Swiss-Webster mouse model measuring ovarian aromatase activity and was found to inhibit aromatase activity by 56% at 25 and 12.5 mg/kg.
- Theaflavin and theaflavin-3,3'-gallate, both isolated from *Camellia sinensis* Kuntze (black tea), were found to strongly inhibit aromatase in microsomes

Kapiszewska M, Miskiewicz M, Ellison PT, Thune I, Jasienska G. Br. J. Nutr. 2006;95:989; Goodin MG, Rosengren RJ. Toxicol. Sci. 2003;76:262; Way TD, Lee HH, Kao MC, Lin JK. Eur. J. Cancer. 2004;40:2165.

Green Tea
Camellia sinensis

Drinking 3-5 cups per day has been reported to be associated with decreased numbers of axillary lymph node metastases in premenopausal women with stage I and II breast cancer and with increased expression of progesterone and estrogen receptors among postmenopausal women.

Zhang M, Holman CD, Huang JP, Xie X. Green tea and the prevention of breast cancer: a case-control study in southeast China. carcinogenesis. 2006 Dec 20. Nagata, C., Kabuto, M., and Shimizu, H. Association of coffee, green tea, and caffeine intakes with serum concentrations of estradiol and sex hormone-binding globulin in premenopausal Japanese women. Nutr Cancer 1998;30(1):21-24. Nakachi, K., Suemasu, K., Suga, K., Takeo, T., Imai, K., and Higashi, Y. Influence of drinking green tea on breast cancer malignancy among Japanese patients. Jpn J Cancer Res 1998;89(3):254-261.

Grape Seed/Skin and Resveratrol

- Grape polyphenols (grape seed/skin/red wine)
  - Inhibit aging of the cell, including brain & heart
  - Improve cardiovascular health, cognitive function, and connective tissue, and cancer preventive
- Significant protection against all chronic diseases, including cancer, heart disease, and cognitive deterioration
- Resveratrol regulates certain age-promoting genes that become activated and induce obesity and diabetes.
- Grapes and wine contain potent phytochemicals that can inhibit aromatase.

Grape seed extract (GSE)

- Contains high levels of procyanidin dimers that have been shown to be potent inhibitors of aromatase.
- GSE was found to inhibit aromatase activity in a dose-dependent manner and reduce androgen-dependent tumor growth in an aromatase-transfected MCF-7 (MCF-7aro) breast cancer xenograft model.
- In another study red wine extract completely abrogated aromatase-induced hyperplasia and other neoplastic changes in mammary tissue.

Kijima I, Phung S, Hur G, Kwok SL, Chen S. Grape seed extract is an aromatase inhibitor and a suppressor of aromatase expression. Cancer Res. 2006 Jun 1;66(11):5960-7;
Eng ET, Williams D, Mandava U, Kirma N, Tekmal RR, Chen S.
Anti-aromatase chemicals in red wine. Ann N Y Acad Sci. 2002 Jun;963:239-46

Grape seed extract clinical trial

- Phase I clinical trials have begun on the botanical dietary supplement IH636 grape seed extract for the prevention of breast cancer in postmenopausal women who are at increased risk of developing breast cancer.
- The IH636 extract has a high concentration of proanthocyanidins and has been shown to inhibit aromatase using *in vitro* and *in vivo* models.

Kijima I, Phung S, Hur G, Kwok SL, Chen S. Cancer Res. 2006;66:5960; Eng ET, Ye J, Williams D, Phung S, Moore RE, Young MK, Gruntmanis U, Braunstein G, Chen S. Cancer Res. 2003;63:8516

Resveratrol (RES)

- The effect of resveratrol on the expression and enzyme activity of aromatase was investigated. By assaying on MCF-7 cells stably transfected with CYP19 (MCF-7aro cells), resveratrol inhibited the aromatase activity with an IC(50) value of 25 microM.

Wang Y, Lee KW, Chan FL, Chen S, Leung LK. The red wine polyphenol resveratrol displays bilevel inhibition on aromatase in breast cancer cells. Toxicol Sci. 2006 Jul;92(1):71-7.

Polyphenols as Modulator of Oxidative Stress in Cancer Disease

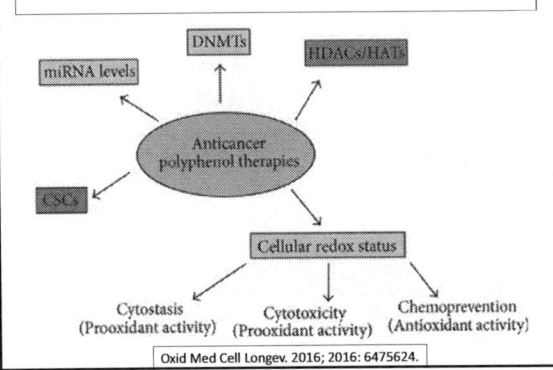

Anticancer polyphenol therapies → miRNA levels, DNMTs, HDACs/HATs, CSCs, Cellular redox status
- Cytostasis (Prooxidant activity)
- Cytotoxicity (Prooxidant activity)
- Chemoprevention (Antioxidant activity)

Oxid Med Cell Longev. 2016; 2016: 6475624.

BERBERINE

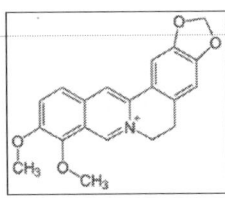

- Is strongly yellow colored, which is why in earlier times Berberis species were used to dye wool, leather and wood. Wool is still today dyed with berberine in northern India.
- Possesses potent insulintrophic and anti-tumor effects.

GOLDENSEAL
(Hydrastis canadensis)

Has a long established history for use as a medicinal plant among the native people of the northeastern United States.
The Native American Indians (Cherokee) and later the Eclectic Physicians used it for treatment of cancer, "general debility," "dyspepsia", to improve appetite and as a tonic and wash for local inflammations.

Coptis spp.
Chinese goldthread, Huang Lian

Coptis is mostly found in the eastern region of Asia, is used in much the same manner as other berberine containing herbs, and is a relative of goldenseal.
Used for infection with excess heat, immune system enhancement, for the treatment of canker sores, poor digestion, liver diseases, mouth sores, diarrhea, bacterial infections, gastrointestinal concerns, and hypertension. It was also used in protecting and keeping the gallbladder and liver healthy.

Coptis extract, or Berberine, with the aromatase inhibitor fulvestrant synergistically suppressing the growth of breast cancer cells

- The research involved testing a combination of treatment with Coptis extract or berberine and fulvestrant,
- Using the combination of Coptis extract or berberine and fulvestrant, a synergistic inhibition of cell growth in MCF-7 cells was significantly enhanced compared to either alone.

Liu J, He C, Zhou K, Wang J, Kang JX Coptis extract enhance the anticancer effect of estrogen receptor antagonists on human breast cancer cells.
Biochem Biophys Res Commun. 2009 Jan 9; 378(2):174-8.

Effects of combined treatment of COP or BER and FUL on the growth of MCF-7 cells.

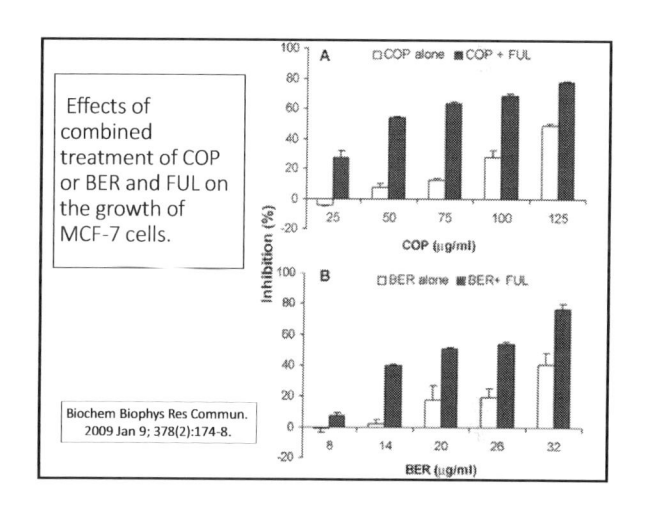

Biochem Biophys Res Commun. 2009 Jan 9; 378(2):174-8.

Anti-tumor targets of various compounds within Coptis

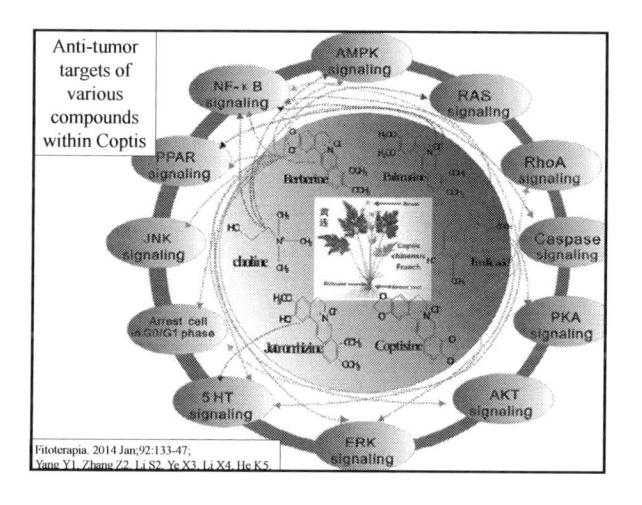

Fitoterapia. 2014 Jan;92:133-47;
Yang Y1, Zhang Z2, Li S2, Ye X3, Li X4, He K5.

Berberine on cell cycle, apoptosis, autophagy and inflammation through the modulation of different targets

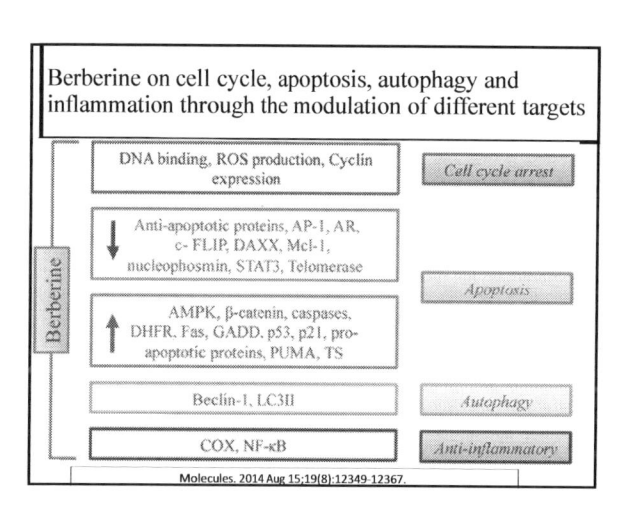

Berberine		
	DNA binding, ROS production, Cyclin expression	*Cell cycle arrest*
	↓ Anti-apoptotic proteins, AP-1, AR, c-FLIP, DAXX, Mcl-1, nucleophosmin, STAT3, Telomerase	*Apoptosis*
	↑ AMPK, β-catenin, caspases, DHFR, Fas, GADD, p53, p21, pro-apoptotic proteins, PUMA, TS	
	Beclin-1, LC3II	*Autophagy*
	COX, NF-κB	*Anti-inflammatory*

Molecules. 2014 Aug 15;19(8):12349-12367.

Licorice (*Glycyrrhiza glabra*), Isoliquiritigenin, flavonoid inhibits Aromatase

- Isoliquiritigenin, was found to be an inhibitor of aromatase enzyme activity'
- When added in diet isoliquiritigenin inhibited significantly the xenograft growth in ovariectomized athymic mice transplanted with MCF-7aro cells.
- Isoliquiritigenin also inhibited aromatase expression in vivo.
- This study indicated that isoliquiritigenin has the potential to be used as a tissue-specific aromatase inhibitor in breast cancer.

Ye L, Gho WM, Chan FL, Chen S, Leung LK: Dietary administration of the licorice flavonoid isoliquiritigenin deters the growth of MCF-7 cells overespressing aromatase. Int J can 2009, 124:1028-1036.

Biochanin A, an Isoflavone isolated from Red clover (*Trifolium pratense*)

- Isoflavones resemble the structure of estrogen, and display agonistic and antagonistic interactions with estrogen receptors.
- Biochanin A significantly inhibited aromatase activity and hampered cell growth attributing to the enzyme activity.

Wang Y, Man Gho W, Chan FL, Chen S, Leung LK. The red clover (Trifolium pratense) isoflavone biochanin A inhibits aromatase activity and expression. Br J Nutr. 2007 Aug 29;:1-8

Hop (*Humulus lupulus*) flavonoids

- Prenylflavonoids xanthohumol, isoxanthohumol and 8-prenylnaringenin have show to suppress breast cancer.
- Prenylflavonoids were able to suppress breast cancer in part by inhibiting aromatase activity.

Monteiro R, Faria A, Azevedo I, Calhau C. Modulation of breast cancer cell survival by aromatase inhibiting hop (Humulus lupulus L.) flavonoids. J Steroid Biochem Mol Biol. 2007 Jun-Jul;105(1-5):124-30. Epub 2007 Jul 23.

Hops (*Humulus lupulus*)

- Traditional usage: Insomnia, Nervous anxiety, irritability, and as Anti-aphrodisiac
- Used quite widely by the Eclectic physicians in a specific medicine known as "Lupulin."
- Sedative, hypnotic, and astringent properties, as well as mild estrogenic constituents.
- As a bitter it was also used for the treatment of gastritis, colitis, and indigestion.
- Active compounds: prenylflavonoids, including prenylnaringenin, xanthohumol, and isoxanthohumol

---

Hops extract suppresses Breast cancer growth in mouse mammary glands

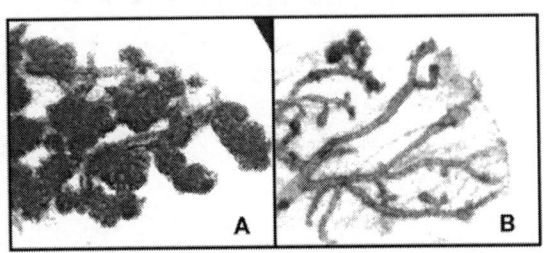

B represents a partial view of a mammary gland incubated with 1.0 μm **xanthohumol**

Gerhauser C et al. Mol Cancer Ther 2002;1:959-969

Vitamin D supplementation prevents Aromatase inhibitor (AI) associated Arthalgia

- Arthalgia (joint pain) is the most common side effect from AI's.
- A prospective cohort of 290 women starting AI also started vitamin D supplementation.
- Vitamin D may help to prevent the development of AI arthralgia but higher loading doses are often required to attain an effective vitamin D level (>40 OH) in women with deficiency at baseline.
- After supplementation (daily 800 IU and additional 16,000 IU every 2 weeks), 50% of them still failed to reach adequate concentrations at 3 months.

Prieto-Alhambra D, Javaid MK, Servitja S, Arden NK, Martinez-García M, Diez-Perez A, Albanell J, Tusquets I, Nogues X. Vitamin D threshold to prevent aromatase inhibitor-induced arthralgia: a prospective cohort study, Breast Cancer Res Treat. 2011 Feb;125(3):869-78. Epub 2010 Jul 28.

Important Foods that Inhibit Aromatase and Suppress Cancer

- Flax seeds (**Lignans**) are precursors of enterolactone, which inhibits aromatase and reduces the ratio of 16-OH over 2-OH estrogen metabolites.
- Mushrooms (**Fatty acids**)
- Olive oil (**Fatty acids, Phenols**)
- Pomegranate (**Ellagic acid**)
- Citrus (**Narigenin and Hespertin**)
- Celery/artichoke (**Apigenin**)
- Red (seeded) grapes, red wine (**Polyphenols, Resveratrol**)
- Artichokes, celery, thyme, green peppers (**Luteolin**)

Flax Seeds

- Best source of phytonutrient lignans which can balance reproductive hormones, lessen peri-menopausal symptoms, and prevent the onset of breast and prostate cancer.
- Lignans in the diet also help prevent type 2 diabetes.
- **Flaxseed reduces prostate cancer proliferation rates in men pre-surgery.**

Cancer Epidemiol Biomarkers Prev. 2008 Dec;17(12):3577-87.

Flax seeds and Enterolactone

- Enterolactone and enterodiol are lignans which are converted in the intestinal flora from dietary foods such as **flaxseeds**, **sesame seeds**, kale, broccoli, and apricots, that impede tumor proliferation by inhibiting activation of NFκB and VEGF.
- Flaxseed-derived enterolactone inhibits tumor cell proliferation in men with localized prostate cancer.
- Flaxseed and its lignans reduce serum estrogens in ER+ breast cancer and inhibit angiogenesis.
- Flax seeds inhibit the growth of human ER+ breast cancer and strengthened the tumor-inhibitory effect of Tamoxifen.
- Flaxseeds are radioprotective.

J Med Food. 2013 Apr;16(4):357-60. doi: 10.1089/jmf.2012.0159; Clin Cancer Res. 2007 Feb 1;13(3):1061-7; Clin Cancer Res. 2004 Nov 15;10(22):7703-11; Biol Ther. 2014 Jul;15(7):930-7.

Mushrooms For Better Health

- White button mushroom, portobello, shiitake maitake, crimini, morel, oyster, etc.
- Potent immune enhancing and cancer inhibiting properties.

- In vitro and in vivo studies with mushrooms and isolated bioactive constituents suggest many beneficial pharmacological effects including anti-tumor, antioxidant, antiviral, cholesterol lowering, and blood sugar lowering effects.
- Several research papers have documented a correlation between dietary mushroom intake and a significant reduction in breast cancer (Shin, et al., 2010; Hong, et al., 2008).
- In one study, the benefits were enhanced when green tea was consumed daily as well (Zhang, et al., 2009).
- White button mushrooms reduce aromatase activity and inhibit the proliferation of breast cancer in vitro and in vivo. (Grube, et al., 2001; *Cancer Res* December 15, 2006 *66;* 12026).

Olives and Olive oil

- Olive oil-rich diet is related to a significant reduction in all-cause mortality.
- Extra virgin olive oil potentiates the effects of aromatase inhibitors

Br J Nutr. 2011 May 17:1-11.

Food Chem Toxicol. 2013 Dec;62:817-24

Extra virgin olive oil potentiates the effects of aromatase inhibitors

- The estrogenic suppressive effects of letrozole and anastrozole were amplified when used in combination with olive oil.
- The employment of aromatase inhibitors in combination with olive oil could orchestrate a reduction in intracellular estrone biosynthesis which feeds ER-positive cells, while simultaneously depleting cancer cells GSH levels and increasing ROS generation, thus releasing cytochrome c and subsequent induction of apoptosis in MCF-7 cells.

Ismail AM, In LL, Tasyriq M, Syamsir DR, Awang K, Omer Mustafa AH, Idris OF, Fadl-Elmula I, Hasima N. Extra virgin olive oil potentiates the effects of aromatase inhibitors via glutathione depletion in estrogen receptor-positive human breast cancer (MCF-7) cells. Food Chem Toxicol. 2013 Dec;62:817-24. doi: 10.1016/j.fct.2013.10.024. Epub 2013 Oct 23

Pomegranates (*Punica granatum*)

- Rich in polyphenolics including ellagic acid, inhibits both prostate, breast and other cancer, has shown to inhibit aromatase activity by 60-80%.

Kim ND. Mehta R. Yu W. Neeman I. Livney T. Amichay A. Poirier D. Nicholls P. Kirby A. Jiang W. Mansel R. Ramachandran C. Rabi T. Kaplan B. Lansky E. Chemopreventive and adjuvant therapeutic potential of pomegranate (Punica granatum) for human breast cancer. Breast Cancer Research & Treatment. 71(3):203-17, 2002 Feb.

Pomegranate

- Cancer suppressing/inhibits cancer angiogenesis
- Anti-obesity - ameliorates metabolic syndrome, activates PPAR gamma and alpha (punicic acid) ameliorates glucose tolerance and suppresses obesity-related inflammation.
- Cardiovascular protective - inhibit the buildup of plaque in cardiac arteries, inhibits LDL oxidation.
- Hormone modulating - contain six compounds that prevent the development of hormone-dependent breast and prostate cancers.

Food Funct. 2013 Jan 19;4(1):19-39. doi: 10.1039/c2fo30034f. Epub 2012 Oct 12.; Nutrition 28 (2012) 595–604; J Am Coll Nutr. 2009 Apr;28(2):184-95; Cancer Research 67, 3475-3482, April 1, 2007; Clin Nutr. 2004 Jun;23(3):423-33; Free Radic Res. 2006 Oct;40(10):1095-104.

Ellagic acid

Is a phytochemical, or plant chemical, found in **pomegranates**, raspberries, strawberries, cranberries, walnuts, pecans, and other plant foods.

Exerts anti-angiogenesis effects
Breast cancer xenografts study revealed that ellagic acid significantly inhibited cancer growth and P-VEGFR2 expression.

Breast Cancer Res Treat. 2012 Aug;134(3):943-55.

Ellagic acid (polyphenol) inhibited VEGFR-2 in animals with breast cancer

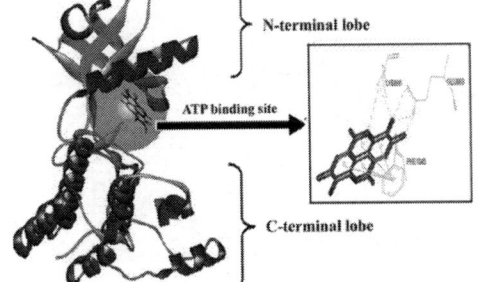

N-terminal lobe
ATP binding site
C-terminal lobe

Breast Cancer Res Treat. 2012 Aug;134(3):943-55.

Naringenin, a flavonoid abundant in citrus fruits

- Cancer suppressing
- Is a weak estrogen agonist that exhibits anti-estrogenic effect in estrogen-rich states and estrogenic activity in estrogen-deficient states
- **Aromatase inhibition**
- Anti-inflammatory properties
- Redox/anti-ox properties
- Anti-viral - hepatitis C virus

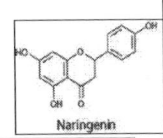

Naringenin

Asian Pac J Cancer Prev. 2012;13:427–436. Environ Health Perspect. 1998 February; 106(2): 85–92. Int J Clin Exp Med. 2013; 6(10): 890–899; J Periodontal Res. 2008;43:400–7; Elem Res. 2012;146:354–9; J Hepatol. 2011 Nov;55(5):963-71.

Citrus flavonone hesperetin inhibits growth of aromatase-expressing MCF-7 tumor in mice.

- Apigenin, naringenin, chrysin and **hesperetin (HSP)** are four of the most potent natural aromatase inhibitors.
- Dietary administration of HSP at 1000 ppm and 5000 ppm significantly deterred tumor growth, cyclin D1, CDK4 and Bcl-x(L) were reduced in the tumors.
- Further study illustrated that plasma estrogen in HSP-treated mice was reduced.

J Nutr Biochem. 2012 Oct;23(10):1230-7.

Apigenin

- Flavonoid found Artichokes, Parsley, Celery, Propolis, Potent multi-mechanistic anti-cancer effects including:
  - Regulate Gene expression, including NF-kB, p53
    - Binds with an estimated 160 proteins in the human body
  - Selective induce apoptosis (pancreatic cancer),
  - Inhibits K-RAS,
  - Inhibits HER2,
  - Inhibits VEGF,
  - Inhibits PI3k-1,
  - Inhibits RANKL,
  - Inhibits Met

Food and Chemical Toxicology, 2013; 60: 83; Biochim Biophys Acta . 2012 February ; 1823(2): 593–604.

Luteolin

- Is a common flavonoid that exists in many types of foods and medicinal herbs including cruciferous vegetables, artichoke, celery, thyme, parsley, peppermint, basil, green peppers, lemons, and chamomile.
- Inhibits TBK1, a signaling enzyme associated with inflammation in the body.
- It inhibits **protein kinase C** and **Src kinase** activities, both of which have been implicated in oncogenic signaling.
- <u>Significantly inhibits HER2 expression</u> and tumor growth in nude mice dose-dependently.

Biomed Res Int. 2014; 2014: 890141, http://www.sciencedaily.com/releases/2010/07/100708141622.htm; Distribution and Biological Activities of the Flavonoid Luteolin, by Miguel López-Lázaro in 2009 (X19149659).

Co-administrating luteolin minimizes the side effects of the aromatase inhibitor letrozole

- This study compared the efficacy of the flavonoid luteolin to the clinically approved AI letrozole (Femara).
- Both letrozole and luteolin are competitive aromatase inhibitors.
- Similar to letrozole, luteolin administration reduced plasma estrogen concentrations and suppressed breast cancer in mice.
- The regulation of cell cycle and apoptotic proteins-such as a decrease in the expression of Bcl-xL, cyclin-A/D1/E, CDK2/4, and increase in that of Bax.
- In contrast to letrozole, luteolin increased fasting plasma high-density lipoprotein concentrations and produced a desirable blood lipid profile.
- These results suggested that the flavonoid could be a co-adjuvant therapeutic agent without impairing the action of AIs.

Li F, Wong TY, Lin SM, Chow S, Cheung WH, Chan FL, Chen S, Leung LK. Coadministrating luteolin minimizes the side effects of the **aromatase** inhibitor letrozole. J Pharmacol Exp Ther. 2014 Nov;351(2):270-7. doi: 10.1124/jpet.114.216754

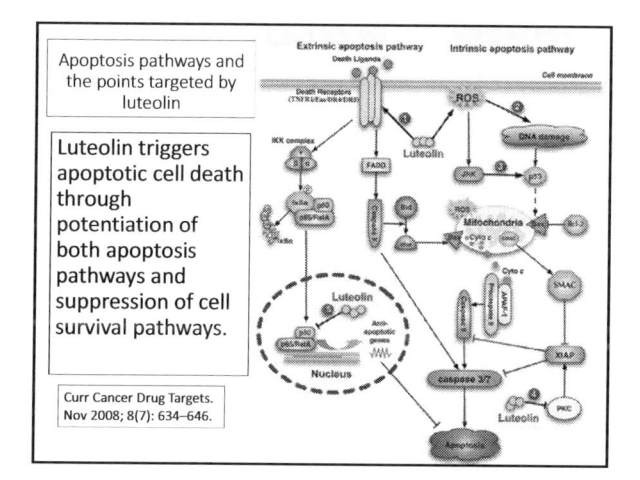

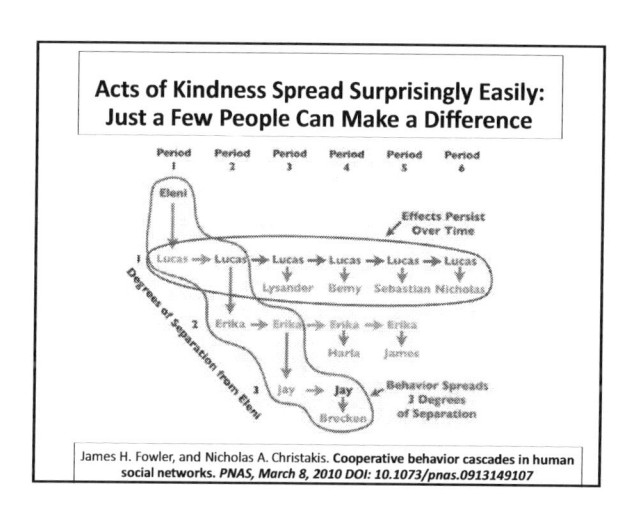

Apoptosis pathways and the points targeted by luteolin

Luteolin triggers apoptotic cell death through potentiation of both apoptosis pathways and suppression of cell survival pathways.

Curr Cancer Drug Targets. Nov 2008; 8(7): 634–646.

Acts of Kindness Spread Surprisingly Easily: Just a Few People Can Make a Difference

James H. Fowler, and Nicholas A. Christakis. Cooperative behavior cascades in human social networks. PNAS, March 8, 2010 DOI: 10.1073/pnas.0913149107

Bonus slides
Hormone positive Breast Cancer

Build Vital Essence

Kidneys (HPAA) **House** Vital Essence

Direct Vital Essence Inward or outward

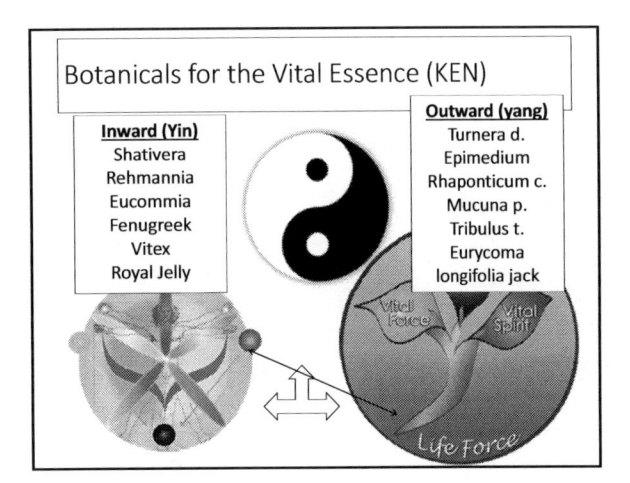

Botanicals for the Vital Essence (KEN)

Inward (Yin)
- Shativera
- Rehmannia
- Eucommia
- Fenugreek
- Vitex
- Royal Jelly

Outward (yang)
- Turnera d.
- Epimedium
- Rhaponticum c.
- Mucuna p.
- Tribulus t.
- Eurycoma longifolia jack

Damiana (*Turnera diffusa*)

- The Greeks named it aphrodisiakos, and it was known as the '"goddess of love.'
- Used traditionally (Mayan Indians), mostly woman, as a aphrodisiaca/sexual tonic
- Increase energy, used to treat impotence as well menstrual problems.
- Selective phosphodiesterase-5 (PDE-5) inhibitor/actives NO
- Antibacterial activity against Gram-positive and Gram-negative bacteria
- Anti-spasmodic/anti-anxiety
- **Significantly suppresses aromatase activity.**
- **Two compounds responsible are pinocembrin and acacetin are attributed to the aromatase inhibition.**

Estrada-Reyes, R. et al. (2009) J Ethnopharmacol 123:423-429J Ethnopharmacol. 2008 Dec 8;120(3):387-93

Botanicals That Enhance Outward Essence (Testosterone)

Plant	Active compound
Rhaponticum carthamoides	Ecdisterones
Tribulus terrestris	Protodioscin
Epimedium brevicornum	Icariin
Eurycoma longifolia jack	Quassinoids
Mucuna pruriens *Pfaffia paniculata* (Suma) *Lepidiummeyenii* (maca)	L-dopa Ecdisterones AA's plus sterols as beta-sitosterol, campesterol, & stigmasterol

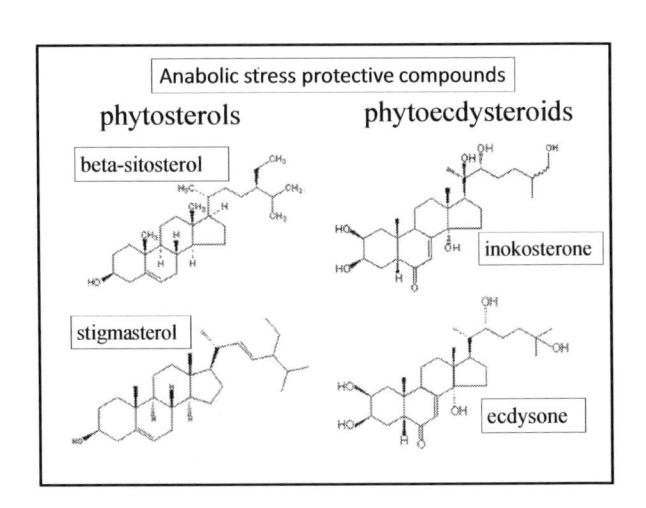

Anabolic stress protective compounds

phytosterols — beta-sitosterol, stigmasterol

phytoecdysteroids — inokosterone, ecdysone

Rhaponticum carthamoides (Leuzea)

- World's strongest natural anabolic agent
- Builds Kidney Essence
- Grows in the alpine and subalpine zones of Southern Siberia
- Parts used: roots (& seeds)
- Chemical constituents include: Phytoecdysterones, flavonoids, glycosides, organic acids, carotenoids, tannins, ether oils, resins

Main Actions of Rhaponticum

- Adaptogenic
- Anti-fatigue (mental and physical)
- Anabolic (Increased protein synthesis)
- Accelerates recovery
- Redox cycling (antioxidative)
- Cardiovascular and Cerebral protective

Main Actions of Rhaponticum (continued)

- Decreased platelet aggregation (stress induced)
- Anti-diabetic / insulintrophic
- Immune system enhancement
- Antimicrobial
- Anticancer
- Chemotherapy protective
- Sexual enhancement and sexual organ development

Tribulus terrestris

- Used for hundreds of years for the treatment of infertility, impotence, liver, kidney, and heart problems
- Known primarily as a natural aid to help impotence, low libido, and male infertility

Tribulus Terrestris Research

- Improves cardiovascular health by reducing angina pectoris, high blood pressure, and fluid retention
- Stimulates the flow of bile and breakdown of fats in the liver, promotes regular bowel patterns & eliminates liver toxins
- Kidney detoxifier and rejuvenator, and a mild diuretic
- Cancer inhibiting, free-radical quenching, anti-diabetic, and immune-enhancing activity
- Protodioscin, is the active compound in Tribulus, and improves sexual desire and enhances erection via the conversion of protodioscin to DHEA/Testosterone/GH

Eurycoma (Eurycoma longifolia jack)

- "Tongkat Ali," Nicknamed – "Malaysian Ginseng"
- Contains a group of compounds called Quassinoids
- Improves athletic performance and energy
- Increases sexual desire and performance
- Increases DHEA & Testosterone
- Modulates negative feedback loop via the hypothalamus and pituitary glands
- Possesses cytotoxic, anti-malarial, anti-ulcer, antipyretic, anti-depressive and mood-balancing effects
- Anti-cancer: Down-regulates Bcl-2 protein

Eurycoma longifolia standardized quassinoids extract anti-cancer activities in vivo against prostate cancer

- Suppressed LNCaP cell growth via G0/G1 phase arrest which was accompanied by the down-regulation of CDK4, CDK2, Cyclin D1 and Cyclin D3 and up-regulation of p21Waf1/Cip1 protein levels.
- Cause G2M growth arrest leading to apoptotic cell death
- Also inhibited androgen receptor translocation to nucleus which is important for the transactivation of its target gene,
- And, resulted in a significant reduction of PSA secretion after the treatment
- Significantly suppressed the tumor growth on mouse

Cissus Quadrangularis (Veld Grape)

- Possesses potent anabolic effects.
- Builds lean muscle mass, insulintrophic, promotes fat lose
- Speeds the remodeling process of the healing bone - increases bone density & strength. Mobilizes fibroblast and chondroblasts to an injured tissue & enhances regeneration.
- Blocks the muscle damaging effect of cortisol (Anti-catabolic).
- Shows significant inhibition in free radical formation, superoxide radical production and lipid peroxide production.
- Nervine effect on central nervous system.

tetracyclic triterpenoids **Ketosterones**, natural calcium

Natl J Maxillofac Surg. 2014 Jan;5(1):35-8.

Goat Weed
(*Epimedium brevicornum or grandiflorum*)

- Enhances androgenic hormone levels
- Can stimulate the growth of the prostate and testes, and raise testosterone levels
- Anabolic – regenerates bone and nerve cells
- Cardiovascular protective – normalizes BP
- Increases peripheral circulatory and vaso-dilating effects
- Immune activating and enhancing
- Supports the HPA axis/stress protective
- Inhibits cancer, including prostate cancer

Epimedium (continued)

- Protects and enhances the HPAA
- Regenerates nerve tissue and bone
- Protection from the catabolic and immune-suppressing effects of steroids such as prednisone

Mucuna
(*Mucuna pruriens*)

- L-dopa rich extract boosts growth hormone and testosterone
- Exerts the growth hormone boosting effects by stimulating the release of hypothalamic GHRH. *Fertility and Sterility.* 92(6), 1934-40.
- Androgenic enhancing
- Serotonin
- Kidney tonic (protective and improves general function)
- **Anti-diabetic/Insulintrophic**
- Protection against snake venom
- Shown to slow down the progression of Parkinson's Disease

Botanicals for Prostate Health that Suppress Cancer

Plant	Active compound
Serenoa repens berry	Fatty acids/Sterols
Urtica dioica root	AA's/Beta sitosterol
Pygeum africanum bark	Sterols
Crataeva nurvala stem bark	Lupeol (pentacyclic triterpene), saponins
Cucurbita pepo (pumpkin seed oil) Pumpkin seed oil has been shown to inhibit 5-alpha reductase and aromatase. *Alternative Medicine.* 2014;2014:7.	Fatty acids

Serenoa repens (Saw Palmetto)
liposterolic extract

- Effective in the treatment of genitourinary problems, including benign prostatic hypertrophy (BPH)
- Suppress prostate cancer
- Other purported uses
  - to increase sperm production
  - to increase breast size in women/PCOS
  - to increase libido
  - mild diuresis
  - Infertility (male & female)
  - Anabolic
  - Lung health
  - Hair and skin (acne) health

Serenoa Pharmacology

- Inhibition of 5-alpha reductase (in vitro)
- Antagonism of DHT at androgen receptors
- Anti-inflammatory actions (COX-2, significant reduction of CCR7, CXCL6, IL-6, and IL-17, STAT-3 expression)
- Inhibition of prolactin
- Inhibition of prostatic cell proliferation, induces prostate cancer cell apoptosis (Bcl-2/Bax, p27, p53)
- Inhibits prostate cancer
- Mediates IGF-1

Integr Cancer Ther. 2006 Dec;5(4):362-72; Int J Cancer. 2005 Mar 20;114(2):190-4; Endocrinology. 2004 Mar 19; BJU Int. 2009 Jan 12; Prostate. 2015 Feb 14; Prostate. J Cell Physiol. 2009 Apr;219(1):69-76. 2015 Feb 14. doi: 10.1002/pros.22953.

Serenoa repens (Saw Palmetto)
liposterolic extract

- Effective in the treatment of genitourinary problems, including benign prostatic hypertrophy (BPH)
- Suppress prostate cancer
- Other purported uses
  - to increase sperm production
  - to increase breast size in women/PCOS
  - to increase libido
  - mild diuresis
  - Infertility (male & female)
  - Anabolic
  - Lung health
  - Hair and skin (acne) health

Saw Palmetto Pharmacology

- Inhibition of 5-alpha reductase (in vitro)
- Antagonism of DHT at androgen receptors
- Anti-inflammatory actions (COX-2, significant reduction of CCR7, CXCL6, IL-6, and IL-17, STAT-3 expression)
- Inhibition of prolactin
- Inhibition of prostatic cell proliferation, induces prostate cancer cell apoptosis (Bcl-2/Bax, p27, p53)
- Inhibits prostate cancer
- Mediates IGF-1

Integr Cancer Ther. 2006 Dec;5(4):362-72; Int J Cancer. 2005 Mar 20;114(2):190-4; Endocrinology. 2004 Mar 19; BJU Int. 2009 Jan 12; Prostate. 2015 Feb 14; Prostate. J Cell Physiol. 2009 Apr;219(1):69-76. 2015 Feb 14. doi: 10.1002/pros.22953.

Pygeum (Prunus) africanum

- Widely used in the therapy of BPH and in combinational therapy for prostate cancer
- Beneficial effects for prostate diseases in clinical trials
- Pygium compounds atraric acid and N-butylbenzene-sulfonamide as antagonists of the human androgen receptor and inhibitors of prostate cancer cell growth.
- Is a potent inhibitor of rat prostatic fibroblast proliferation in response to direct activators of protein kinase C, the defined growth factors bFGF, EGF and IGF-I.

Mol Cell Endocrinol. 2011 Jan 30;332(1-2):1-8. Epub 2010 Oct 19; J Urol 1997 Sep;158(3 Pt 1):889.

Crateva (Crataeva nurvala)
an ancient herb used traditional in Ayurvedic medicine

- Effective for prostate enlargement and bladder sensitivity
- Maintain a healthy urinary tract and bladder function, increasing bladder tone.
- Cleanses the kidney of stones (calcium & uric)
- Also possess anti-diabetic/insulintrophic effects
- Lupeol, a pentacyclic triterpene isolated from the root bark of crateva, has been shown to significantly minimize the deposition of stone-forming constituents in kidneys.

Journal of Scientific Research in Plant Medicine 3, 2/3, 75--79. 1982; Indian J Med Res. 1982; 76 (Suppl): 46-53; Bioallied Sci. 2010 Jan;2(1):18-21 ; J Ethnopharmacology. 1991;31:67-73.

Lupeol
a Androgen Receptor Inhibitor for Prostate Cancer

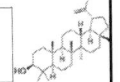

- A very potent inhibitor of androgen receptor (AR) in vitro and in vivo.
- Induces fas-mediated apoptotic death of androgen-sensitive prostate cancer cells and inhibits tumor growth in a xenograft model.
- Inhibits proliferation of human prostate cancer cells by targeting beta-catenin signaling.
- Inhibit tumor growth in a melanoma-bearing mouse model.
- Possesses broad-spectrum anti-inflammatory and anti-

Clin Cancer Res; 17(16); 5379–91. _2011 AACR; Cancer Letters 285 (2009) 109–115; Biomed Rep. 2013 Jul;1(4):641-645. Epub 2013 May 28.; Carcinogenesis. 2009 May;30(5):808-17 Cancer Res. 2005 Dec 1;65(23):11203-13.

Nettle (*Urtica dioica* L.)

- Active Parts for prostate Roots & seeds
  - Phenylpropanes and lignans
  - Scopoletin, steryl derivatives, lignan glycosides, flavonol glycosides
  - B, C, and K vitamins, sitosterol and other steroid related compounds
- Root extract significantly inhibited on Adenosine Deaminase (controls to control nucleotide and stimulates plasminogen activation promoting prostate cancer) activity in prostate tissue from patients with prostate cancer

Cancer Biol Ther. 2004 Sep 18;3(9).

Problem: Diet rich in refined sweeteners, grains, and fats

- Foods are not only "fast" foods but "fast release" foods
  - American diet is high in calorie-dense, insulin-provoking refined carbohydrates (e.g., flour, sugar, corn syrup etc.)
  - Loss of nutrients and fiber
  - 98% of grain products consumed in the US are refined and contain **GMOs** (wheat, corn, soy etc.)
  - Refined grains: blood sugar and insulin responses 2-3 times greater than whole grains or coarse-milled products
  - **Endocrine-disrupting-chemicals (EDCs) also called Xenohormones** (PCBs, BPA, Alkylphenols etc).
- Loss of micronutrients involved in glucose regulation
  - vanadium, zinc, chromium, copper, iron, and nickel

Model of the endocrine systems targeted by EDCs.

Major endocrine organs are vulnerable to endocrine disruption, including the HPA axis, reproductive organs, the pancreas, and the thyroid gland.
EDCs are also known to impact hormone-dependent metabolic systems and brain function.

J Steroid Biochem Mol Biol. 2011 November; 127(3-5): 204–215.

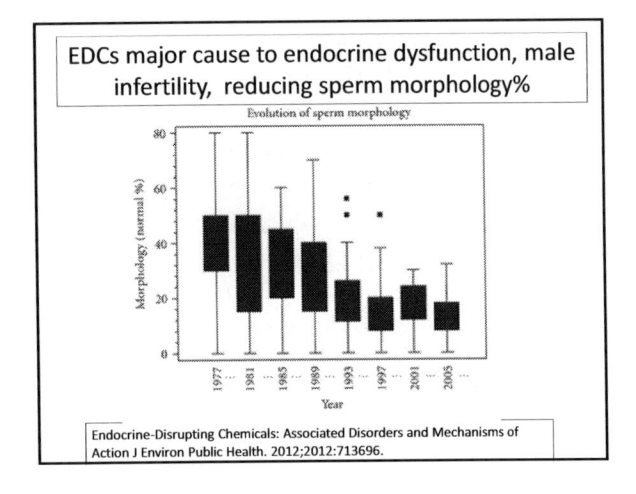

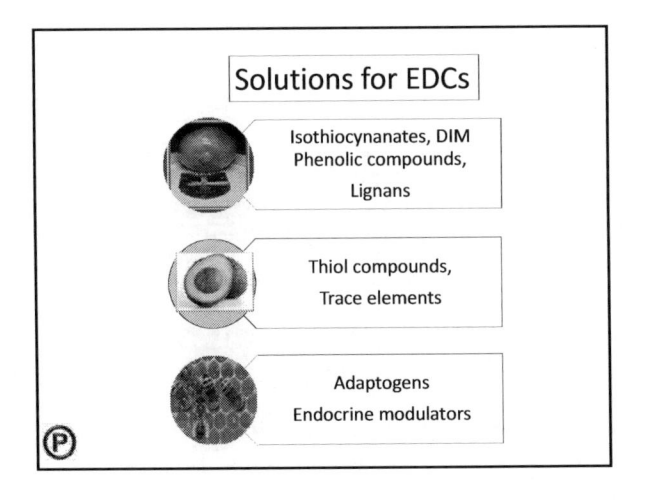

EDCs major cause to endocrine dysfunction, male infertility, reducing sperm morphology%

Evolution of sperm morphology

Endocrine-Disrupting Chemicals: Associated Disorders and Mechanisms of Action J Environ Public Health. 2012;2012:713696.

Solutions for EDCs

- Isothiocynanates, DIM Phenolic compounds, Lignans
- Thiol compounds, Trace elements
- Adaptogens Endocrine modulators

Nrf2

Regulation of the Nrf2-mediated pathways by natural phytochemicals, providing multiple modes of resistance to EDC and other chemical induced carcinogens.

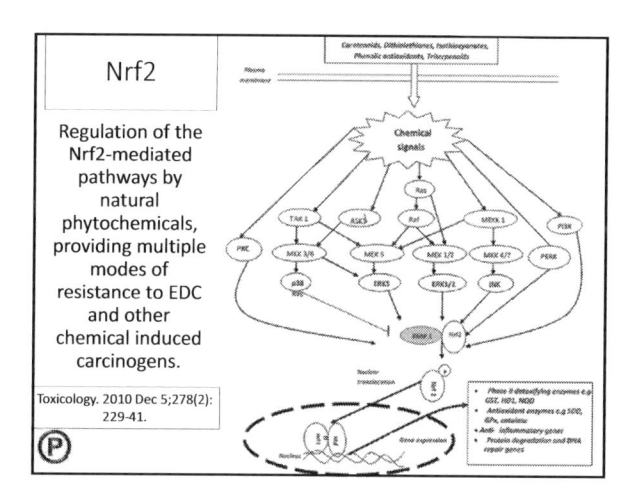

Toxicology. 2010 Dec 5;278(2): 229-41.

Thyroid hormones influences Insulin, Leptin, Estrogens, Mitochondrial Energy, and Hepatic detoxification

- Dysfunctional thyroid (low T-3), contributes to general endocrine imbalances, and resistant hormones including insulin, leptin, and estrogen.
- Leptin resistance, which is strongly associated with breast and other cancers, is a link between obesity and alterations of thyroid hormones.
- Leptin concentrations influence TSH release.
- Low T-3 also causes low cellular energy production and mitochondrial weakness.
- Hyperthyroidism is associated with breast and other cancers and poor outcome in breast cancer.

Mol Cell Endocrinol. 2010 Mar 25;316(2):165-71. doi: 10.1016/j.mce.2009.06.005. Epub 2009 Jun 18.; Endocrinology. 1997 Oct;138(10):4485-8.
Int J Clin Exp Med 2012;5(4):358-362

Combining Low dose Endocrine and Biologics with Botanical Medicine

Estrogen Receptor- Mediated Signalling Pathways in Breast Cancer

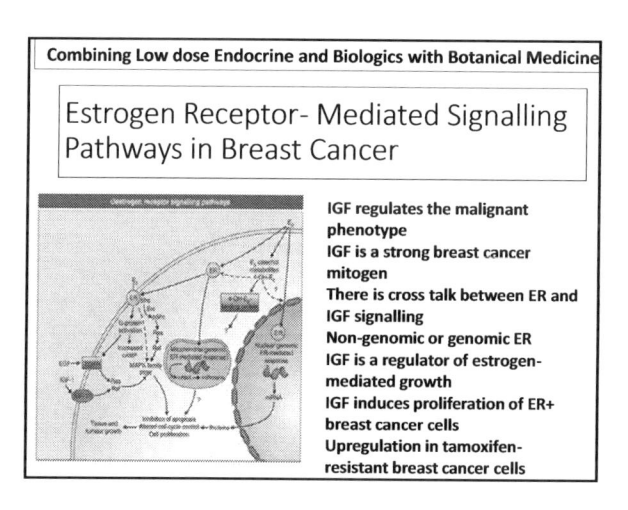

- IGF regulates the malignant phenotype
- IGF is a strong breast cancer mitogen
- There is cross talk between ER and IGF signalling
- Non-genomic or genomic ER
- IGF is a regulator of estrogen-mediated growth
- IGF induces proliferation of ER+ breast cancer cells
- Upregulation in tamoxifen-resistant breast cancer cells

Estrogen Receptor- Mediated Signalling Pathways in Breast Cancer

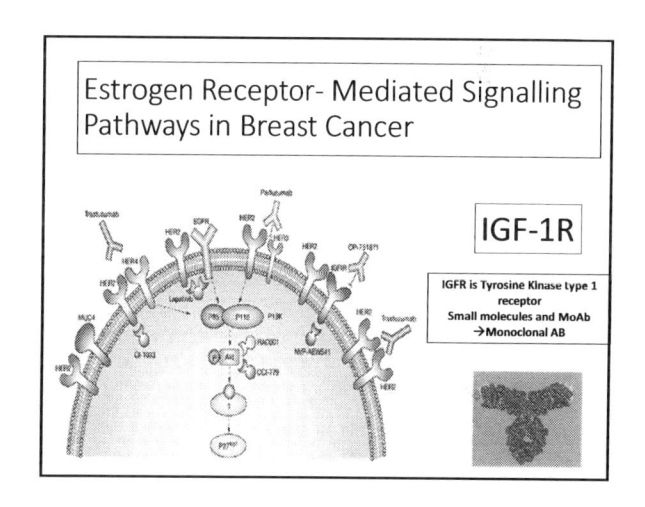

IGF-1R

IGFR is Tyrosine Kinase type 1 receptor
Small molecules and MoAb
→Monoclonal AB

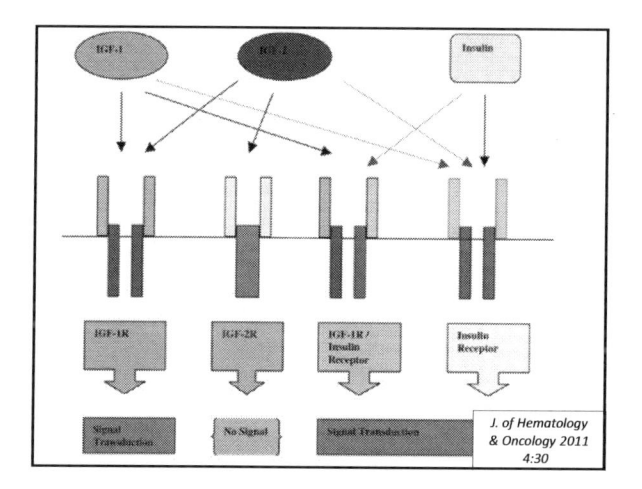

J. of Hematology & Oncology 2011 4:30

Insulin & Insulin Growth Factors (IGFs)

- In cancer, IGFs promote cell proliferation and inhibit apoptosis
- Higher levels are associated with a **4-fold** greater risk of developing certain cancers
- IGF binding proteins (IGFBPs), <u>act as natural inhibitors</u> of IGF-1
- IGF-1 is a known mitogen (stimulator of cell division and tumor growth).
- IGF-1 also acts as an angiogenic growth (switch) factor
- IGF-1 receptors are found on primary cancer cells as well as on osteoblasts in bone metastasis.
- Insulin & IGF-1 stimulates cancer cells to make uPA (urokinase-type plasminogen activator), a cell product implicated in the invasiveness and metastasis of cancer.

Mol Carcinog. 2000 Jan;27(1):10-7, Cancer Res. 2001 Feb 15;61(4):1367-74.

Pathways & Mechanisms Whereby Glucose and Insulin Promote Cancer

- Insulin receptor impairment ➔ causes a desensitization of the IGF-binding proteins (I, II & most importantly III), enabling circulating insulin and IGFs to proliferate cancer
- increases stimulation of the IGF1R by increasing IGF1 bioavailability
- Increases uPA and PAI-1 ➔ Fibrinogen ➔ Thrombosis
- Increases aromatase enzyme ➔ increases estrogen ➔ reduces estrogen clearance
- Increases oxidative damage, particularly Advanced Glycation End products (AGEs)
    ➔ increases glucose uptake ➔ cancer-related hypoxia (restrict ATP production to glycolysis) ➔ HIF-1a ➔ angiogenesis, chemo & radiation resistance *Otto Warburg*

BMC Cancer 2009, 9:241, J Nucl Med 42 (2001), pp. 170–175, J. Nucl Med 37 (1996), pp. 502–506, Br J Cancer. 2003 September 1; 89(5): 877–885.

Pathways Whereby Glucose and Insulin Promote Cancer (...continued)

- Hepatic stress/stagnation, fatty liver (disrupts detoxification)
- Reduced mitochondrial biogenesis - Mitochondrial dysfunction - nutrient oxidation inefficiency and increased generation of ROS.
- Increase levels of Leptin (resistance)
- Increases cancer cell glucose transporter activity (GLUT-1)
- Increases levels of pro-inflammatory cytokines (TNF-a, IL-6 etc.)
- Gene mutations such JAK-2, p53
- Impairment of AMPK/cyclic AMP
- c-MYC activation
- mTOR/PI3-k activation

BMC Cancer 2009, 9:241, J Nucl Med 42 (2001), pp. 170–175, Nucl Med 37 (1996), pp. 502–506, Diabetes. 2013;62:743-752, Circulation Research.2008; 102: 401-414

GLUT-4 and Insulin Resistance

- GLUT4 is a glucose transporter in fat and muscle cells.
- When an insulin receptor is activated, it induces the GLUT4 protein to move from reserves (inside cells) to active (outside cells).
- Deficient GLUT-4 translocation to plasma membranes in response to insulin can cause a glucose/insulin traffic jam, leading to insulin resistance.
- In insulin resistance GLUT4 transporter no longer moves to the cell membrane to let in insulin,
- However cancer cells up-regulate GLUT-4 and other GLUT transporter letting in larger amounts of insulin and glucose to feed the proliferation and growth.

Metabolism. 2004 Mar;53(3):382-7.
Horm Metab Res. 2012 Jun;44(6):436-41. doi: 10.1055/s-0031-1301301. Epub 2012 Feb 20.

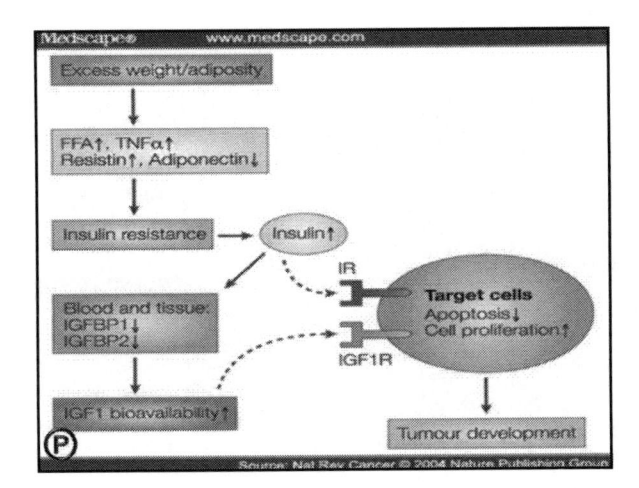

Cancer Cells Contain a Range of distinguishing mutations and characteristics

- Drivers – Promote cancer
- Passengers
    - Some assist the driver
    - Others are just with the driver
- Example: **c-MYC drives glutamine into the cancer cells (glutamine is not the problem)**, mutated PTEN is likely "driver" that activates NF-kB

Vitamin D is a potent down regulator of c-MYC and is a key nutrient for the suppression of cancer.

Endocrinology. Proc Natl Acad Sci, 2012 Nov 13;109(46):18827-32, 2009 May; 150(5): 2046–2054.

CDK (cyclin-dependent kinases) 4/6 inhibitors

- Are a novel class of therapeutics that target the CDK 4/6 kinases that promote transition through the cell cycle.
- Currently, palbociclib (PD0332991, Pfizer), abemaciclib (LY2835219, Lilly) and ribociclib (LEE011, Novartis) are being investigated in clinical trials.
- CDK4/6 inhibitors have shown promising preclinical activity in sarcomas, glioblastoma, renal and ovarian cancer models as well.

Curr Opin Obstet Gynecol. 2015 Dec 4.

Cyclin-dependent kinase 4/6-Rb protein: a key pathway in cell cycle progression

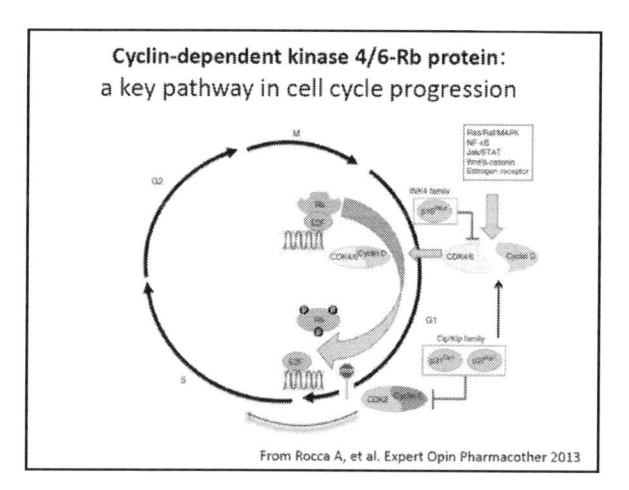

From Rocca A, et al. Expert Opin Pharmacother 2013

Gene expression alterations associated with outcome in aromatase inhibitor (AIs) -treated ER+ early-stage breast cancer patients

- Although AIs improve overall survival, resistance is still a major clinical problem, thus additional biomarkers predictive of outcome of ER+ breast cancer patients treated with AIs are needed.
- Twenty-six genes, including TFF3, DACH1, RGS5, and GHR, were shown to exhibit altered expression in tumors from patients with recurrence versus non-recurrent (fold change ≥1.5, $p < 0.05$) TFF3, which encodes for trefoil factor 3 and is an estrogen-responsive oncogene shown to play a functional role in tamoxifen and AI resistance
- **CDK 4 and/or 6** and PI3-K mutations are major contributors to AI resistance as well.

Breast Cancer Research and Treatment (Nov 2015)

Novel Drug Approved for Breast Cancer (2/2015): Palbociclib (Ibrance)

- Palbociclib (Ibrance) is indicated for use with the aromatase inhibitor letrozole as first-line treatment in postmenopausal women with metastatic breast cancer that is estrogen receptor (ER)-positive and human epidermal growth factor receptor 2 (HER2)- negative.
- The new drug acts as an inhibitor of CDK 4 and 6, which are involved in promoting the growth of cancer cells.
- The results from this phase 2 trial — the PALOMA-1/TRIO-18 study — were recently published in the January issue of The Lancet Oncology, and were reported by Medscape Medical News at the time.
- Palbociclib More Than Doubled Progression-Free Survival in Phase 3 Trial for Patients With HR+, HER2- Metastatic Breast Cancer

Clinical Cancer Research, 2014; DOI: 10.1158/1078-0432.CCR-14-2258
Curr Oncol Rep. 2015 May;17(5):443. doi: 10.1007/s11912-015-0443-3;
Lancet Oncol. 2015 Jan;16(1):25-35. doi: 10.1016/S1470-2045(14)71159-3. Epub 2014 Dec 16.

CDK 4/6 Inhibitor Palbociclib (PD0332991) for Rb+ Advanced Breast Cancer:

- Palbociclib was given at 125 mg orally on days 1 to 21 of a 28-day cycle.
- Biomarker assessment includes Rb expression/localization, KI-67, p16 loss, and CCND1 amplification.
- Single-agent palbociclib is well tolerated and active in patients with endocrine resistant,
- HR+ , **Rb-positive** breast cancer.
- Cytopenias were uncomplicated and easily managed with dose reduction

Clin Cancer Res. 2014 Dec 11.

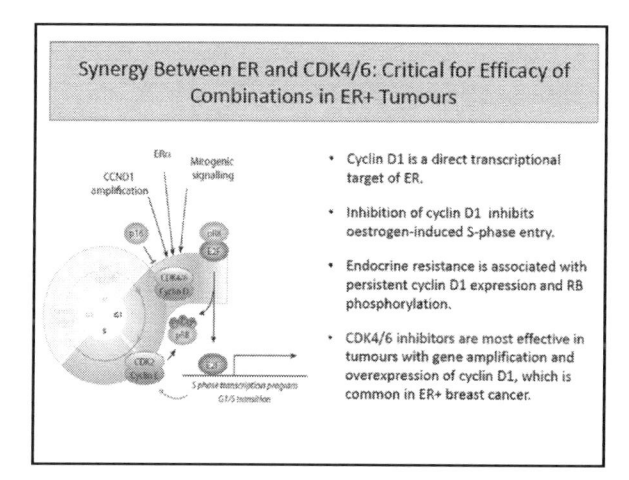

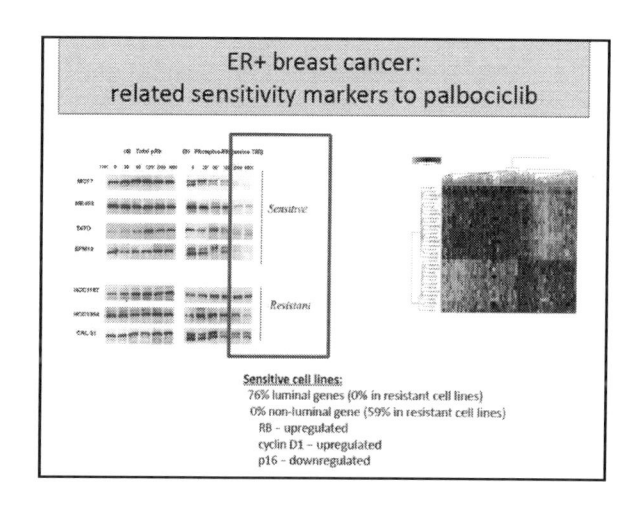

Synergy Between ER and CDK4/6: Critical for Efficacy of Combinations in ER+ Tumours

- Cyclin D1 is a direct transcriptional target of ER.
- Inhibition of cyclin D1 inhibits oestrogen-induced S-phase entry.
- Endocrine resistance is associated with persistent cyclin D1 expression and RB phosphorylation.
- CDK4/6 inhibitors are most effective in tumours with gene amplification and overexpression of cyclin D1, which is common in ER+ breast cancer.

ER+ breast cancer: related sensitivity markers to palbociclib

Sensitive cell lines:
76% luminal genes (0% in resistant cell lines)
0% non-luminal gene (59% in resistant cell lines)
RB - upregulated
cyclin D1 - upregulated
p16 - downregulated

Palbociclib - Predictive biomarkers
Rb nuclear score

Clark AS, et al. SABCS 2013

Palbociclib predictive markers
% p16 nuclear staining

Clark AS, et al. SABCS 2013

Progression-Free Survival

IR and IGF-IR signaling, trigger the activation of: Ras/Raf/Mek/Erk /mTOR and PI3K pathways.

Front Endocrinol (Lausanne). 2011; 2: 93.

IGF-IR Signaling Pathway

Samani, A. A. et al. Endocr Rev 2007;28:20-47

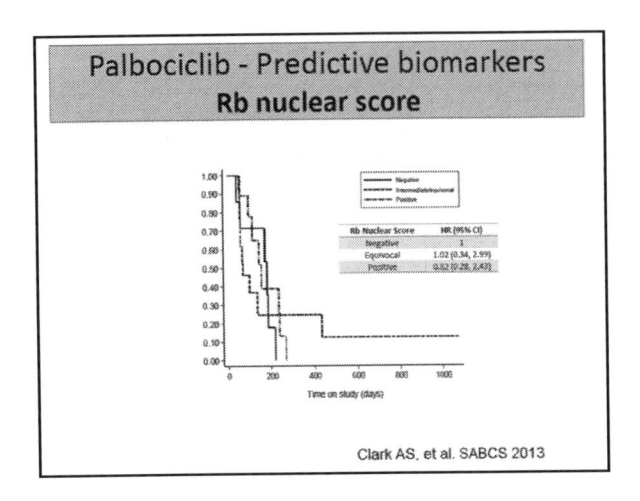

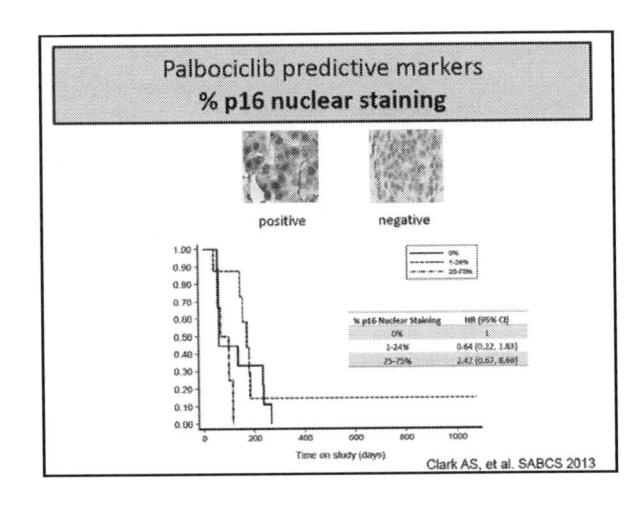

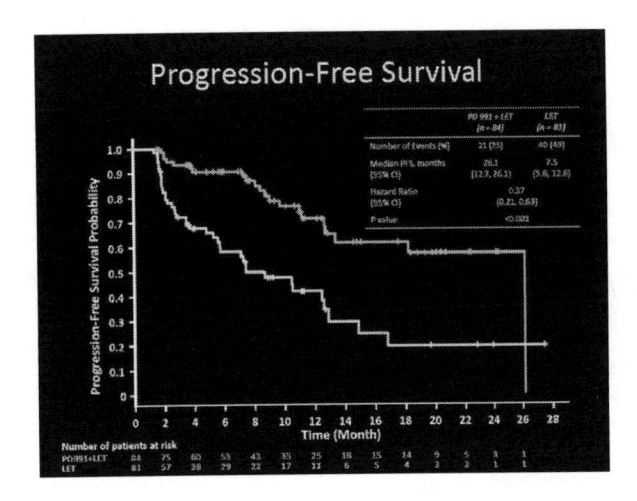

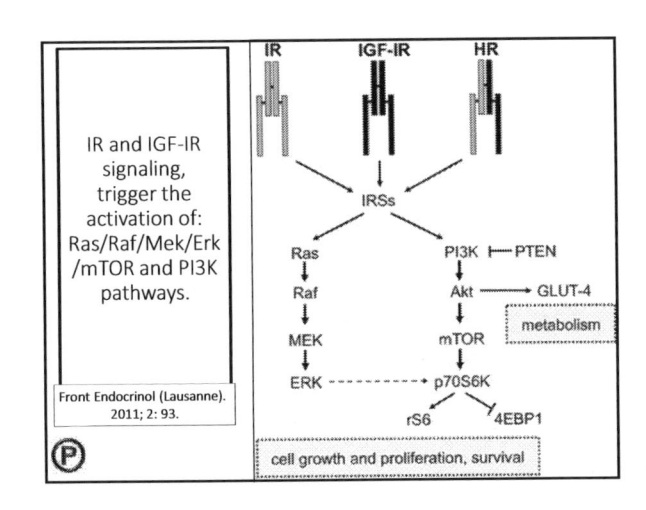

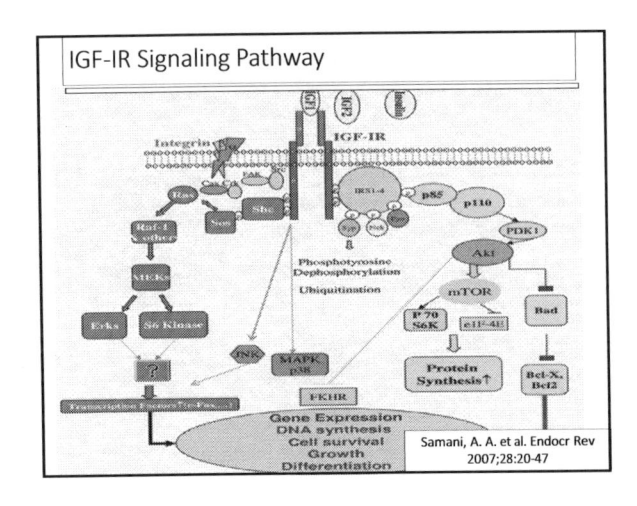

IGF Binding Proteins

- There are also at least six IGF-binding proteins (IGFBP-1-6).
- Altered levels of IGF-I, IGFBP-2 and **IGFBP-3** have been associated with the occurrence of malignancies.
- **IGFBP-3 exerts antitumor effects** via IGF-independent mechanisms which involve activation of caspase-dependent apoptosis and cross-talk with NF-κB signaling.

Nat. Rev. Cancer 4 (2004), pp. 505–518, Clin. Chem. Lab. Med. 42 (2004), pp. 654–664, Endocr. Rev. 16 (1995), pp. 3–3, Growth Horm IGF Res. 2008 Jun 10., Cell Physiol. 183 (2000), pp. 1–9, Cancer Lett. 2011 Aug 28;307(2):200-10.

Bitter melon (*Momordica charantia*)
Main actions on the anti-diabetic effects

- "vegetable insulin"
- Increase glucose utilization by the liver,
- Decrease gluconeogenesis via inhibition of two key enzymes (glucose-6-phosphatase and fructose-1,6-bisphosphatase),
- Improve glucose oxidation through the shunt pathway by activating glucose-6-phosphate dehydrogenase.
- Enhance cellular uptake of glucose, promote insulin release and potentiate its effect,
- Increase the number of insulin-producing beta cells in the pancreas of diabetic animals.

M. M. Lolitkar and M. R. Rajarama Rao (1962), Journal of the University of Bombay, volume 29, pages 223-224, Sridhar MG, Vinayagamoorthi R, Arul Suyambunathan V, Bobby Z, Selvaraj N (2008-04-01). *British Journal of Nutrition* 99 (04): 806

Momordica extract (ME) possesses profound anti-tumor effects

- Induces cycle arrest and apoptosis without affecting normal cell growth.[1]
- Chemopreventive effect against DMBA induced skin tumorigenesis, melanoma tumor & cytogenicity.[2]
- Modulates signal transduction pathways for inhibition of breast cancer cell growth.[3]
- IV of ME to nude mice resulted in a 100% survival compared with 80% in the controls.
- Anti-metastatic effect, both in vitro and in vivo.

1. Pharm Res. 2010 Jun;27(6):1049-53. Epub 2010 Mar 3. 2. *Asian Pacific J Cancer Prev*, 11, 2010, 371-375. 3. Cancer Res. 2010 Mar 1;70(5):1925-31. Epub 2010 Feb 23
4. Cancer Sci. 2010 Oct;101(10):2234-40

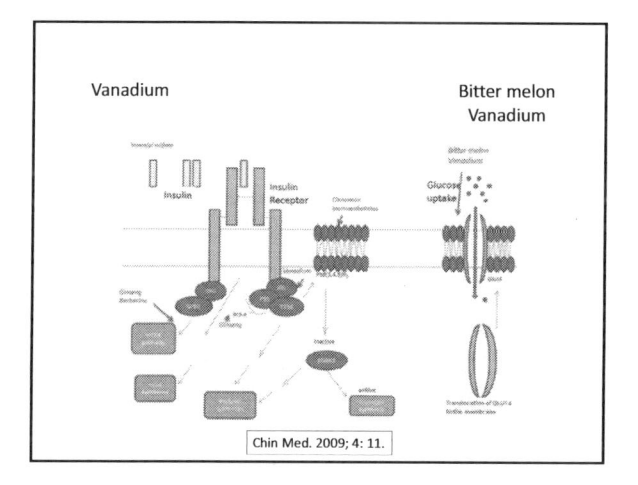

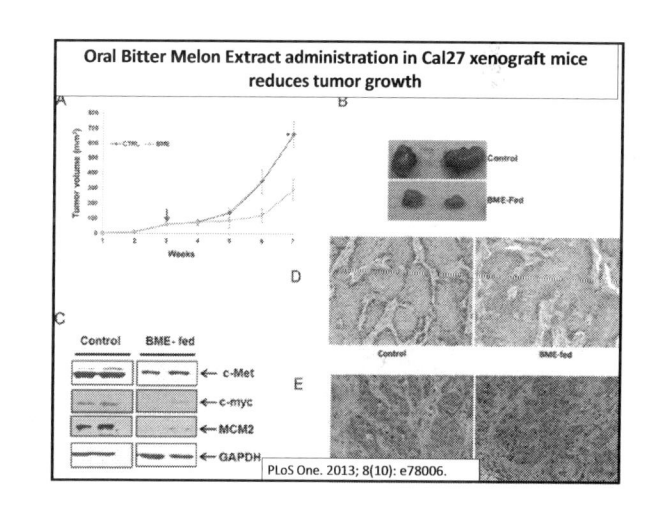

Vanadium — Bitter melon Vanadium

Chin Med. 2009; 4: 11.

Oral Bitter Melon Extract administration in Cal27 xenograft mice reduces tumor growth

PLoS One. 2013; 8(10): e78006.

Src

- Is a non-receptor tyrosine kinase involved in signaling and crosstalk between growth-promoting pathways
- Is over-expressed in many cancer types
- Src activation participates in herceptin mechanisms of resistance and indicates poor prognosis, mainly in HER2/neu hormone receptor-negative breast cancer.
- Inhibiting Scr may be beneficial in those patients.

British Journal of Cancer (2014) 111, 689–695. doi:10.1038/bjc.2014.327

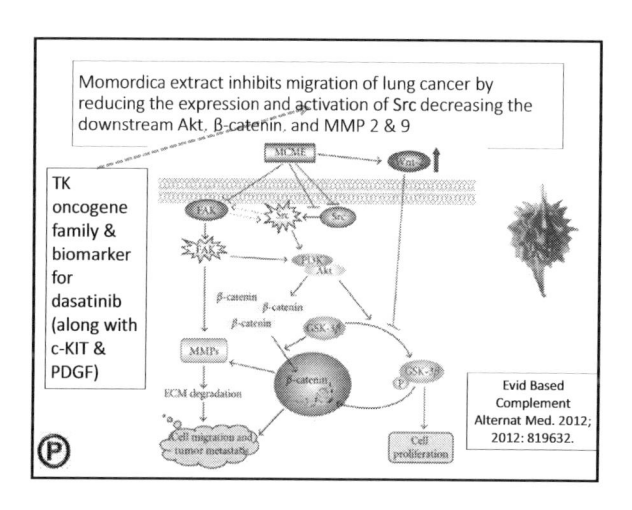

Momordica extract inhibits migration of lung cancer by reducing the expression and activation of Src decreasing the downstream Akt, β-catenin, and MMP 2 & 9

TK oncogene family & biomarker for dasatinib (along with c-KIT & PDGF)

Evid Based Complement Alternat Med. 2012; 2012: 819632.

Fenugreek Seed
(Trigonella foenum-graecum)

- Member of pea family.
- Traditionally used to treat diabetes – insulin like effect.
- Sooths mucous membranes of the sinuses, lungs, and digestive tract. Externally used as drawing agent.
- Improves glucose, insulin & lipids and decreases insulin resistance in type-2 diabetics,
- **Protodioscin**, purified from fenugreek seed inhibits leukemia through an induction of apoptosis
- Intra-peritoneal administration of the alcohol extract in mice produced more than 70% inhibition of tumor cell growth.
- Inhibits breast and gastric cancer, activates antioxidant defense system

Journal of the Association of Physicians of India. 49:1057-61, 2001 Nov, *Phytotherapy Res.* 2001;15:257-59, *Int J Mol Med* 2003;11:23-26. *Journal of Ethnopharmacology.* 81(3):393-7, 2002 Aug. Asian Pac J Cancer Prev. 2011;12(12):3299-304. Toxicol Int. 2012 Sep;19(3):287-94.

Galega officinalis (Goat's rue)

- Has been traditional used to lower blood sugar levels, and to treat diabetes.
- Has a novel weight reducing action
- Metformin, a biguanide, was developed from galegine, a guanidine derivative in Galega.
- Anti-melanoma effects

Metab Cardiovasc Dis. 2005 Jun;15(3):149-60, J Pharm Pharmacol. 1999 Nov;51(11):1313-9 Clin Pharmacokinet. 2011 Feb 1;50(2):81-98

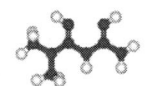

Nigella sativa seeds

- Anti-inflammation, hypoglycemic, antihypertensive, antiasthmatic, antimicrobial, antiparasitic, antioxidant and anticancer effects. Am J Chin Med. 2011;39(6):1075-91.
- Generally enhances immunity and cancer inhibiting.
- Has specifically been used traditionally for treating diabetes. Journal of Endocrinology and Metabolism, Vol. 1, No. 1, Apr 2011
- Inhibits intestinal glucose absorption and improves glucose tolerance in rats. J Ethnopharmacol. 2009 Jan 30;121(3):419-24.
- A human study indicated that a dose of 2 gm/ day of is beneficial in type 2 diabetic patients. Journal of Endocrinology and Metabolism, ISSN 1923-2861, 1923-287, April, 2011
- Also shown to significantly improve lipid profiles and fasting blood glucose. Int J Diabetes Dev Ctries 2008;28(1):11-14.
- I use the CO_2 super critical extract (2-5 mls daily)

Nigella s. (thymoquinone) extract potent cancer inhibitor

- Mitigates all obesity-promoted diseases including cancer. Plant Foods Hum Nutr. 2012 Jun;67(2):111-9.
- Activates AMPK, a master metabolic regulating enzyme. Diabetes Obes Metab. 2010 Feb;12(2):148-57. Epub 2009 Sep 25.
- Redox/antioxidant role, improves body's defense system, induces apoptosis and controls Akt pathway and is a HDAC inhibitor. Afr J Tradit Complement Altern Med. 2011;8(5 Suppl):226-32.
- Chemo-sensitizer: Potent enhancer of the cytotoxic effects of chemotherapy. Int J Cancer. 2010 Jun 21, J Pharm Belg 1998 Mar-Apr;53(2):87-93
- Does not add toxicity to health cells and is generally protective to vital organs such as the kidneys, heart and liver.J Ethnopharmacol. 1999 Nov 1;67(2):135-42, Br J Biomed Sci. 2010;67(1):20-8
- Extremely effective for withdrawal from opiates. J Ayub Med Coll Abbottabad. 2008 Apr-Jun;20(2):118-24.

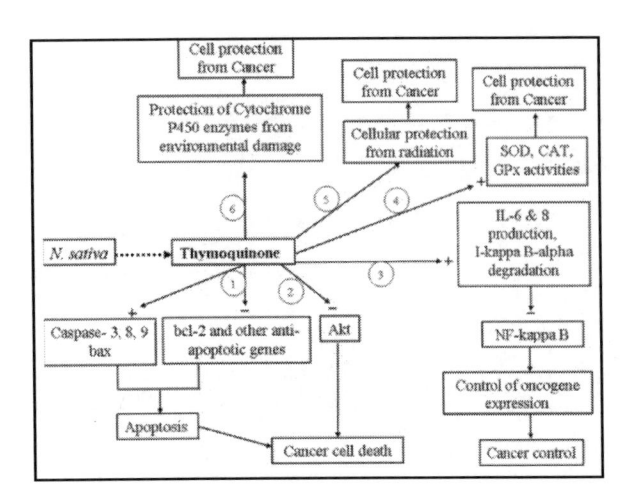

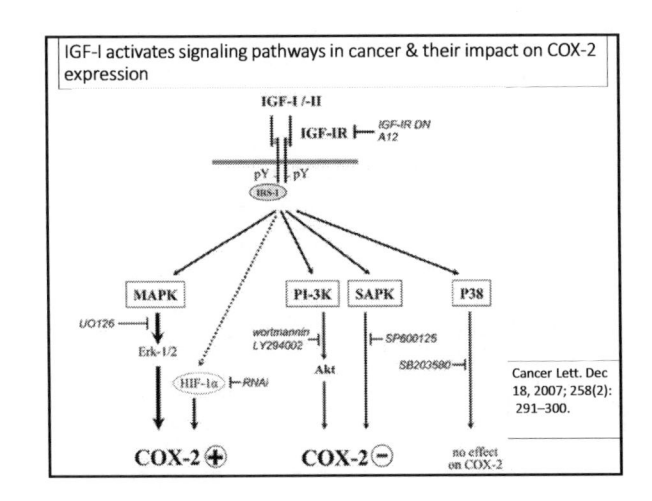

IGF-I activates signaling pathways in cancer & their impact on COX-2 expression

Cancer Lett. Dec 18, 2007; 258(2): 291–300.

Effects of COX-2 inhibition (Celebrex) on secretion of VEGF and PGE2

Mol Biol Rep. Jul 2012; 39(7): 7743–7753.

Herbal Compounds that inhibit COX-2

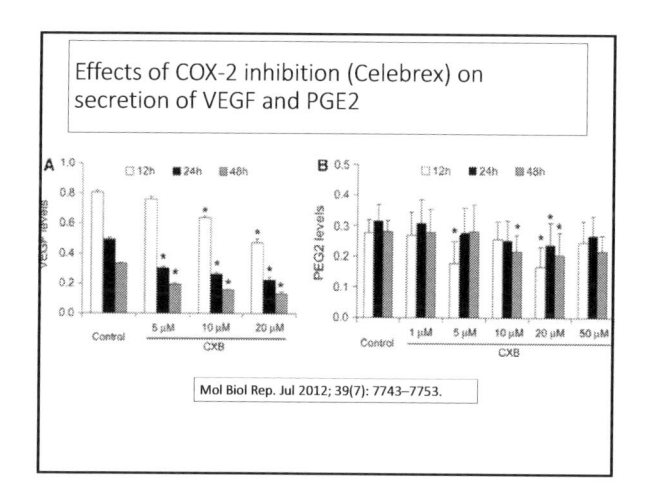

Herbal compound	Source & Reference
Grape seed	Concentrated OPC rich extract Mol Cancer Ther. 2010 Mar;9(3):569-80
Honokiol	*Magnolia grandiflora/officinalis* Int J Oncol. 2011 Mar;38(3):769-76
Berberine	*Hydrastis* (Goldenseal) PLoS One. 2013; 8(7): e69240
Myricetin	Flavonoid found in berries J Agric Food Chem. 2007 Nov 14;55(23):9678-84. Epub 2007 Oct 19
Quercetin	Flavone found in plants & foods PLoS ONE 6(8): e22934. doi:10.1371/journal.pone.0022934; Cancer Chemother Pharmacol. 2006 Mar 22
Petasites hybridus (Butterbur)	Whole plant extract Planta Med. 2005 Jan;71(1):12-9

Herbal Compounds that inhibit COX-2

Herbal compound	Source & Reference
Pinolenic acid	Pine seed oil Food Chem Toxicol. 2014 Apr;66:122-33.
6-(methylsulfinyl) hexyl isothiocyanate	Isothiocynate found in Wasabi Oncol Rep. 2007 Jan;17(1):233-8
Sulforaphane isothiocyanate	Isothiocynate found in Broccoli Biochimie 94 (2012) 1754e1763; Ai Zheng. 2006 Apr;25(4):432-7
Ursolic acid	Common sage Mol Nutr Food Res. 2008 Nov;52(11):1349-57
White willow bark (*Salix alba*)	Concentrated extract Mol Nutr Food Res. 2008 Nov;52(11):1349-57
Wogonin	*Scutellaria baicalensis* Mol Nutr Food Res. 2008 Nov;52(11):1349-57
Zinc	Carcinogenesis. 2011 Apr;32(4):554-60. Epub 2011 Jan 18

Herbal Compounds that inhibit COX-2

Herbal compound	Source & Reference
Baicalein and baicalin	*Scutellaria baicalensis* Biochem Pharmacol. 2000 Jun 1;59(11):1445-57.
Oroxylin A	*Scutellaria baicalensis* Biochem Pharmacol. 2000 Jun 1;59(11):1445-57
Wogonin	*Scutellaria baicalensis* Mol Nutr Food Res. 2008 Nov;52(11):1349-57
Gingerols and shogaols	Phenolic compounds ginger (*Zingiber officinale*) Fitoterapia. 2011 Jan;82(1):38-43.
Arctiin	*Forsythia suspensa* J Inflamm (Lond). 2011 Jul 7;8(1):16. doi: 10.1186/1476-9255-8-16.
Atractylochromene	*Atractylodes lancea* J Nat Prod. 1998 Mar;61(3):347-50.
Bacopasides	*Bacopa monnieri* Curr Med Chem. 2012 Dec 3.

Exercise can also alter autonomic nervous system function by increasing parasympathetic nervous system activity, the effects of which may regulate the inflammatory reflex

Graeme J. Koelwyn, MSc, Erik Wennerberg, PhD, Sandra Demaria, MD, and Lee W. Jones, PhD
Exercise in Regulation of Inflammation-Immune Axis Function in Cancer Initiation and Progression
Review Article | December 15, 2015 | Oncology Journal, Integrative Oncology

HERB PHARM
supports the work of the Southwest College of Naturopathic Medicine and Health Sciences.

Since 1979 HERB PHARM has been committed to providing the highest quality herbal extract products possible, educating people on the safe and effective use of medicinal herbs, and inspiring a love for plants and a respect for Mother Nature.

We support the sustainability of wild herb populations through our support of a variety of environmental organizations like United Plant Savers, and through our research and development of organic agricultural methods for cultivating threatened wild herb species.

As herbalists, we know that the quality of our herbal products directly affects the quality of our customers' health and well-being, and that our environmental approach contributes to the health of our planet for generations to come.

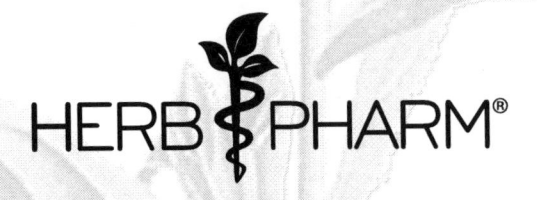

HERB PHARM®

800-348-4372 *tel* • 800-545-7392 *fax*
www.herb-pharm.com • Box 116, Williams, Oregon 97544 USA

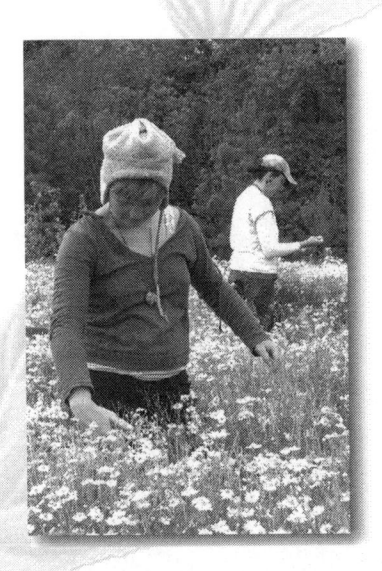

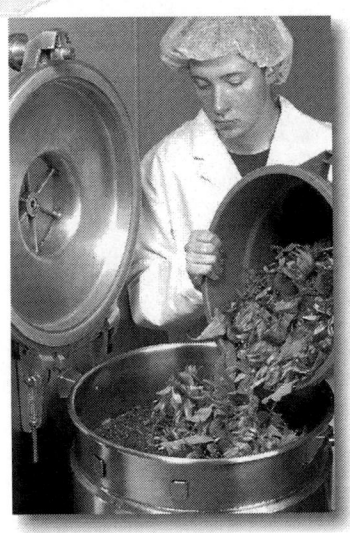

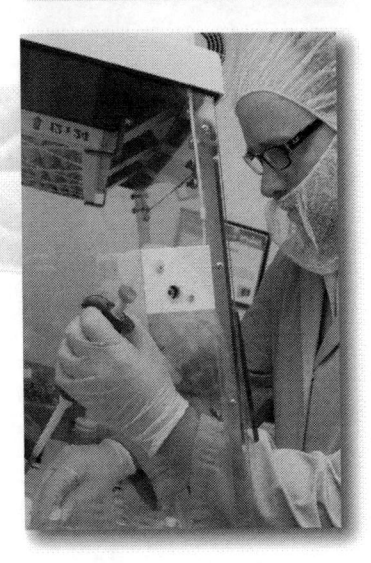

At Kan, Quality is a Way of Life.

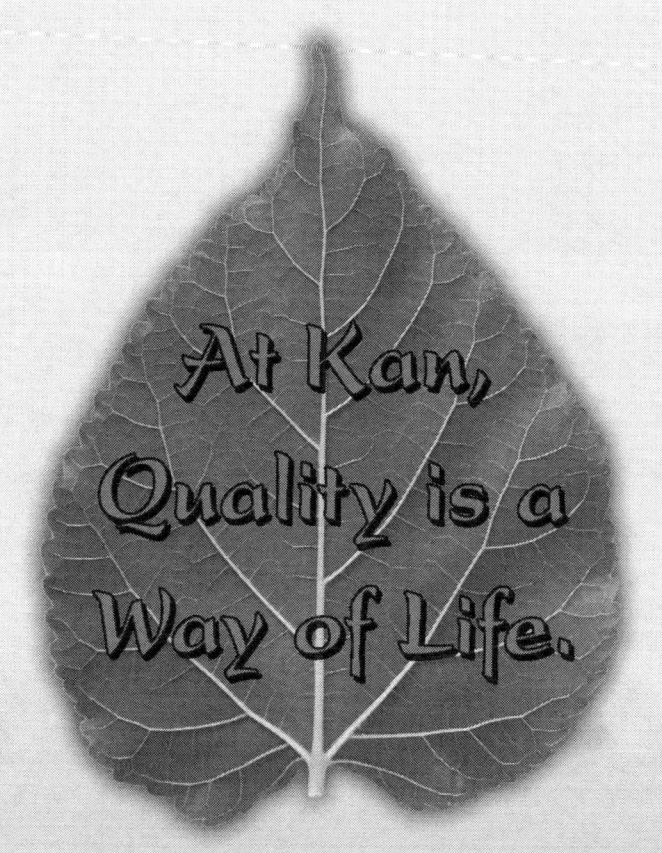

Our Extensive Chinese Herbal Formula Line Includes:

Kan Herbals
Kan Traditionals
Kan Essentials
Chinese Modular Solutions
Gentle Warriors
Sage Solutions
Jade Woman/Jade Man Herbals
MycoHerb
Alembic Herbals
Kan Singles

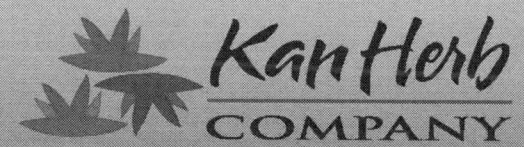

Kan Herb COMPANY
CHINESE HERBAL PRODUCTS YOU CAN TRUST

380 Encinal Street, Suite 100 ▸ Santa Cruz, CA 95060
800.543.5233 ▸ customer@kanherb.com ▸ www.kanherb.com

Scientifically Assured Quality, Consistency, Potency and Purity.

All formulas are manufactured and tested exclusively in the USA.

Only the freshest and highest quality herbs are procured, many of them organic when possible.

Identity testing is performed to ensure that the right herb is being used every time.

Quality control tests and examinations are performed on all incoming ingredients.

Quality control tests and examinations are performed at every stage of production.

Because we manufacture our product from beginning to end at our state of the art facility in California, we ensure that the quality of our products is guaranteed every time.

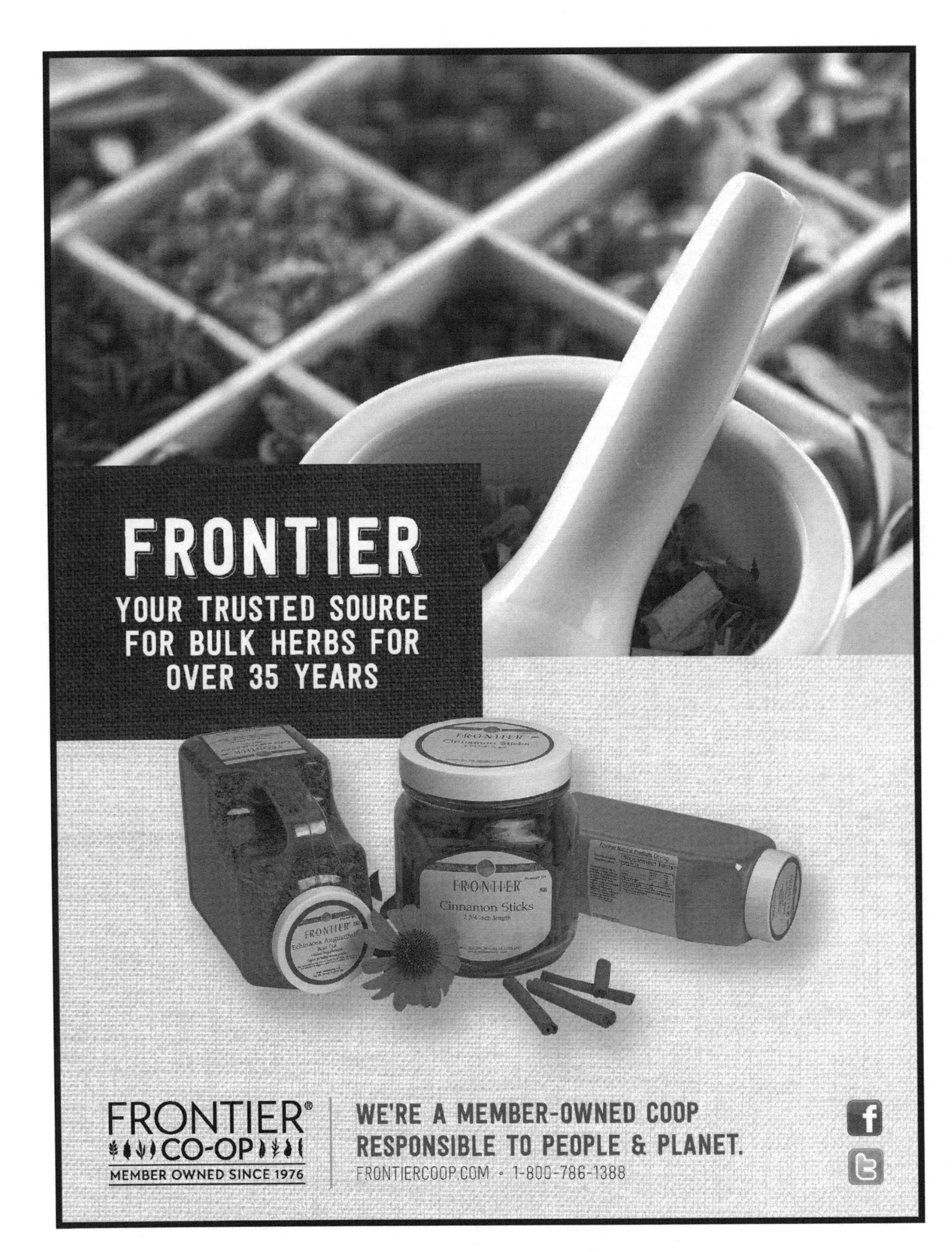

FRONTIER
YOUR TRUSTED SOURCE FOR BULK HERBS FOR OVER 35 YEARS

FRONTIER® CO-OP
MEMBER OWNED SINCE 1976

WE'RE A MEMBER-OWNED COOP
RESPONSIBLE TO PEOPLE & PLANET.
FRONTIERCOOP.COM • 1-800-786-1388

KEEP YOUR PATIENTS ON THE RIGHT TRACT.

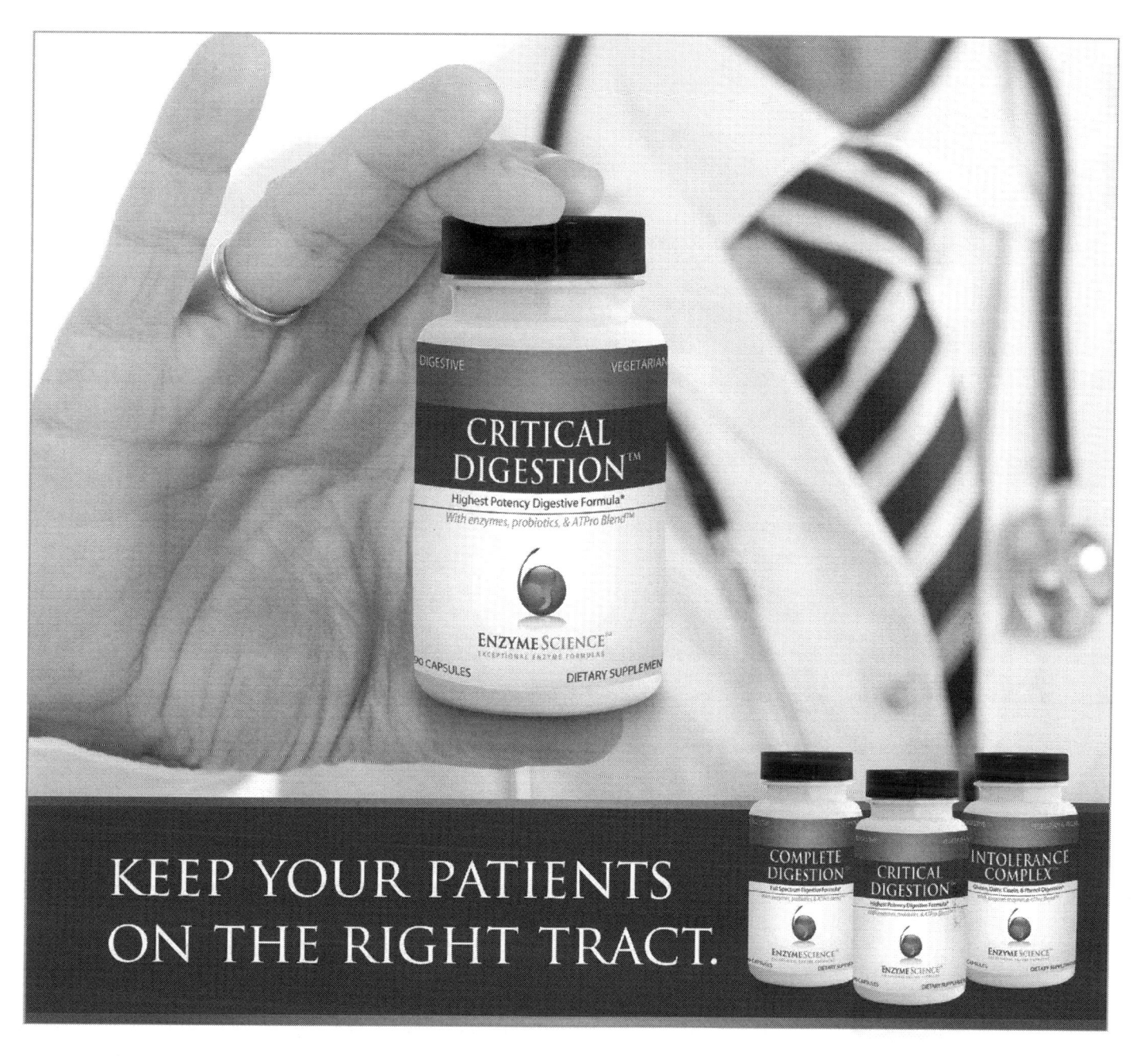

EXCEPTIONAL GI SUPPORT FOR BETTER DIGESTION*

Enzymes are the most effective tools made by the body to aid digestion and assimilation of nutrients. Nutrients supplied to the body are utilized as energy for various biological processes. When there is an insufficient quantity of digestive enzymes present in the body, undigested food may pass into the large intestine and be acted upon by intestinal flora. Byproducts of bacterial digestion and yeast fermentation include hydrogen, carbon dioxide and methane gas. The consequence of such combinations can result in familiar symptoms of occasional gas and bloating, and may negatively impact gut integrity. Enzyme supplementation encourages healthy digestion of proteins, fats, fibers and carbohydrates, in addition to promoting an optimally functional GI tract.*

* These statements have not been evaluated by the Food and Drug Administration. This product is not intended to diagnose, treat, cure or prevent any disease.

A division of
ENZYMEDICA
The Enzyme Experts

ENZYME SCIENCE™
EXCEPTIONAL ENZYME FORMULAS
855-281-7246 · www.EnzyScience.com

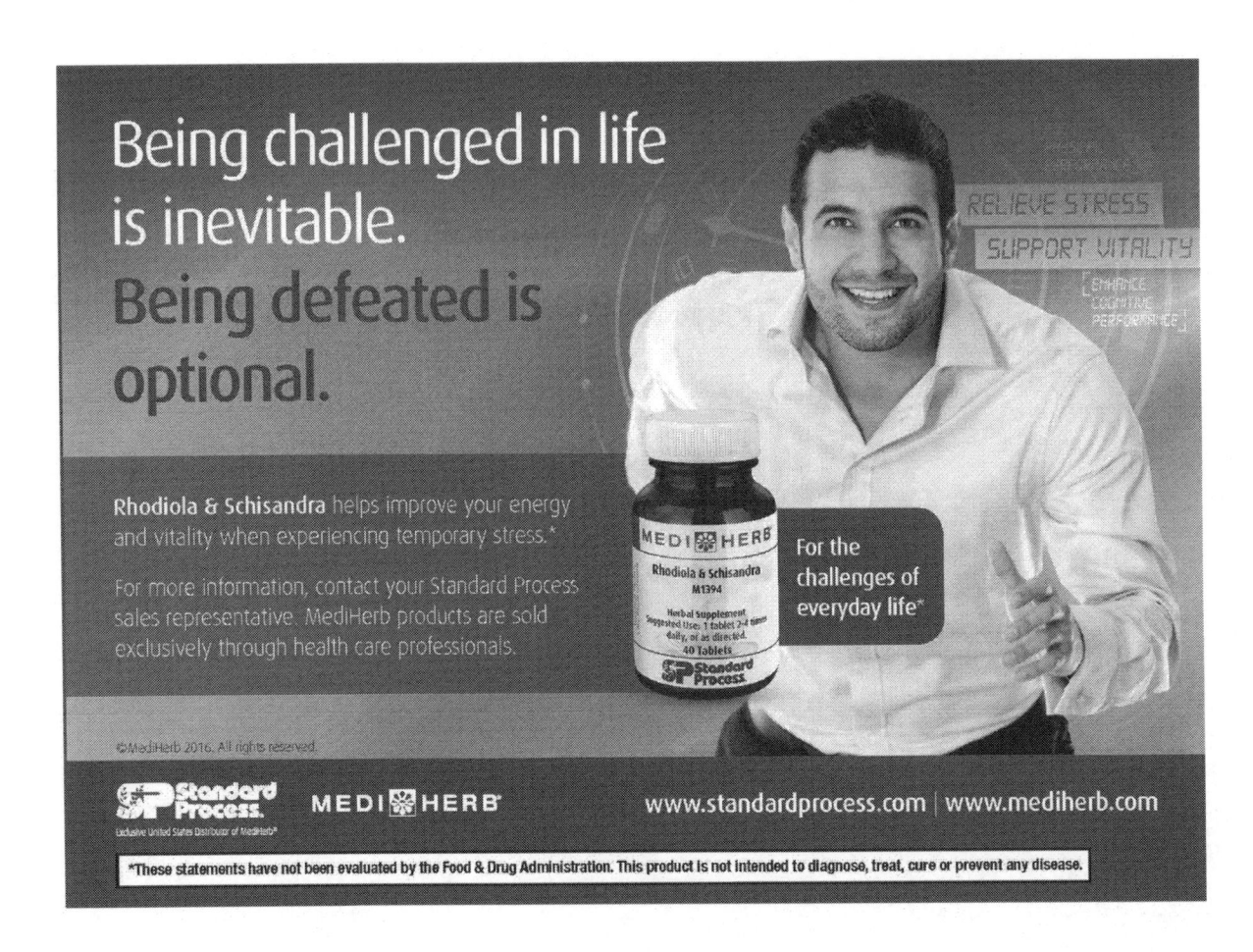

Being challenged in life is inevitable. Being defeated is optional.

Rhodiola & Schisandra helps improve your energy and vitality when experiencing temporary stress.*

For more information, contact your Standard Process sales representative. MediHerb products are sold exclusively through health care professionals.

©MediHerb 2016. All rights reserved.

RELIEVE STRESS
SUPPORT VITALITY
ENHANCE COGNITIVE PERFORMANCE

For the challenges of everyday life*

Standard Process — Exclusive United States Distributor of MediHerb®   MEDIHERB®   www.standardprocess.com | www.mediherb.com

*These statements have not been evaluated by the Food & Drug Administration. This product is not intended to diagnose, treat, cure or prevent any disease.

INTEGRATIVE THERAPEUTICS®

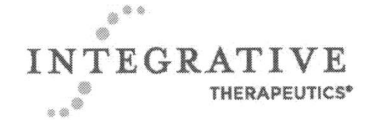

ACT FAST WITH ALLQLEAR.

Using a unique ingredient with a unique mechanism of action, new AllQlear from Integrative Therapeutics™ offers fast-acting seasonal support.* Extracted from a proprietary blend of quail eggs, ovomucoids act as a trypsin inhibitor to quickly stabilize mast cells, supporting healthy respiratory function in response to unavoidable seasonal and environmental sensitivities.* **To request a free sample visit integrativepro.com/allqlear**

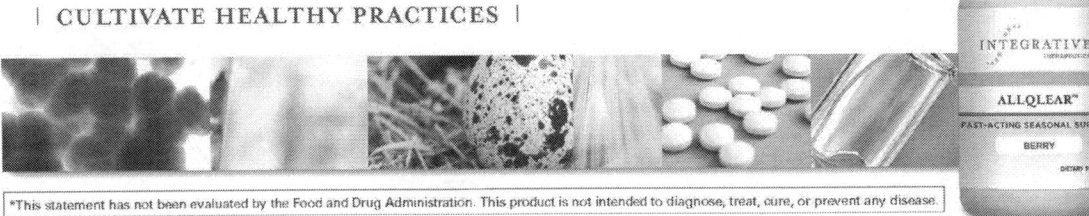

| CULTIVATE HEALTHY PRACTICES |

*This statement has not been evaluated by the Food and Drug Administration. This product is not intended to diagnose, treat, cure, or prevent any disease.

© 2016 Integrative Therapeutics, LLC

Zero Compromises.
Pure Results.

pure encapsulations®
Nothing But Pure

Pure Encapsulations® products are made using hypoallergenic ingredients, are scientifically validated by third-party laboratories and are designed to deliver predictable results.*

Visit us online to see what's in our products and **what's not**.

[ZERO HYDROGENATED FAT]
[ZERO ARTIFICIAL SWEETENERS]
[ZERO GLUTEN]
[ZERO COATINGS]
[ZERO MAGNESIUM STEARATE]
[ZERO ARTIFICIAL COLORS]

800-753-2277 | PureEncapsulations.com
©2016 Pure Encapsulations, Inc. All Rights Reserved

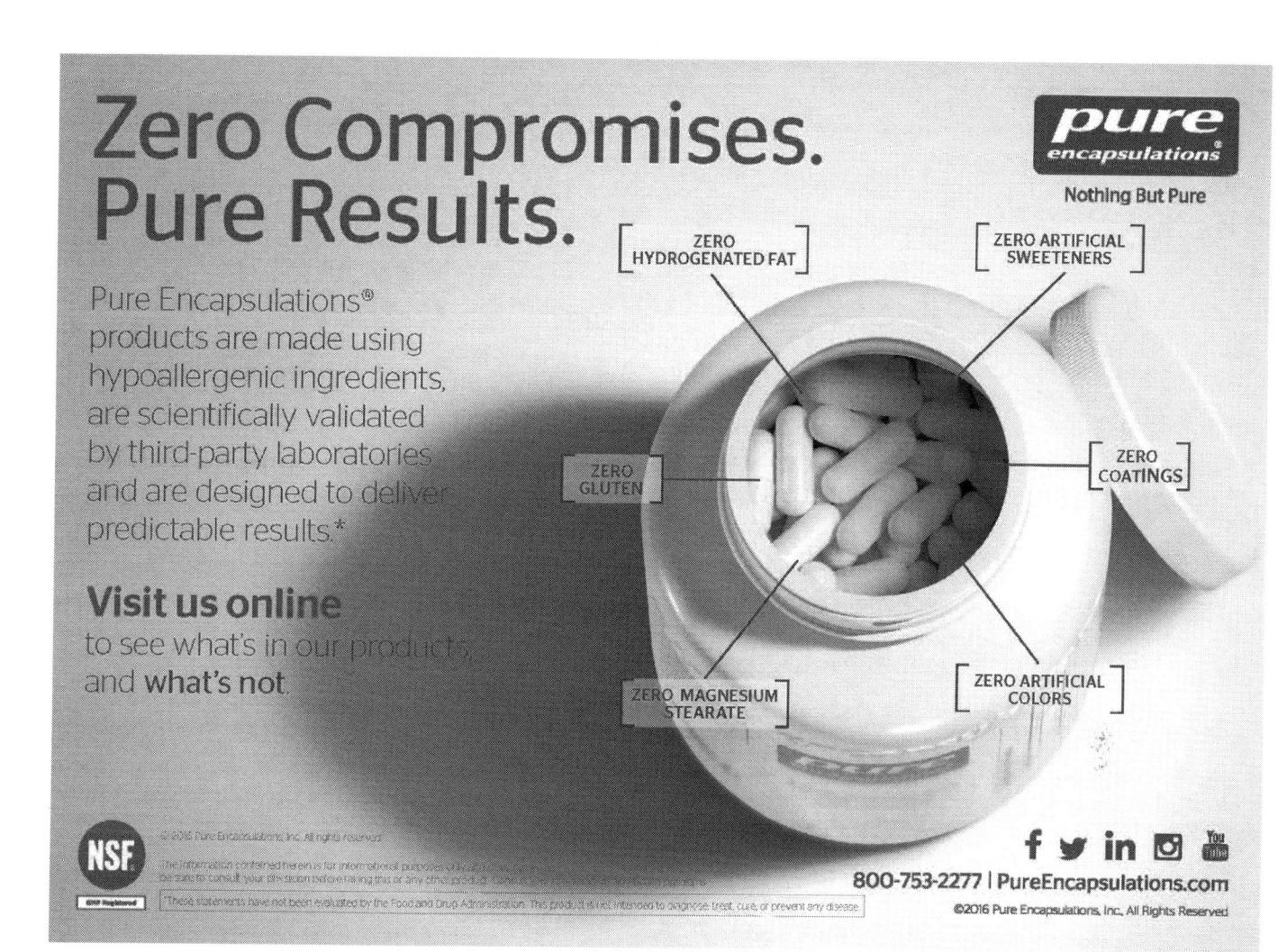

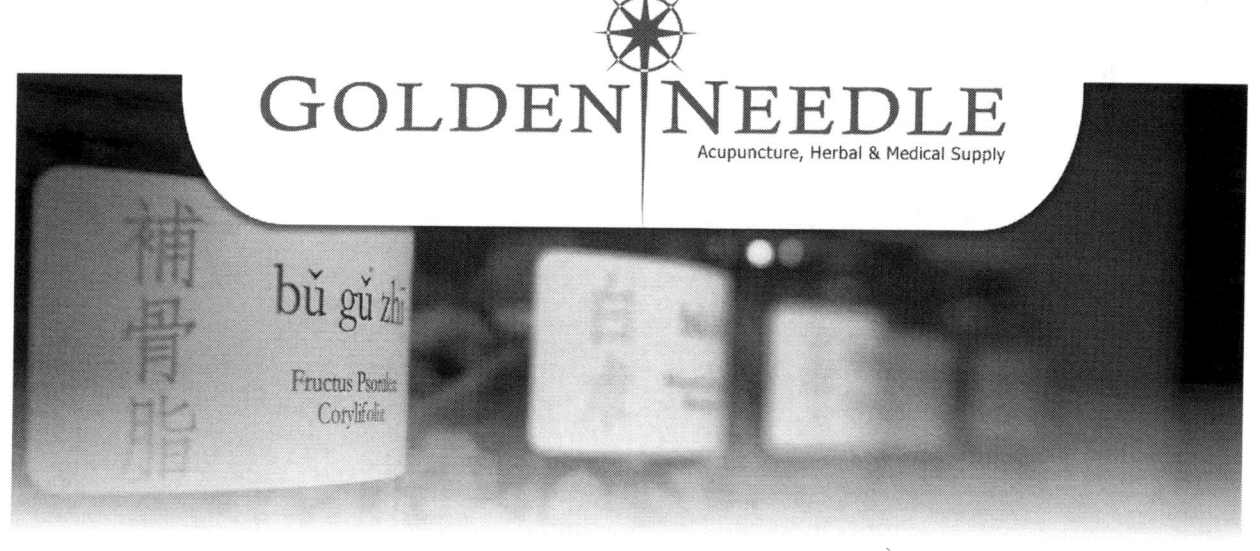

GOLDEN NEEDLE
Acupuncture, Herbal & Medical Supply

bǔ gǔ zhī
Fructus Psoralea Corylifolia

One of the largest online selections with over 17,000 items including:

{ Chinese & Western Herbs | Homeopathics | Nutraceuticals
Clinical Supplies | Acupuncture Needlees }

10% Discount for Students and Schools

Standard 1-2 Day Shipping

20% OFF your next order
Use coupon code: SOUTHWEST
Expires 5/10/2016

GoldenNeedleOnline.com   toll free 866.222.2999

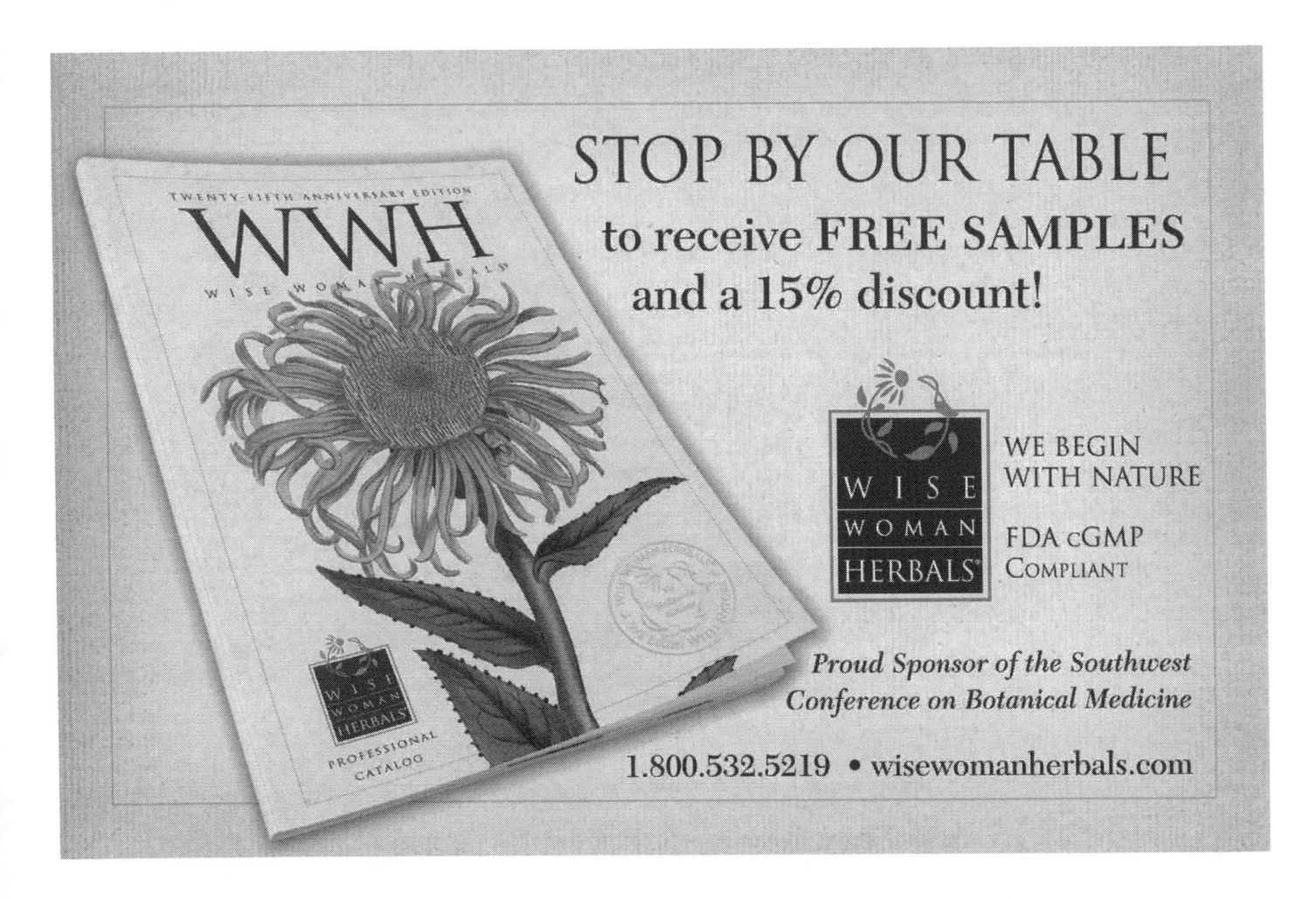

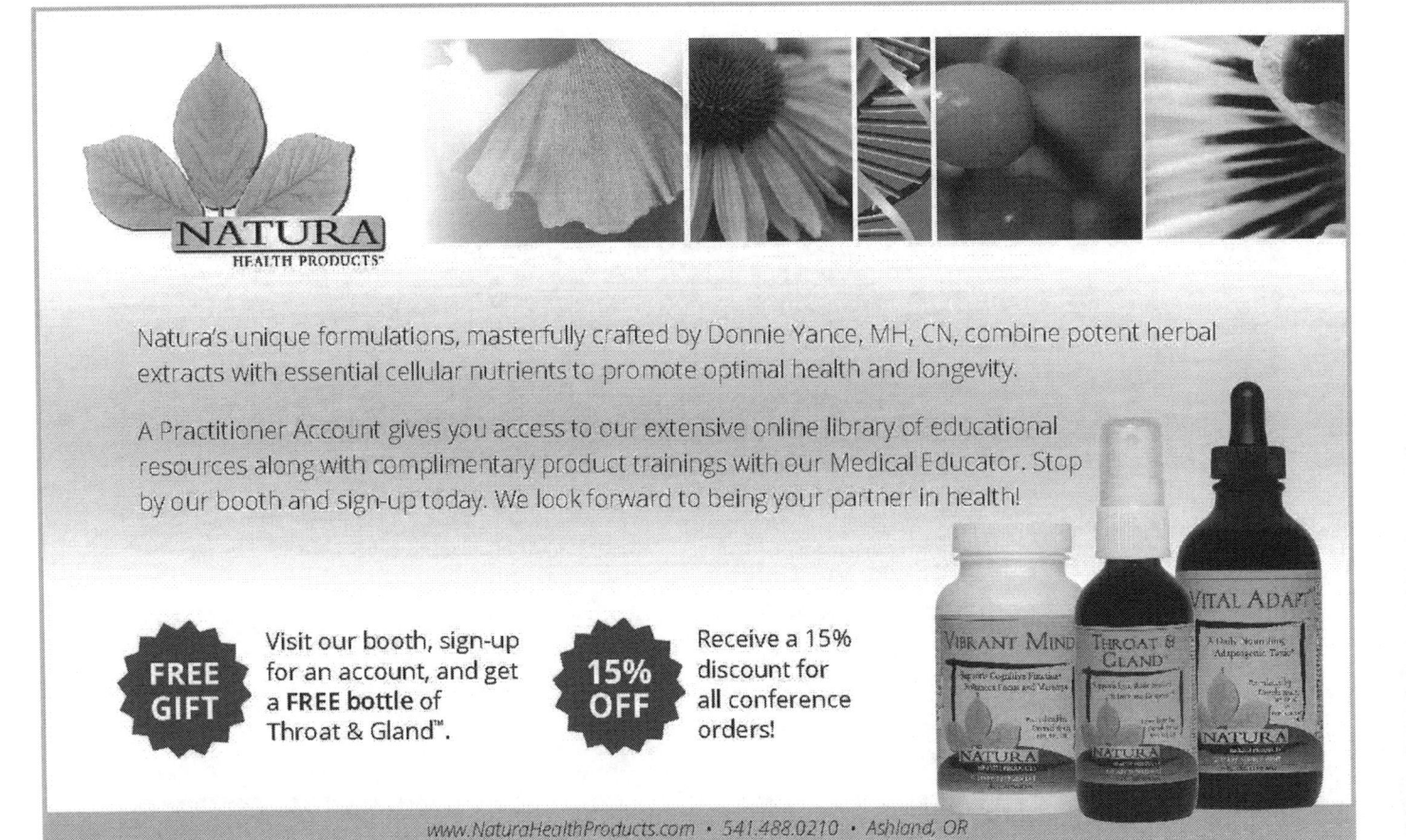

STOP BY OUR TABLE
to receive FREE SAMPLES and a 15% discount!

WISE WOMAN HERBALS

WE BEGIN WITH NATURE

FDA cGMP COMPLIANT

Proud Sponsor of the Southwest Conference on Botanical Medicine

1.800.532.5219 • wisewomanherbals.com

NATURA HEALTH PRODUCTS

Natura's unique formulations, masterfully crafted by Donnie Yance, MH, CN, combine potent herbal extracts with essential cellular nutrients to promote optimal health and longevity.

A Practitioner Account gives you access to our extensive online library of educational resources along with complimentary product trainings with our Medical Educator. Stop by our booth and sign-up today. We look forward to being your partner in health!

FREE GIFT — Visit our booth, sign-up for an account, and get a **FREE** bottle of Throat & Gland™.

15% OFF — Receive a 15% discount for all conference orders!

www.NaturaHealthProducts.com • 541.488.0210 • Ashland, OR

JOIN THE LEADING EDGE IN MEDICINE...
BECOME A NATUROPATHIC PHYSICIAN

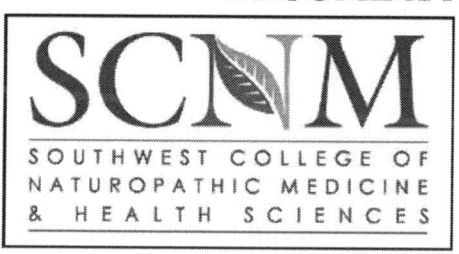

SCNM
SOUTHWEST COLLEGE OF NATUROPATHIC MEDICINE & HEALTH SCIENCES

- Join the growing national movement toward natural medicine.
- Clinical emphasis in a four year academic program.
- Federal financial aid available.
- Learn nutrition, botanical and homeopathic medicine, manipulation and acupuncture.

APPLY NOW FOR FALL 2016

For more information:
Southwest College of Naturopathic Medicine
2140 E. Broadway Rd.
Tempe, AZ 85282
(480) 858-9100
www.scnm.edu

Medical Herbalism
A Clinical Newsletter for the Herbal Practitioner

- In-depth discussion of herbal controversies
- Case studies
- Commentaries by clinical experts
- Scientific reviews
- Clinical tips from Eclectic Medicine
- Clinical news for Europe and Asia
- Book reviews
- Educational resources

Subscriptions
US- 1 year $45/ 2 years $80
Overseas- $50 per year

Back issues available in a binder- $99

Medical Herbalism • PO Box 13758 • Portland, OR 97213
(720) 841-3626   http://medherb.com

HERBAL EDUCATIONAL SERVICES

BotanicalMedicine.org

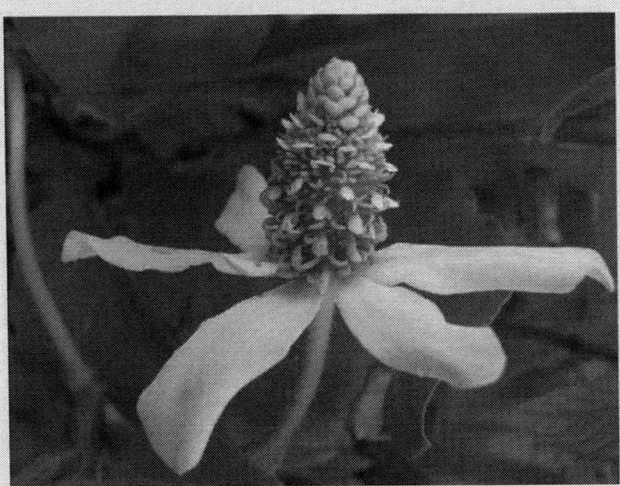

Yerba Mansa by Mimi Kamp

Our goal is to offer the highest quality information on herbal medicine through conferences, audio recordings and books.

NEW! Download 2016 conference MP3s just a few days after they are recorded:

    Southwest Conference on Botanical Medicine

    Medicines from the Earth Herb Symposium

Organizing and recording conferences since 1993
Herbal Educational Services
www.botanicalmedicine.org

Thank you to our conference sponsors

Traditional Medicinals
www.traditionalmedicinals.com

Herb Pharm
www.herb-pharm.com

Frontier Co-op
www.frontiercoop.com

Enzymedica
www.enzymedica.com

Herbalist and Alchemist
www.herbalist-alchemist.com/

Thank you!

Made in the USA
San Bernardino, CA
26 March 2016